ATHLETIC TRAINING
EXAM REVIEW

A STUDENT GUIDE TO SUCCESS

Sixth Edition

ATHLETIC TRAINING EXAM REVIEW

A STUDENT GUIDE TO SUCCESS

Sixth Edition

LYNN VAN OST, MED, RN, PT, ATC
University Orthopaedic Associates
Somerset, New Jersey

KAREN LEW FEIRMAN, DHSC, LAT, ATC
University of West Florida
Pensacola, Florida

KAREN MANFRÉ, LAT, RETIRED
Hunterdon Central High School
Flemington, New Jersey

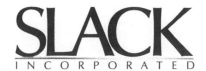

SLACK
INCORPORATED

www.Healio.com/books

ISBN: 978-1-63091-364-9

Copyright © 2017 by SLACK Incorporated

Lynn Van Ost, *Karen Lew Feirman*, and *Karen Manfré* have no financial or proprietary interest in the materials presented herein.

Athletic Training Exam Review: A Student Guide to Success, Sixth Edition includes ancillary materials specifically available for faculty use. Included are Test Bank Questions. Please visit www.efacultylounge.com to obtain access.

The procedures and practices described in this publication should be implemented in a manner consistent with the professional standards set for the circumstances that apply in each specific situation. Every effort has been made to confirm the accuracy of the information presented and to correctly relate generally accepted practices. The authors, editors, and publisher cannot accept responsibility for errors or exclusions or for the outcome of the material presented herein. There is no expressed or implied warranty of this book or information imparted by it. Care has been taken to ensure that drug selection and dosages are in accordance with currently accepted/recommended practice. Off-label uses of drugs may be discussed. Due to continuing research, changes in government policy and regulations, and various effects of drug reactions and interactions, it is recommended that the reader carefully review all materials and literature provided for each drug, especially those that are new or not frequently used. Some drugs or devices in this publication have clearance for use in a restricted research setting by the Food and Drug and Administration or FDA. Each professional should determine the FDA status of any drug or device prior to use in their practice.

Any review or mention of specific companies or products is not intended as an endorsement by the author or publisher.

SLACK Incorporated uses a review process to evaluate submitted material. Prior to publication, educators or clinicians provide important feedback on the content that we publish. We welcome feedback on this work.

Published by: SLACK Incorporated
                 6900 Grove Road
                 Thorofare, NJ 08086 USA
                 Telephone: 856-848-1000
                 Fax: 856-848-6091
                 www.Healio.com/books

Contact SLACK Incorporated for more information about other books in this field or about the availability of our books from distributors outside the United States.

Library of Congress Cataloging-in-Publication Data

Names: Van Ost, Lynn, author. | Lew Feirman, Karen, author. | Manfré, Karen, author.
Title: Athletic training exam review : a student guide to success / Lynn Van
   Ost, Karen Lew Feirman, Karen Manfré.
Description: Sixth edition. | Thorofare, NJ : Slack Incorporated, [2017] |
   Includes bibliographical references. | Description based on print version
   record and CIP data provided by publisher; resource not viewed.
Identifiers: LCCN 2017010950 (print) | LCCN 2017011785 (ebook) | ISBN
   9781630913656 (epub) | ISBN 9781630913663 (web) | ISBN 9781630913649 (pbk.
   : alk. paper)
Subjects: | MESH: Physical Education and Training | Physical Fitness |
   Exercise | Examination Questions
Classification: LCC RC1210 (ebook) | LCC RC1210 (print) | NLM QT 18.2 | DDC
   617.1/027076--dc23
LC record available at https://lccn.loc.gov/2017010950

Printed in the United States of America.

Last digit is print number: 10   9   8   7   6   5   4   3   2

DEDICATION

This edition is dedicated to an author, an editor, an educator, a visionary, an athletic trainer, a mentor, and one amazing person who loves, lives, and laughs more than anyone......Karen Manfré, this one is for you! Thank you for all of the time, energy, and effort you have put into this project since the beginning.

CONTENTS

Preface

A Winner's Creed
If you think you are beaten, you are,
If you think you dare not, then you won't.
If you like to win, but you think you can't,
It is almost certain you won't.
If you think you'll lose, you're lost.
For out of the world we find,
Success begins with a fellows will.
It's all in the state of mind.
If you think you are outclassed, you are.
You've got to be sure of yourself before
You can ever win a prize.
Life's battles don't always go to the stronger or faster man,
But sooner or later the man who wins
Is the man who thinks he can.
—*Author Unknown*

The first edition of this book came about by questioning, "Why can't we write a guide to assist athletic training students in preparing for the BOC examination?" After all of the times that we had informally guided former students to prepare for this examination, we felt that we could put together such a study guide. Thus began an amazing journey.

My mentors and colleagues throughout my career (38 years) were the type of individuals who would always challenge me, but make themselves available for my questions. They pushed me to my maximum, but did so knowing it would only make me a better athletic trainer. To each of them, I am grateful for their unwavering guidance and support. I wanted to pay that forward. The evolution of this study guide is a result of that desire.

Preparation is one of the keys to success. We as authors have put together a great number of questions and answers in multiple formats to help you challenge yourself and be successful in passing the BOC examination. The intention was not to "spoon-feed" you, but to make you think and problem solve. My favorite story is of Rikki Tikki Tavi. It is a story of a mongoose who is curious and always searching for answers. I relate to this story because I have such a passion for this great profession and the only way I could become better at my craft was to "run and find out" like the mongoose in this story. It has to come from within. No professor can teach that.

We have spent countless hours reviewing material and keeping abreast of new topics relevant to the profession to assure the book is as up-to-date as possible. Of course, at the time of printing, other topics may evolve that we can only address in future editions. Believe me, it is a formidable task to keep up with all of the changes in this profession; but that means growth and that is a good thing.

For over 15 years, *Athletic Training Exam Review: A Student Guide to Success* has provided students with a comprehensive manuscript in preparing for the BOC examination. This latest edition provides over 1350 questions with a new section on Evidence-Based Practice.

As authors, we hope to provide a study guide that will help alleviate most of the trepidations of this examination. We tried to provide a "roadmap" for you to follow that would make this entire experience easier to swallow. Chapters 1 and 2 are specifically dedicated to providing you with that pathway. Those chapters are dedicated to giving you a feel of the format of the examination and how to approach studying for it.

The book is divided up into several sections, including Knowledge Assessment, Applied Decision Making, Skills Assessment, and Critical Thinking. All of the questions/scenarios have the corresponding answers in the back section of the book, with the majority of the information coming directly from the most up-to-date BOC reference list. In addition, we felt it was necessary to go the extra step to provide in-depth explanations for each question/scenario to provoke further thought.

In conclusion, the late Pat Summit, University of Tennessee's former women's head basketball coach, said it best: "It's what you learn after you know it all that counts the most."

Karen Manfré, LAT, Retired

INTRODUCTION

This study guide for the Board of Certification (BOC) exam was inspired and developed as a result of a strong passion for our profession. Athletic training is a unique health care profession in that the athletic trainer is often in the position of experiencing the results of his or her efforts. The patients' victories are our victories, and their losses, our losses. We become friends, mentors, counselors, teachers, guardians, protectors, and healers. It takes a special individual to become a proficient and dedicated professional athletic trainer. Long hours are spent in the athletic training facility, classroom, and field experience venues preparing for the final exam that will allow you to place the letters "ATC" behind your name.

Our intent in writing this study guide is to assist you in accomplishing that final goal of passing the BOC exam. It is an accumulation of dedicated research and past experience. We have included a section on study techniques to assist you in your preparation for the exam and a general overview of the exam format to help you organize your thoughts.

This guide has been divided into 7 chapters: Study Techniques and Test-Taking Strategies, General Information and the Examination Format, Knowledge Assessment, Applied Decision Making, Skills Assessment, Critical Thinking, and What to Do if You Do Not Pass the First Time.

The multiple choice and true/false questions in Chapter 3 have been organized according to the BOC's *Practice Analysis* (7th ed) Educational Domains and are also subdivided into related athletic training subjects to allow you to assess specific subjects in which you may be weak and those in which your strengths lie. Although this study guide will assist you in preparing for the certification exam, it should not be used in place of your textbooks or other sources of study from your academic program. It is not intended to be a "practice" exam; it is meant only to be used as an adjunct source of information and to tie everything you have learned in the classroom and during your clinical education experiences together.

In Chapters 1 and 2, we have provided some specific tools to help you organize yourself up to 6 months prior to the examination. Chapter 3, Knowledge Assessment, consists of more than 1300 study questions. The majority of the multiple choice and true/false questions is a "mixed bag" of subjects derived from the BOC's *Practice Analysis* Educational Domains, and the balance covers most of the related subject matter of athletic training, as previously mentioned. Chapter 4, Applied Decision Making, tests your ability to make appropriate judgment calls and improve your problem-solving skills. Each problem presents a specific scenario with several possible options that you can choose to follow. Chapter 5, Skills Assessment, is composed of 26 problems that are designed to test your manual athletic training skills. Chapter 6, Critical Thinking, is composed of scenario-based problems designed to test your ability to develop differential diagnoses. Chapter 7 is directed at helping you if your test results are not favorable. We have included some suggestions on how to deal with the immediate difficulties not passing may cause and how to begin the process of developing a new approach for your next attempt. Provided you have applied the information you have learned in the classroom and on the field to the study strategies we have offered in this manual, you will not need to read this final chapter.

The *Sixth Edition* also features an online component with a variety of questions. You can test your knowledge with these exams and receive the results for each when completed. Also, at the end of each sample exam, you will be able to review the questions along with the correct answers for a complete and comprehensive review. We wish you luck and look forward to welcoming you as a colleague.

Study Techniques and Test-Taking Strategies

The most obvious question that comes to mind when preparing for the Board of Certification (BOC) exam is "Where do I start?" Just the thought of studying for this examination can be overwhelming. There seems to be so much information and so little time to absorb it all. The good news is that none of this information should be new to you, so consider this a review of what you already know.

The purpose of this text is to be a comprehensive review of previously learned material. Our goal is for you to utilize this as a study guide and assessment tool. In using this as a review method, you can assess areas of strengths, as well as weaknesses. As you progress through this book, you can document areas that you need to focus on or research more information. The information contained throughout this text should serve as an excellent guide in your preparations for the BOC exam, as well as for your final evaluations within your athletic training program.

The best way to prevent yourself from feeling overwhelmed and to develop the motivation to study is to begin by taking small steps toward your goal. The first step is to learn new study strategies or improve the ones you currently find effective. Learning how to concentrate and organize your time in an efficient manner is the basis of good study skills. Remember, it is not necessarily the **quantity** of time you spend, but the **quality** of time that counts. Many people use a variety of study strategies, and it is up to you to find what works best for you. It is best that you do not rely on others' study strategies but rather create your own, so they are reflective of what is best for you.

IMPROVING CONCENTRATION

Concentration may be defined as the ability to focus on the task at hand. Here are some suggestions to improve your ability to concentrate while studying.

Eliminate Environmental Distractions

- Select 1 or 2 special study areas, preferably a place that is quiet and secluded (eg, library, park, computer lab, coffee shop).
- Agree with those with whom you live (eg, roommates, spouses, relatives, children) on times when you will be free to socialize and times when you will study. Convey the importance of adhering to your schedule and setting up a routine.
- Hang a "Do Not Disturb" sign on your door, wear a specific item of clothing, or tie a brightly colored ribbon to the door as your signal to others that you do not wish to be interrupted. In order to avoid disturbances, make the determination that you will not let anything interfere with your study time. Add a post to your Twitter or Facebook account letting others know you are studying and not to disturb you.
- Inform those who find it necessary to interrupt you during your study time on a regular basis that it is important they do not talk to you until you are ready to do so. Make sure you send a clear but tactful message, as they might not be aware that they are interfering with your ability to concentrate.

Van Ost L, Lew Feirman K, Manfré K. *Athletic Training Exam Review:
A Student Guide to Success, Sixth Edition* (pp 1-4).
© 2017 SLACK Incorporated.

- Ignore distracting sights and sounds, such as your cell phone, television, social media, or loud music. Although some students state that they study better with music in the background, a silent room will provide no distractions at all. It is best to use voicemail so you are not tempted to answer the phone. While studying, make sure that your computer and cell phone are turned off. Having all electronic devices out of sight will allow for less interruption. Having mp3 players, cell phones, and games accessible deters from your studying.

Reduce Mind Wandering

- Stand up and walk away from your material when you find your mind wandering. Then come back and try again.
- Concentrate only on the material you are reviewing. If you have errands or something suddenly pops into your mind, write it down on a note pad and tackle it at a later time. This is very helpful if you think of topics you might want to add to your review list or study points.
- Make sure you stay in good shape, both physically and mentally. It is important to eat, sleep, and exercise routinely. You cannot concentrate or perform adequately if you are hungry or are a victim of sleep deprivation. Get out and exercise; it will relax you and clear your mind.
- If you have other major concerns about which you are currently worrying, such as personal problems at home or at work, make sure you attend to them when you are not studying. Try to find a way to resolve the problems as soon as possible so they do not distract you from the goal at hand.
- Remember to reward your studying with a social event or some quiet time alone to do an enjoyable activity that requires little focused concentration. Set a goal for your reward, such as reviewing a particular subject completely and to your satisfaction. Be careful not to set up your "time off" as your goal.

Improve Your Concentration

- Develop a good attitude toward the subject you are studying. Have an inquisitive mind; ask yourself additional questions and search your books and notes for the answers. Skim through the textbook before reviewing a subject, or create games for yourself. Try to make your study time as exciting and challenging as you can. The power of positive thinking will help you "ride the tide."
- Break down major areas into smaller components for study (eg, instead of tackling anatomy, try a smaller subject, like the muscles of the lower extremity).

- When you get tired, take a break. Get something to drink or eat or take a stroll around the neighborhood. Try to become more aware of the amount of time you are able to adequately concentrate. It is probably best to study for only 2 to 3 hours at a time before taking a 10- to 20-minute break. Everyone needs a break during studying, so remember to give yourself time as it will help you to focus when you return to what you are doing.
- Make sure you do not vary your study spots. The areas you have chosen for studying should be utilized only to study. Try to select a specific time to study and do not get involved in any other activity in that area until you are done. Being consistent with both the time and place you choose to study will train you to be more efficient.

ADDITIONAL STUDY SUGGESTIONS

- *Form or attend a study group.* Make sure the individuals you ask to join the group are eager learners and are willing to participate on a regular basis. This will assure everyone that each person is contributing his or her fair share of work. Make sure the goals of the group are clearly defined so time is not wasted, and that everyone has an equal role in accomplishing those goals.
- *Textbook review.* Only refer to your textbooks when it is necessary to review areas on which you are weak or to study a topic in more detail. Trying to read any of your textbooks from beginning to end is completely ineffective and will only cause you to panic. Use "subject-focused books" (eg, a book on modalities or anatomy) rather than "general" athletic training books (eg, sports injury management or sports medicine). The BOC offers a list of references that are used in question development for its exam, and it is helpful to utilize these textbooks when reviewing material. The list of references can be found under the exam development section and also in the educators section of the BOC website.
- *Examination review courses.* Some schools will offer review courses for the examination. These courses are often given in the summer when the school curriculum is less intense.
- *Class notes.* Your notes from your classes should be composed of the majority of your study materials. The subjects outlined by the BOC as requirements for candidates planning to take the certification examination should have been sufficiently covered in your curriculum. If you are unsure of anything that was covered in a particular class, contact the professor so that he or she might help clear up your questions.

- *Audiovisual aids.* Audiovisual aids may help to clarify a confusing topic. It sometimes helps to be able to see or hear how a task is performed and have the ability to rerun the task several times to fully understand how it is done. If you learn better by hearing and seeing, ask your instructor or supervisor where you might obtain websites or instructional videos (eg, handling an unconscious athlete, strength training techniques). You may also want to create your own video with friends or an instructor.
- *Practice with a buddy.* If you find you do not work well in groups but need to practice specific skills, enlist the assistance of a friend, especially another candidate whose needs are similar to yours. Feedback is important for accuracy and timing, and only someone familiar with what you are trying to accomplish can give you helpful insight. Working with someone "in the same boat" can also help alleviate your anxieties. You may also recruit a certified athletic trainer whom you are comfortable with to help you practice a skill in which you may be particularly weak.
- *Flash cards.* Make up flash cards with questions and answers and carry them with you. This technique works especially well when studying factual information, such as anatomy, kinesiology, or therapeutic modalities. They are easy to carry and allow you to study in bits and pieces anytime, anywhere.
- *Multimedia.* Use DVDs, webinars, online practice tests offered by the BOC, and podcasts (eg, anatomy, goniometry, or manual muscle testing) to study from and clarify questions or utilize the Internet and explore helpful websites.

TIME MANAGEMENT

- It is essential that you learn to organize your time and develop some specific test-taking techniques. Careful planning of your time will allow you to work more efficiently. Developing a purposeful calendar of events will allow you to prioritize your tasks and accomplish them step by step. Preparation is the key to success. Time spent organizing and planning in advance will reduce your anxiety and allow you to think straight under pressure. The following ideas might be of help if you find either one or both of the previously mentioned areas to be a source of frustration.
- Plan a schedule for studying by creating a chart dividing the months into weeks and weeks into days and hours (see Appendix A). You may also try using a day planner, calendar, or to-do list on your phone or a computer-based calendar program that is part of your email.
- Fill in this chart with your planned study times, activities, and "down time." Keep a record of your study pattern and review it on a weekly basis. If you are not spending enough time studying, where are you spending the time?
- When scheduling study times, be sure to allow yourself additional time for your harder topics. This will help you to avoid cramming, which is ineffective.
- Concentrate your study efforts on clinical situations, diseases, or areas with which you are not as familiar. For example, if you have never dealt with an athlete with a thoracic injury or a life-threatening allergic reaction, focus a bit more on those topics. Get more information until you are satisfied that the topic is well covered.
- Know the date and location of your examination and make sure all of the preliminaries are taken care of ahead of time (eg, you have turned in your application materials, your CPR card is current). This will help you organize your calendar.
- Think about the following questions and answer them to identify how you manage your time:
  - When are you most alert—in the morning, afternoon, or evening? What time is optimal for you to study?
  - How much sleep do you require to be most alert and able to concentrate?
  - When do you prefer to have your meals?
  - How much time do you like to exercise? What time is optimal for exercising?
  - How much time do you allow for relaxation or fun activities when you study?
  - What other priorities do you have in your life, and when are the best times to address them?

SPECIFIC TEST-TAKING STRATEGIES

By following a few simple guidelines when you actually sit down to take the test, you may eliminate a number of unnecessary mistakes that can easily be made as a result of being too anxious.

- Review the instructions given to you for the computer-based exam.
- Read all test instructions thoroughly before starting.
- Budget your time; note how many questions you must answer and how much time you have for the exam. Estimate how much time you have to answer each question.
- Make sure you read the entire question and all of the answers to the question before deciding which choice is best.
- If you are unsure of an answer, go with your first choice.
- Utilize your critical thinking in choosing the best answer.

- Keep track of your time during the examination with your watch or a wall clock.
- Rephrase difficult questions in your own words, but be sure not to change the meaning of the question.
- Answer all of the questions even if you have to guess. Do not leave any question unanswered.
- For multiple choice questions, if you have a question that has "choose all that apply" or "choose only one" as possible answers, go through each of the other answers and place a true or false next to it. If all of the answers are true or false, then choose all that apply, or if there is only one choice, select the correct answer.
- When you are taking the exam, you will be given scratch paper or a dry erase board. Utilize these items when you are studying for the exam so you are prepared and comfortable during your actual exam.

DECREASING YOUR TEST ANXIETY

Everyone feels some level of anxiety before taking a test; it is a normal response to feeling challenged. However, it is important to take control of your feelings so they do not overwhelm you and paralyze your thought process. Here are some ideas you might try to make you more comfortable.

- Prepare early, approximately 6 months prior to the exam. Check to make sure you have everything in order to apply to take the test. If you are well prepared before the actual examination, it will be one less thing about which to worry. Assuming you have met all of the requirements, this is the time to start organizing your study plan.
- Know the location of the test site and leave enough time to get there early. Make sure to check the weather reports the night before to allow for any changes in planning. If you live a good distance away, stay at a hotel the night before. If you are staying in the city or town in which the examination is being given, take the time to drive the route from your hotel to the examination site to avoid increasing your anxiety about specific directions or timing the next morning. Go to the actual building and room where the exam is being given to ensure you will not get lost. Also, when you are doing your trial run, identify where you will park. Many testing locations are on college campuses, and a visitor's pass may be required.
- Try to relax the night before the examination. Go out to dinner or take in a fun movie with friends. This will help you to sleep well the night prior to the examination. Just be sure not to stay up late! You will want to be very alert the next morning.
- Eat a good meal prior to the examination. You will not be able to concentrate if you are hungry, and you need fuel to stay alert.

- Make sure to dress comfortably. Wear clothing that is loose but neat, and wear layers of clothing so you can make adjustments if the room temperature is not to your liking. It is best to appear professional and avoid wearing athletic apparel, such as a sweatsuit. Do not wear a hat or bandana on your head, as this may attract attention, and it is advisable not to wear clothing with a school or clinic logo.
- Do not cram the morning of the examination; this will only cause further stress. It might help to scan through 1 or 2 small topics prior to the test, but in general, you will know all you are going to know by that time anyway.
- While waiting for the test, try stretching a bit and practice focusing. If you know how to do progressive relaxation (ie, progressively tensing and relaxing your muscles from head to toe), feel free to try it. Locate the bathroom and water fountain in case you need them later.
- Close your eyes and take some deep breaths; try to think positively and confidently. Remember, you have prepared yourself for this! If you go "blank" or find yourself panicking during the test, put your pencil down, close your eyes, and take a deep breath. Count to 10 or until you can focus again.
- Do not rehash your performance after the examination. What is done is done. Try to forget it for a couple of days. Plan to do something fun and stress-free after it is over.
- Do not compare yourself to your friends. You did the best you could, and every candidate's test scores will vary. Do not allow your score to be a measure of your self-worth.

WHAT TO BRING TO THE EXAMINATION

Be sure to bring the following items with you on the day of the examination:

- A map to the test site with written directions (or use an online road map service/GPS)
- Telephone numbers for the test site, the test administration company, and BOC
- Your test appointment/email confirmation
- A photo ID (driver's license or passport)
- Your confirmation notice from the BOC/testing center
- A watch (stopwatch capabilities may be useful)
- Tissues
- Reading glasses, if necessary
- Proof of change of address or name change, if applicable

General Information and the Examination Format

GOALS OF THIS TEXT

The purpose of the *Sixth Edition* of this book is to be a comprehensive review of previously learned material that will assist the candidate in highlighting his or her individual strengths and weaknesses, as related to the domains of athletic training and associated subjects. The *Sixth Edition* features a variety of changes that reflect current trends in academic testing, patient evaluation, and critical thinking. It also serves to help a student prepare for final examinations within an athletic training educational program.

It is the intent of the authors to present a text that will act as an **adjunct** to material distributed by the students' own academic faculty or that information presented in a review course in preparation for the BOC exam. It is designed strictly to be a self-evaluative tool. The authors have kept the structure very similar to prior editions to make it easy for the candidate to understand. This text is not meant to be a "practice" BOC exam and has been formatted in such a way to be user friendly and thought provoking. It is not designed to exactly mimic the BOC exam in either content or presentation.

ELIGIBILITY AND APPLYING FOR THE BOC EXAM

The National Athletic Trainers' Association Executive Committee for Education (NATA-ECE) was originally formed by the BOC to monitor the curriculum and field experiences provided by those schools offering athletic training programs. It was this committee's responsibility to ensure that all programs designed to prepare students to become certified athletic trainers met and maintained the academic and clinical standards set by the BOC. The NATA-ECE is charged with setting the guidelines for the academic and clinical education of those students enrolled in accredited athletic training programs as well as ensuring improved patient care using an evidence-based practice approach to patient care.

Since it is not within the scope of this manual to include all of the current policy changes being made by the NATA-ECE regarding athletic training education, nor is it the intent of the authors to have this manual used as a complete source of these changes, it is best to obtain information pertaining to these developments directly from the NATA-ECE if you have specific questions or concerns.

Those candidates who are eligible to take the BOC exam must have completed a program of study in athletic training that is accredited by the Commission on Accreditation of Athletic Training Education (CAATE). A CAATE-accredited athletic training program is divided into 2 components: didactic education and clinical experience. The didactic education component incorporates academic courses or academic credit that meets the requirements of the CAATE guidelines. These courses are designed to teach the athletic training student the clinical skills of the profession and provide a venue in which he or she may practice those skills. It has been recommended by the NATA-ECE that these courses provide an academic syllabus and/or a clinical instruction manual that outlines the educational

Van Ost L, Lew Feirman K, Manfré K. *Athletic Training Exam Review: A Student Guide to Success, Sixth Edition* (pp 5-7).
© 2017 SLACK Incorporated.

objectives and clinical skill outcomes. These outcomes are derived from the entry-level athletic training clinical proficiencies. The individual university or college determines the amount of academic credit assigned to a given course according to the institution's individual guidelines. Clinical academic coursework may include an internship, externship, or clinical laboratory class in addition to, but not in lieu of, formal academic clinical courses. Athletic training students are assigned to a designated preceptor who is responsible for on-site daily supervision and the evaluation of the student's global performance.

The accredited athletic training program no longer requires a minimum number of hours. A student graduating from an accredited program will have had to successfully complete all of the athletic training education competencies and clinical integrated proficiencies, which must be performed under the supervision of a BOC-certified athletic trainer or a qualified preceptor. If a student is also preparing to take a state licensure examination, he or she must check with the specific state to ensure that he or she will meet all of the requirements of the state's governing board. These competencies and proficiencies will be fulfilled throughout the student's progression through the athletic training program under the direct supervision of a certified athletic trainer. Many of these competencies and clinical integrated proficiencies will be done in an athletic training facility, physician's office, or hospital. These facilities provide comprehensive athletic health care services (such as prepractice and pregame preparation, emergency and rehabilitative services, etc) to an active population. Athletic training students may also experience a variety of settings, such as a sports medicine center, emergency room, high school, performing arts, military setting, or physician's office.

Candidates who have entered an accredited athletic training curriculum must have successfully completed the athletic training program in no less than 2 academic years and must have received their degree from the college or university at which they completed their coursework. All eligible candidates may take the examination during the semester or quarter prior to graduation provided all of the prerequisites have been met. All candidates must be endorsed prior to registering for the exam.

The endorsing athletic trainer is the program director. All endorsements are now done by the program director on the BOC website. It is up to the student to register and begin the application process to sit for the exam. The application process can be found using the BOC Central application on the BOC website, www.bocatc.org. Students should access the BOC website and fill out their candidate information. The student is responsible for the entire registration process through the BOC. Following a student's registration, an email of verification and endorsement will be sent to the student program director. Once the student is endorsed, the process can continue. For further details, refer to the BOC website (www.bocatc.org).

A current candidate must fulfill the requirements for eligibility to take the BOC examination. The following basic requirements must be met in order to apply:

- Proof of graduation from an accredited college or university
- Electronic endorsement by the candidate's program director

An approved curriculum candidate may apply to take the certification examination prior to graduation as long as he or she has completed all of the required academic and clinical requirements outlined by the BOC. The examination may be taken during the final semester of the candidate's anticipated date of graduation.

Candidates are required to register online utilizing the BOC Central option. BOC Central allows the user to register and submit the information needed to determine a candidate's eligibility. Once the BOC office in Omaha, Nebraska, receives the information from the candidate, the BOC will notify the candidate of approval. After the candidate receives the approval notification, he or she may continue with the registration process. The application, once approved, is good for only 1 year. The test is offered 5 times per year all over the country at select testing centers, and the candidate is able to see what sites are available in real time. Having the ability to choose your own site, based on availability, is a huge benefit.

It is advisable to register for the certification examination 5 months prior to the test so that you have plenty of time to make sure you have all of your requirements completed and that any necessary forms are properly filled out and submitted in a timely fashion. You will choose your test date and site according to availability. We also suggest that you become a NATA member if you have not done so, as it will impact your application fee. The fee must be paid by credit or debit card, check, or money order and will cost less if you are an NATA member. Be sure to check with the BOC for current application fees. Be sure to complete your online application prior to the published deadline for the test date for which you are intending to sit. Applying early will help to ensure that it is accepted by the deadline. If you must postpone or cancel your test for any reason, you must request this in writing electronically with the BOC and Castle testing services. If you wish to reschedule your test date to a date other than your originally scheduled date, a $40 fee may be charged. Candidates may reschedule within the same exam window up to 4 business days prior to their scheduled appointment by going onto the Castle website. Rescheduling your test during the open window is allowed according to availability at the selected test site. For a $100 fee, candidates who have a scheduled exam appointment may reschedule to a different exam window up to 4 business days prior to their scheduled appointment.

DEVELOPMENT OF THE BOC EXAM

The development and administration of the BOC exam is the sole responsibility of the BOC. This private, nonprofit organization is governed by an 8-member board of directors consisting of 5 certified athletic trainers, a physician director, a public director, and a corporate/educational director. Within the organizational structure of the BOC are 7 committees, each responsible for addressing various areas that are pertinent to the function of the BOC. Two of these committees—the Examination Administration Committee and the Examination Development Committee—are directly involved in the procedural aspects and design/validation of the examination. The questions for the test are developed, validated, and edited by certified athletic trainers. These questions are scrutinized to meet the specifications of the *Role Delineation Study/Practice Analysis* that were validated by the BOC. The *Seventh Edition* of the *Practice Analysis* will be implemented beginning with the April 2017 test and the January 2018 continuing education cycle. All test questions developed for the examination are based on the following 5 domains of athletic training:

1. Injury/Illness Prevention and Wellness Protection
2. Clinical Evaluation and Diagnosis
3. Immediate and Emergency Care
4. Treatment and Rehabilitation
5. Organizational and Professional Health and Well-Being

THE BOC EXAM FORMAT

The first certification examination given by the NATA in 1967 included 150 written questions and a practical section consisting of 5 questions. The original test was administered and manually scored by 3 athletic trainers. The certification examination has come a long way since that time and has experienced numerous changes. Currently, the test is one comprehensive exam. The exam consists of 175 questions, including both scored and unscored (experimental) questions, in which the candidate has 4 hours to complete the examination. The examination is scored by computer, and candidates can expect to receive their results within 2 to 4 weeks. The examination questions are in a variety of formats, including multiple choice, drag and drop, multiselect, and focused testlets.

SECTIONS WITHIN THIS BOOK

This book is now divided into 4 sections: Knowledge Assessment, Applied Decision Making, Skills Assessment, and Critical Thinking. The Knowledge Assessment section contains more than 1300 multiple choice questions and 95 true/false questions. This section allows the candidate to review the basic "building blocks" of athletic training on which all other skills and professional decisions are based and assess which areas the candidate must focus on when studying for the BOC examination.

Although there is no longer a "practical" portion offered in the current BOC exam, the authors feel that the importance of "hands-on" practice of athletic training skills and tasks cannot be understated. The Skills Assessment section of this book will help guide the candidate through tasks commonly encountered by the athletic trainer in the field or clinical setting. There are 26 problems offered in this section, allowing the candidate to navigate through a broad spectrum of tasks in front of his or her peers.

The Critical Thinking section aims at having the candidate process information at a higher level, "putting it all together," so to speak. This section requires the athletic training candidate to absorb and process information presented to him or her and then draw a specific conclusion. The problems also reflect a wider patient population, in line with the direction in which our profession is progressing.

Knowledge Assessment

MULTIPLE CHOICE QUESTIONS

ATHLETIC TRAINING DOMAINS

Injury/Illness Prevention and Wellness Protection

1. A sphygmomanometer is a device that measures which of the following?
   A. Grip strength
   B. Body fat percentage
   C. Intra-abdominal pressure
   D. Blood pressure
   E. None of the above

2. A Q-angle of > 25 degrees may predispose a patient to what postural deviation?
   A. Excessive genu varus
   B. Excessive genu valgus
   C. Genu recurvatum
   D. Coxa valgus
   E. Coxa vara

3. All of the following are factors in lower extremity overuse syndromes in runners except:
   A. Poor footwear
   B. Poor posture
   C. Change in surface
   D. Short strides
   E. A and B

4. All of the following questions are significant when screening a young patient for an underlying cardiac abnormality except:
   A. Does the patient have chest pain with activity?
   B. Does the patient have a family history of sudden cardiac death in a family member under age 50 years?
   C. Does the patient have numbness or tingling in either or both hands in cold weather?
   D. Does the patient have a history of a "racing heart?"
   E. Does the patient have a history of heart problems?

5. During a preparticipation physical, the team physician comes across a basketball player with the following profile: The athlete is tall with an arm span greater than his height, pectus carinatum or excavatum, high-arched palate, and myopia. What is the probable diagnosis?
   A. Paget's disease
   B. Milch disease
   C. Addison's disease
   D. Gigantism
   E. Marfan syndrome

Van Ost L, Lew Feirman K, Manfré K. *Athletic Training Exam Review: A Student Guide to Success, Sixth Edition* (pp 9-129).

6. A patient's pulmonary function is tested via spirometry. Several measurements are taken during this test. What is the maximum amount of air that can be expired after a maximum inspiration called?
    A. Maximum expiratory flow rate
    B. Forced expiratory volume
    C. Vital capacity
    D. Tidal volume
    E. Residual volume

7. During a preparticipation physical, a patient is diagnosed with myopia. What is this patient's problem?
    A. Double vision
    B. Farsightedness
    C. Blindness in one eye
    D. Nearsightedness
    E. None of the above

8. All of the following are functions of the liver except:
    A. Carbohydrate metabolism
    B. Detoxification of blood
    C. Protein synthesis
    D. Detoxification of urine
    E. Bile production

9. All of the following functions contribute to the athlete's ability to maintain a steady state during periods of increased metabolic needs while exercising except:
    A. Pulmonary diffusion
    B. Vascular adaptation
    C. Physical condition of the involved muscles
    D. A high-protein pre-event meal
    E. A and C

10. One method of estimating body fat has been through the use of skin-fold measurements at 4 sites. These 4 sites include all of the following except:
    A. Biceps
    B. Triceps
    C. Suprailiac
    D. Suprascapular
    E. None of the above

11. In hot, wet environments, the patient's ability to adjust to a significantly increased cardiovascular workload is limited by which factor?
    A. Hypoxia
    B. Hypervolemia
    C. Dehydration
    D. Hypernatremia
    E. Inability to dissipate heat by evaporation

12. When testing the physical conditioning of a patient, the coach asks the patient to sprint 50 yards. What does this test?
    A. Aerobic endurance
    B. Vital capacity
    C. Lower extremity power
    D. Power
    E. Anaerobic capacity

13. What is the definition of power?
    A. Power = work x force
    B. Power = speed x distance
    C. Power = force x distance
    D. Power = work x velocity
    E. Power = work x distance

14. During prolonged, intense training and conditioning of a patient, what cardiac change may occur over a period of time?
    A. Development of heart murmurs
    B. Development of premature ventricular contractions
    C. Increase in heart size
    D. Decrease in heart size
    E. Mitral valve prolapse

15. If it was determined that a 25-year-old patient should work at 80% of his maximal heart rate, what would be his target heart rate?
    A. 170 BPM
    B. 156 BPM
    C. 145 BPM
    D. 140 BPM
    E. 130 BPM

16. How long (generally) should a "warm-up" be to adequately prepare the body for athletic performance?
    A. 5 to 10 minutes
    B. 35 to 45 minutes
    C. 60 minutes
    D. 10 to 15 minutes
    E. 45 to 60 minutes

17. On the average, a college athlete expends between _____ to _____ calories per day.
    A. 4000 to 5000
    B. 2000 to 3000
    C. 2500 to 3000
    D. 2200 to 4400
    E. 1000 to 1800

18. An athlete's diet should consist of approximately _____ protein, _____ fat, and _____ carbohydrate.
    A. 12% to 15%, 40% to 50%, 55% to 70%
    B. 10% to 20%, 30% to 40%, 50% to 70%
    C. 5% to 10%, 30% to 45%, 60% to 80%
    D. 25% to 35%, 55% to 65%, 70% to 90%
    E. 45% to 55%, 10% to 20%, 45% to 55%

19. The pre-event meal should be planned by whom?
    A. The coach
    B. The athlete
    C. The athletic trainer
    D. A and B
    E. All of the above

20. The pre-event meal should be eaten ____ before competition to ensure proper digestion.
    A. 2 to 3 hours
    B. 3 to 4 hours
    C. 5 to 6 hours
    D. 6 to 8 hours
    E. 1 to 2 hours

21. How many glasses of water should an athlete consume on a daily basis?
    A. No more than 8
    B. 2 to 3
    C. 8 or more
    D. 5 to 7
    E. 4 to 6

22. How much calcium should a female athlete who shows signs of low bone mass consume a day?
    A. 500 to 700 mg
    B. 750 mg
    C. 1000 mg
    D. 1500 mg
    E. 1200 mg

23. When monitoring a carbohydrate-loading program for an endurance athlete, what should the athlete do the day prior to competition?
    A. Eat a high-carbohydrate meal and perform little or no exercise
    B. Eat a low-carbohydrate meal and participate in a regular amount of exercise
    C. Eat a high-carbohydrate meal and participate in a regular amount of exercise
    D. Hyperhydrate and rest the day before competition
    E. Eat a low-protein diet and participate in a regular amount of exercise

24. When working on a bleeding patient, what should the athletic trainer always do?
    A. Avoid touching the bloody areas
    B. Wash hands before treatment
    C. Wear gloves
    D. Wear eye protection
    E. Elevate the body part

25. Alpine skiing world championships are scheduled in Japan. Jet lag is bound to occur as a result of crossing several time zones. What should the athletic trainer recommend to the team members prior to their flight to combat the jet lag effect?
    A. Upon arrival, adjust all training, eating, and sleeping schedules to the local time of the country in which they are competing
    B. Consume caffeine only when traveling east
    C. Reset watches to the new time zone 3 days in advance to get used to the time change
    D. When traveling west, it is important to have a large breakfast in the morning to carry the athlete through the day
    E. Make sure the team trains late in the day prior to the trip

26. The NATA's position statement on exertional heat illness recommends which of the following?
    A. Ensure that the appropriate medical care is available and the rescue personnel are familiar with exertional heat illness prevention, recognition, and treatment
    B. Plan rest breaks to match environmental conditions and the intensity of the activity
    C. Weigh high-risk athletes (in high-risk conditions, weigh all athletes) before and after practice to estimate the amount of body water lost during practice and to ensure a return to prepractice weight before next practice
    D. Allow athletes to practice in shaded areas or use electric or cooling fans to circulate air when feasible
    E. All of the above

27. How is pediculosis spread between individuals?
    A. Coughing and sneezing
    B. Poor hand washing/hygiene
    C. Close sexual contact
    D. Contact with open sores
    E. Sharing eating utensils

28. When selecting and fitting protective gear and sports equipment, the athletic trainer should do which of the following to minimize liability?
    A. Buy protective gear or equipment from a reputable manufacturer
    B. Ensure that the individual who assembles the equipment is competent to do so
    C. If the athlete is wearing a cast, brace, or other type of immobilization device, ensure that it does not violate the rules of the sport
    D. Ensure the equipment is not defective
    E. All of the above

29. Which of the steps below are correct when fitting a football helmet?
    I.   Place the helmet over the head, tilt it backward, and rotate it forward into position
    II. Try to turn the helmet side-to-side with the head in a stationary position
    III. Check to make sure the helmet sits 3 finger-breadths above the eyebrows
    IV. Press straight down on the crown of the helmet to see if the pressure is at the crown of the head
    V.   Check to see if the jaw pads fit snugly against the jaw
    VI. Check the chin strap adjustment for a tight fit
    A. I, II, IV, V, VI
    B. I, II, III, VI
    C. I, III, IV, V
    D. I, III, IV, VI
    E. I, III, IV, V, VI

30. All of the following conditions would disqualify a patient from athletic competition except:
    A. Renal disease
    B. Uncontrolled hypertension
    C. Acute mononucleosis
    D. The absence of one testicle
    E. HIV

31. The _____ and _____ should be involved with the athlete and athletic trainer in selecting and maintaining the athlete's protective equipment.
    A. Coach, team physician
    B. Coach, equipment manager
    C. Equipment manager, team manager
    D. Team physician, coach
    E. Team physician, school nurse

32. Which of the following organizations certifies football helmets to make sure they are able to withstand repeated blows of high mass and low velocity?
    A. FDA
    B. NSA
    C. NATA
    D. NFL
    E. NOCSAE

33. Football helmets may fall into 1 or 2 categories. These 2 types are known as _____ or _____.
    A. Air- or fluid-filled, padded
    B. Gel-filled, padded
    C. Plastic, fiberglass
    D. Standard, adjustable
    E. Molded, nonmolded

34. When is maximum protection provided by a properly fitting mouthguard?
    A. When it is made of a flexible, resilient material and is form fitted to the teeth and upper jaw
    B. When it is made of a rigid, plastic material that is fitted to both the upper and lower jaw
    C. When it is certified by the National Operating Committee on Standards for Athletic Equipment
    D. When it is certified by the National Collegiate Athletic Association
    E. When it contains titanium fibers

35. Properly fitting shoulder pads should adequately cover the shoulder complex. Which structure should the epaulets and cups completely cover?
    A. The scapula
    B. The deltoids
    C. The pectoralis major
    D. The trapezius
    E. The pectoralis minor

36. A flak jacket is a piece of equipment designed to protect the athlete after what type of injury?
    A. Scapular injury
    B. Hip pointer injury
    C. Abdominal injury
    D. Rib injury
    E. Clavicle injury

37. Which of the following organizations sets the standards for eye protection for racquet sports?
    A. ACSM
    B. NATA
    C. FDA
    D. ASTM
    E. NOCSAE

38. Of the following pieces of equipment, which is not an NCAA-mandated piece of equipment?
    A. Wrestling—ear guards
    B. Men's lacrosse—protective gloves
    C. Baseball—double ear flap helmet for batting
    D. Gymnastics—palm protectors for the uneven parallel bars
    E. Women's lacrosse—protective eyewear

39. A female gymnast is complaining of symptoms of premenstrual syndrome, such as irritability, anxiety, depression, and bloating. Which of the following vitamins might be helpful in alleviating these symptoms?
    A. Vitamin B_6
    B. Vitamin B_{12}
    C. Vitamin K
    D. Vitamin A
    E. Vitamin C

40. While discussing general nutrition principles with a female swimmer who is a strict vegetarian, the athletic trainer should be aware that her diet might lack what mineral?
    A. Choline
    B. Iron
    C. Niacin
    D. Folate
    E. Potassium

41. Which type of drink would not be appropriate prior to a long-distance run?
    A. Water
    B. Regular soda
    C. Gatorade
    D. Water with lemon juice added
    E. Any drink containing sodium

42. A megadose of which of the following vitamins is potentially very dangerous?
    A. Thiamin
    B. Vitamin B_6
    C. Vitamin C
    D. Vitamin B_{12}
    E. Vitamin A

43. Under what condition(s) is a patient likely to experience a stress fracture of a bone?
    A. After a few high loads or many small loads are applied to the bone
    B. After a large traumatic insult to the bone
    C. After a traumatic incident that is quickly followed by a few small loads to the bone
    D. After 1 or 2 small loads are applied to the bone
    E. None of the above

44. Which of the following should be included in a pre-participation physical examination?
    I. Height and weight
    II. Orthopedic screening
    III. Vital signs
    IV. Ear/nose/throat exam
    V. Blood work
    A. I, II, V
    B. II, IV, V
    C. I, II III, IV
    D. I, III, V
    E. All of the above

45. Which of the following can cause an indirect sports fatality?
    A. Contact sports
    B. A blow to the head
    C. Blunt chest trauma
    D. Rodeo riding
    E. Heat stroke

46. One of your patients has just purchased a bicycle helmet and found a crack in the shell. To which organization should the manufacturer of the helmet report this defect?
    A. NATA
    B. CPSC
    C. NOCSAE
    D. USOC
    E. NASM

47. During a preparticipation physical examination, what type of assessment should be utilized to document the maturity of an athlete's secondary sexual characteristics?
    A. Tanner's 5 stages of assessment
    B. HOPS assessment scale
    C. Glasgow scale
    D. Erickson's hierarchy
    E. Maslow's maturity scale

48. During a preparticipation physical examination, what should the team physician and athletic trainer do jointly?
    A. Perform blood tests
    B. Perform Sentinel's test
    C. Review each examination for the final approval to participate
    D. Perform an orthopedic screening
    E. Perform psychological fitness assessments

49. According to the NATA position statement, Pre-participation Physical Examinations and Disqualifying Conditions, who should make the final decision regarding an athlete's participation in a sport?
    A. Athletic trainer
    B. School nurse
    C. Team physician and institution
    D. Parents
    E. Athletic director

50. Which of the following individuals is most susceptible to heat stroke and, therefore, must be carefully educated regarding the importance of adequate fluid intake during activity in hot, humid weather?
    A. Basketball guard
    B. A wrestler
    C. Female gymnast
    D. Swimmer
    E. A defensive lineman in football

51. When using an ice pack at home to decrease pain and swelling of an injured limb, what should the athletic trainer recommend to the athlete to prevent a cryotherapy injury?
    A. Add acetone to the ice at a 3:1 ratio
    B. Keep the injured limb elevated while using ice
    C. Place a damp towel between the athlete's skin and the ice pack
    D. Leave the ice pack on the body part between 20 to 40 minutes at a time
    E. All of the above

52. One of your athletes has been diagnosed with impetigo. What should the athletic trainer recommend to the athlete to prevent spread of the infection to other individuals?
    A. Clean his clothing daily with bleach
    B. Wear gloves
    C. Practice safe sex
    D. Prevent others from borrowing his clothing or using his towels
    E. Cover his mouth when coughing and avoid socializing in large crowds

53. A wrestler comes to the athletic training facility inquiring about a "drug that will make him lose weight quickly." He mentions a diuretic. Which of the following drugs has been banned by the International Olympic Committee and causes diuresis?
    A. Furosemide
    B. Salbutamol
    C. Caffeine (< 12 mcg/mL)
    D. Salicylates
    E. None of the above

54. A baseball player complains of recurrent ingrown toenails. What might the athletic trainer suggest to prevent this problem?
    A. Have the athlete put a small amount of cotton under his nails
    B. Have the athlete wear shoes with a large toe-box
    C. Have the athlete trim his toenails in a rounded shape parallel to the border of the cuticle
    D. Have the athlete trim his toenails weekly and cut them straight across
    E. Have the athlete purchase larger shoes

55. When advising an athlete about the proper construction of a running shoe, which of the following criteria will help prevent foot and ankle injuries?
    I. The midsole should be somewhat soft, but should not easily flatten out with pressure
    II. The shoe should have good forefoot flexibility
    III. The heel counter should be shallow and firm
    IV. The heel counter should be strong and fit well around the foot
    V. The upper should be constructed of quality leather or rubber
    A. I, II, IV
    B. I, III, IV, V
    C. II, III, IV
    D. II, IV, V
    E. I, II, III

56. To prevent the feeling of sedation during the day while taking medications for allergic rhinitis, the athletic trainer should suggest the athlete not take which of the following medications until he or she is ready to go to bed?
    A. Expectorants
    B. Antihistamines
    C. Decongestants
    D. NSAIDs
    E. Antipyretic agents

57. Why is it important for an active individual to follow a varied diet that reflects the Dietary Guidelines for America?
    A. The individual will be making smart choices from every food group
    B. The individual will get the most nutrition out of calories
    C. The individual will stay within daily calorie needs
    D. All of the above
    E. None of the above

58. To prevent the possibility of an acute compartment syndrome, the athletic trainer should advise his or her field hockey players to wear which of the following pieces of equipment?
    A. Thigh pads
    B. Mouthguards
    C. Helmets
    D. Gloves
    E. Shin guards

59. The dangers of possible hypothermia during exercise in very cold weather are significantly pronounced by _____ and _____.
    A. Light clothing, low chill factor
    B. Wind, wet weather
    C. Layered clothing, dry weather
    D. Wind, dry weather
    E. Heavy clothing, wind

60. A female athlete should choose a sports bra that is supportive enough to prevent stretching of which structure?
    A. The skin
    B. The pectoralis major
    C. Cooper's ligaments
    D. The nipples
    E. Ligamentum pectoris

61. When instructing a patient in the proper technique of applying an elastic wrap to control pain and edema of an extremity, the athletic trainer should instruct the patient to remove the wrap if all except the following occurs at the distal end of the extremity:
    A. Numbness
    B. Coolness
    C. Tingling
    D. Cyanosis
    E. Pink hue to the skin

62. When counseling an athlete about the adverse effects of anabolic steroids on females, all of the following effects should be included except:
    A. Severe acne
    B. Increased libido
    C. Increased body fat
    D. Development of a deep voice
    E. Change in menstrual cycle

63. What should the athletic trainer advise his or her athletes to do to minimize the negative effects of jet lag?
    A. Drink an adequate amount of fluids, especially water, to avoid dehydration
    B. Keep watches set to their "home" time zone
    C. Get up and go to bed 2 to 3 hours earlier for each time zone crossed
    D. Wear warm clothing to avoid getting cold while on the plane
    E. Get at least 8 hours of sleep at night the week before the flight

64. You are aware of the general use of smokeless tobacco among your high school baseball players. You decide to develop a seminar for the coaches and players to discourage its use. Which of the following are effects of the chronic use of chewing tobacco?
    I. Leukoplakia
    II. Mouth and throat cancer
    III. Increased aggression
    IV. Bad breath
    V. Mood swings
    VI. Gynecomastia

    A. I, II, IV
    B. III, V, VI
    C. I, II, III
    D. II, III, IV
    E. II, III, IV, V

65. One of your basketball players comes into the athletic training facility insisting that his ankles need to be taped even though he has no known injury. The athlete should be advised of which of the following?
    A. To let the athletic trainer know if he starts developing any knee problems
    B. An elastic or neoprene ankle brace is more effective than taping in preventing an injury
    C. For the ankle taping to be effective, the athlete should rely on ankle-strengthening exercises rather than prophylactic taping if there is no injury present
    D. Advise the athlete to contact his family physician to evaluate his ankles
    E. None of the above

66. It is well known that many athletes will utilize nutritional supplements in an effort to enhance performance. An athlete asks you to explain the action of an antioxidant. Which of the following best describes the role of an antioxidant?
    A. A nutrient that protects the cell from the detrimental effects of substances that may cause health problems, such as premature aging
    B. A mineral that is known to protect the body from cancer
    C. A vitamin that is known to protect the body from heart disease
    D. A substance that is found in vegetables and dairy products and prevents certain types of cancer and osteoporosis
    E. None of the above

67. In order to prevent medial epicondylitis, all of the following actions should be avoided via technique modification except:
    A. Too much wrist flexion at follow-through during a golf swing
    B. Excessive elbow valgus when throwing a javelin
    C. Hyperextension of the wrist when performing a backhand shot in tennis
    D. Excessive wrist flexion during a racquetball forehand shot
    E. A and B

68. Which of the following patients should avoid high-volume, high-intensity plyometric exercises?
    A. Patients who weigh more than 220 pounds
    B. Premenstrual female patients
    C. Patients who weigh less than 75 kg
    D. Diabetic patients
    E. Asthmatic patients

69. All of the following free-weight exercises require one or more spotters except:
    A. Free-weight exercise in which the bar passes over the face
    B. Free-weight exercise in which a bar moves over the head
    C. Free-weight exercise in which a bar curls up in front of the chest
    D. Free-weight exercise in which the bar is positioned on the back
    E. Free-weight exercise in which the bar moves over the chest

70. Keratoderma can be prevented by all of the following except:
    A. Wearing 2 pairs of socks
    B. Applying a lubricant to the skin to prevent friction
    C. Using an antifungal ointment
    D. Using a glove or moleskin
    E. Wearing properly fitting shoes

71. How may an urinary tract infection be avoided in a female athlete?
    A. Drinking fluids that are acidic, such as orange juice
    B. Practicing sanitary bowel and bladder habits
    C. Avoiding food high in magnesium
    D. Avoid wearing colored underwear
    E. None of the above

72. A torus fracture is the result of what kind of force?
    A. Shearing
    B. Traction
    C. Compressive
    D. Twisting
    E. Bending

73. How many servings of fruit should an athlete have as a minimum daily requirement?
    A. 2 to 6 servings
    B. 5 to 7 servings
    C. 2 to 4 servings
    D. Number of servings are according to the athlete's age
    E. Number of servings are according to the athlete's height and weight

74. At the secondary school level, the athletic training student should be involved in the educational efforts involving bloodborne pathogens. These educational items should include all of the following except:
    A. Education on the availability of herpes testing
    B. Education/training in the use of universal precautions and wound care
    C. Education on access to hepatitis B virus vaccinations and testing
    D. Education of parents and guardians regarding the students' risk of infection
    E. Education on the modes of infection and risk of infection from the athletes they care for

75. According to the American College of Sports Medicine, when performing flexibility exercises, how long should a stretch be held for optimal results?
    A. 5 to 10 seconds; after 10 seconds, minimal/no results are achieved
    B. 10 to 30 seconds; only as long as it feels comfortable
    C. 45 to 60 seconds; no less than 45 seconds
    D. 60 to 90 seconds; until the athlete feels some mild discomfort
    E. A minimum of 1½ to 2 minutes

76. A diet that is very low in carbohydrates may result in all of the following except:
    A. Fatigue
    B. Hypoglycemia
    C. Ketosis
    D. Very high blood pH levels
    E. Headaches

77. Which of the following is not a neural effect of resistance training?
    A. Increased motor unit activation and recruitment
    B. Increased discharge frequency of motoneurons
    C. Increased muscle capillary density
    D. Decreased neural inhibitions
    E. Increased neuromuscular efficiency

78. General maintenance and cleaning tasks of the athletic training facility and activities areas of an athletic facility should include all of the following except:
    A. Wood flooring should be kept free of splinters, holes, protruding nails, uneven boards, and screws
    B. All areas should be swept, vacuumed, and mopped according to designated cleaning schedules
    C. Check to make sure that athletic uniforms/equipment are properly stored and inventoried on a regular basis
    D. Lighting apparatuses should be checked and changed on a regular basis
    E. Check to see that ground fault interrupters are working and appropriately located

79. To prevent a hazardous electrical problem in the athletic training facility, _____ and _____ should never be used.
    A. Multiple adapters, extension cords
    B. Ground fault interrupters, 3-pronged wall outlets
    C. Ground fault interrupters, fluorescent lights
    D. Hanging lights, 3-pronged wall outlets
    E. Equipment with electrical cords, equipment that conforms to National Electrical Code guidelines

80. During a preparticipation physical examination that utilizes stations, which of the following personnel is able to perform an examination for adenopathy, abnormalities of the genitalia, and hernias in an athlete?
    A. Athletic training student
    B. Physician or physician assistant
    C. Physical therapist
    D. Certified athletic trainer
    E. School nurse

81. "Counting the number of seconds from lightning flash until the sound of thunder divided by 5" describes the "flash-to-bang" method utilized by athletic trainers to roughly calculate which of the following?
    A. How far away thunder is occurring
    B. The amount of time before play is resumed
    C. How far away lightning is occurring
    D. The intensity of the thunder
    E. None of the above

82. When is it best to have athletes practice outdoors in an urban environment?
    A. Early in the morning
    B. In the middle of the afternoon
    C. Early afternoon
    D. Very late afternoon/early evening
    E. Never

83. There are 2 types of heel cups that are designed to help prevent heel bruises. Of these 2 heel cups, which has an elevated heel that can compress downward so that the heel never actually makes contact with the interior of the shoe?
    A. A rubberized padded cup
    B. A rigid plastic cup
    C. A jelly-filled cushion cup
    D. An air-filled cushion cup
    E. All of the above

84. What is the primary purpose of the Achilles tendon tape job?
    A. To give support and help prevent inversion ankle sprains
    B. Used with acute ankle sprains to help prevent swelling if an elastic wrap is not available
    C. To prevent the medial foot from flattening
    D. To restrict the amount of dorsiflexion at the ankle
    E. A and C

85. Which of the following is not recommended for the prevention of heat-related illnesses?
    A. Check the humidity and temperature daily
    B. Drink 20 ounces of water every 15 minutes
    C. Wear layers of lightweight clothing
    D. Acclimatize
    E. All of the above

86. Which of the following is not a preventive measure for fungal skin infections?
    A. Use powders to absorb moisture
    B. Wear the same pair of shoes everyday
    C. Shower frequently
    D. Avoid contact with contaminated surfaces
    E. Towel off completely following a shower

87. All of the following are measures for preventing infectious diseases except:
    A. Appropriate diet, recovery time between workouts, and sleep
    B. Use individual water bottles, towels, uniforms, and personal equipment
    C. Frequent laundering of uniforms
    D. Use water to clean contaminated surfaces or equipment
    E. B and C

88. Which of the following stages of disease prevention focuses on early detection and appropriate referral?
    A. Primary stage
    B. Secondary stage
    C. Initial stage
    D. Tertiary stage
    E. None of the above

89. All of the following are predisposing conditions to heat illness except:
    A. Medications
    B. Age
    C. Conditioning level
    D. Hydration status
    E. Small body mass

90. All of the following symptoms are considered "red flags," requiring urgent referral to a physician, except:
    A. Persistent headaches
    B. Constant pain
    C. Insomnia
    D. Malaise, fatigue
    E. Hunger

91. All of the following are effects of immobilization on muscle except:
    A. Increase in muscle contraction time
    B. Increase in muscle tension produced
    C. Decrease in muscle fiber size
    D. Decrease in total muscle weight
    E. Decrease in neuromuscular efficiency

92. All of the following types of infection are transmitted through the air except:
    A. Meningitis
    B. Pneumonia
    C. Tuberculosis
    D. Scarlet fever
    E. Malaria

93. Which of the following is a type of exercise that involves a muscle contraction in which the length of the muscle is changing while the contraction is performed at a constant velocity?
    A. Isokinetic
    B. Isotonic
    C. Isometric
    D. Progressive resistance
    E. PNF

94. A shoe with _____ and _____ cleats has been shown to reduce the risk of knee injuries.
    A. Longer, fewer
    B. Shorter, more
    C. Longer, more
    D. Shorter, fewer
    E. Longer, sharper

95. What type of stretching is not recommended because of the potential for causing muscle soreness and possible injury when done over a period of time?
    A. Ballistic
    B. PNF
    C. Static
    D. Concentric
    E. None of the above

96. When exercising in cold temperatures, what should be done by the athlete to prevent hypothermia?
    A. Keep his or her clothes dry
    B. Warm-up exercises and remain active
    C. Wear warm clothing
    D. All of the above
    E. None of the above

97. Sixty-five percent of the heat produced by the body during exercise is lost through what?
    A. Convection
    B. Conduction
    C. Evaporation
    D. Radiation
    E. None of the above

98. Where is the most heat lost from the body in cold weather?
    A. Hands
    B. Feet
    C. Torso
    D. Head and neck
    E. A and B

99. What does a sunscreen SPF of 5 represent?
    A. An individual can be exposed to ultraviolet light 5 times longer than he or she could without having the sunscreen on before his or her skin turns red
    B. An individual will be protected from the sun 105%
    C. Nothing
    D. The sunscreen contains 5% of SPF
    E. The number of applications it takes for 100% protection

100. All of the following are signs and symptoms of dehydration except:
    A. Sunken, soft eyes
    B. High specific gravity of urine
    C. Weight loss
    D. Thirst
    E. Seizures

101. Athlete's foot (tinea pedis) may be prevented by all of the following except:
    A. Dusting the feet daily with powder
    B. Completely drying feet after getting them wet, including between toes
    C. Wearing sandals when showering in a public facility
    D. Washing the feet on a regular basis
    E. Sharing shoes with teammates

102. All of the following are items used to prevent internal ear damage from excessive noise except:
    A. Ear plugs
    B. Ear muffs
    C. Semi-aural devices
    D. A headband
    E. B and C

103. Which of the following is not a cause of a weight-training injury?
    A. The use of a "spotter"
    B. Barbell or platform defects
    C. Poor technique
    D. Not properly warming up before lifting weights
    E. C and D

104. All of the following are intrinsic factors of injury except:
    A. Flexibility
    B. Weather
    C. Age
    D. Weight
    E. C and D

105. A soccer player sustains a strain to the quadriceps muscle group. You are trying to prevent atrophy during rehabilitation. What method of treatment would you use?
    A. Ultrasound and TENS
    B. Interferential current
    C. Stretching
    D. High-volt galvanic stimulation
    E. Russian stimulation

106. Which of the following is a D2 pattern of an extremity?
    A. External rotation with flexion and abduction to internal rotation with extension and adduction
    B. External rotation with flexion and adduction to internal rotation with flexion and abduction
    C. External rotation with adduction and flexion to internal rotation with abduction and flexion
    D. External rotation with abduction and extension to internal rotation with adduction and flexion
    E. None of the above

107. An athlete reports to you that another member of the women's gymnastics team has a recognizable problem with eating. She reports that the athlete binge eats, followed by self-induced vomiting. What is this athlete suffering from?
    A. Anorexia nervosa
    B. Amenorrhea
    C. Bulimia nervosa
    D. B and C
    E. None of the above

108. Which of the following is a condition that is associated with the enlargement of the spleen?
    A. Graves' disease
    B. Constipation
    C. Appendicitis
    D. Hepatitis
    E. Mononucleosis

109. All of the following are true when fitting shoulder pads except:
    A. Axillary straps should not be very tight but just enough to be snug around the chest to keep the shoulder pads in place
    B. Shoulder pads should stop at the midsternum
    C. Acromioclavicular joint should have a channel of foam padding
    D. Lateral flaps should cover down to the deltoid tuberosity
    E. The neck opening must allow the athlete to raise the arm overhead, but not allow the pad to shift

110. When an athletic trainer is performing CPR, certain steps should be taken to minimize the risk of disease transmission via bloodborne pathogen. Which of the following should be used according to OSHA guidelines to protect the athletic trainer?
    A. Gloves
    B. An eye shield
    C. Barrier mask
    D. New AED pads
    E. Striker bag

111. Which of the following minerals decreases the risk of osteoporosis and increases the density of the bone?
    A. Zinc
    B. Folate
    C. Molybdenum
    D. Iron
    E. Calcium

112. All of the following are signs of anorexia nervosa except:
    A. Dramatic weight loss
    B. Obsession with weight gain
    C. Social isolation
    D. Reaching competitive weight and continuing to lose weight in off-season
    E. Significant weight gain during the off-season

113. When trying to decrease the chance of injury during activity, one should stretch thoroughly. Which one of these stretches represents bouncing type movement to achieve a stretch?
    A. Ballistic
    B. Dynamic
    C. Static
    D. Active
    E. PNF-slow-reverse hold

114. While assisting an athlete in stretching exercises, the athletic trainer should follow some guidelines. Which one of the following is not true?
    A. The athlete should be relaxed
    B. The stretch should be stopped when the athlete reports mild discomfort
    C. The stretch should be unilaterally administered
    D. The body part should be stretched for up to 30 seconds
    E. All of the above

115. Athletes can prevent lower leg injuries by all of the following except:
    A. Stretching
    B. Proper footwear
    C. Proprioceptive training
    D. Strength training
    E. All of the above

116. Which of the following is not a way for a throwing athlete to prevent injuries while training?
    A. Minimizing the effects of microtrauma during training
    B. Maintaining cardiovascular and lower extremity conditioning
    C. Good communication between the athlete, athletic trainer, coach, and physician during training
    D. All of the above
    E. B and C

117. Prevention of a chronic or debilitating illness or injury through appropriate care and rehabilitation is called what?
    A. Primary prevention
    B. Secondary prevention
    C. Tertiary prevention
    D. Luminary prevention
    E. Bimodal prevention

118. _____ refers to the concept of dividing the annual training plan into smaller segments, phases, or cycles.
    A. Specificity
    B. Frequency
    C. Duration
    D. Segmental division
    E. Periodization

119. Extrinsic risk factors of athletic injury include which of the following?
    A. Training errors
    B. Poor or inappropriate coaching
    C. Improper technique
    D. All of the above
    E. None of the above

120. _____ states that muscle strength, power, endurance, and hypertrophy increase only when muscles perform workloads greater than those loads previously encountered.
    A. PRE principle
    B. The DAPRE principle
    C. The strength-duration curve
    D. The power training principle
    E. The overload principle

121. A patient with mononucleosis should not play sports until the symptoms subside because of which of the following problems?
    A. Enlarged spleen
    B. Stress on the liver
    C. Possible kidney complications
    D. Malaise and fatigue
    E. Possible gallbladder rupture

122. How soon after a patient sustains a concussion should he or she be allowed to return to competition or practice?
    A. Immediately
    B. Following evaluation and clearance by a physician or designee specifically trained and experienced in concussion evaluation and management
    C. When the patient feels he or she is ready
    D. 12 hours later
    E. 7 days

123. When a football player has a possible cervical injury, which of the following should you do first?
    A. Remove the shoulder pads (only)
    B. Remove the helmet (only)
    C. Remove the shoulder pads then the helmet
    D. Place the athlete on a spine board
    E. Assess level of consciousness

124. A patient presents to you with a suspected shoulder dislocation. What should you do?
    A. Evaluate the injury then reduce the dislocation as soon as possible
    B. Evaluate the shoulder motion and send the patient to the hospital
    C. Tell the patient to sit and wait until you have time to deal with it
    D. Check the neurovascular status of the upper extremity, including dermatomes and myotomes
    E. Immediately immobilize the joint and refer the patient to the team physician

125. Shoulder pads provide protection for which type of injury?
    A. Acromioclavicular joint separation
    B. Glenohumeral joint separation
    C. Rotator cuff tendinitis
    D. Impingement
    E. Brachial plexus injuries

126. Under which of the following environmental conditions would an undiagnosed patient with sickle-cell trait be at most risk?
    A. Hot, humid environment
    B. Cold, dry environment
    C. High-altitude environment
    D. Cold, humid environment
    E. A and C

127. Patients with Down syndrome are restricted from participating in sports such as gymnastics, diving, soccer, and the high jump without documented medical clearance because of the possible presence of which of the following conditions?
    A. Atlantoaxial instability
    B. Strabismus
    C. Slipped capital epiphysis
    D. Aortic aneurysm
    E. Talar subluxation

128. Immunization against the hepatitis B virus will also prevent the manifestation of which of the following viruses?
    A. Hepatitis A
    B. Hepatitis C
    C. Hepatitis D
    D. HIV
    E. Human papillomavirus

129. Which of the following is true regarding the hepatitis B immunization?
    A. It is a series of 3 shots given over 3 months
    B. The one injection will be effective for a lifetime
    C. The immunization may be given as an injection or nasal spray
    D. It is not effective in children
    E. It is a series of 3 shots given over a course of 9 months

130. Genital warts are caused by which of the following?
    A. HIV
    B. Herpes I virus
    C. Herpes II virus
    D. Chlamydia
    E. Human papillomavirus

131. The MMR vaccine is given in protection against which of the following diseases?
    A. Mononucleosis, meningitis, rubella
    B. Meningitis, mononucleosis, rubeola
    C. Mumps, meningitis, rubeola
    D. Measles, mumps, rubella
    E. Mumps, measles, rhabdomyolysis

132. Which of the following is the most common type of cerebral palsy?
    A. Flaccid
    B. Spastic
    C. Dyskinetic
    D. Ataxic
    E. Atrophic

133. A patient who ignores his or her diagnosis of cardiac hypertrophy and continues to exercise at an intense level risks which of the following?
    A. Commotio cordis
    B. Pulmonary hypertension
    C. A fatal cardiac event
    D. Aortic rupture
    E. Stroke

134. The function of the pituitary gland is to do all of the following except:
    A. Increase the levels of calcium in the blood
    B. Increase thyroid function
    C. Increase estrogen release (in females)
    D. Increase testosterone release (in males)
    E. Increase water absorption in the kidneys

135. Screening for Marfan syndrome includes musculoskeletal and eye exams. Which of the following tests is also part of the screening process?
    A. Urinalysis
    B. Echocardiogram
    C. Pulmonary function test
    D. Electrocardiogram
    E. Complete blood count

136. All of the following arrhythmias require limitation of activity (in asymptomatic patients without structural heart disease) except:
    A. Atrial flutter
    B. Atrial fibrillation
    C. Ventricular tachycardia
    D. Short QT syndrome
    E. Long QT syndrome

137. Which of the following statements is true about hypertrophic cardiomyopathy (HCM)?
    A. The incidence of sudden death from HCM is 2 to 3 times higher in children and adolescents than in adults
    B. The incidence of sudden death from HCM is 2 to 3 times higher in adults than in teenagers
    C. The incidence of sudden death from HCM is 4 to 6 times higher in Black males than in White males
    D. The incidence of sudden death from HCM is 4 to 6 times higher in males than females
    E. The incidence of sudden death from HCM is 4 to 6 times higher in females than males

138. The label on a dietary supplement must contain all the following elements except:
    A. Name and location of the manufacturer
    B. Distributor
    C. A complete list of ingredients
    D. The contents of the product
    E. The date of initial packaging

139. Which of the following medications can contribute to heat-related illnesses?
    A. Proton pump inhibitors
    B. Antiemetics
    C. Beta-blockers and antihistamines
    D. Anti-inflammatories
    E. Antibacterials

140. Bismuth subsalicylate (Kaopectate, Pepto-Bismol) should not be taken by a patient for whom use of _____ is a precaution or contraindicated.
    A. Penicillin
    B. Albuterol
    C. Prednisone
    D. Aspirin
    E. Claritin

141. The athletic trainer should be aware of which of the following when setting up an exercise regime for an individual who is taking beta-blockers for hypertension?
    A. Extreme drowsiness
    B. Exercise fatigue
    C. Sudden onset of vertigo
    D. Inattentiveness
    E. Diaphoresis during aerobic exercise

142. According to the NATA's position statement on the prevention of pediatric overuse injuries, full effort throwing limits for players 9 to 14 years old should be as follows:
    A. 90 pitches/game, 800 pitches/season
    B. 75 pitches/game, 600 pitches/season
    C. 25 pitches/game, 350 pitches/season
    D. 50 pitches/game, 500 pitches/season
    E. There are no pitching limits for those players participating in a year-round sport

143. The NATA's position statement on the prevention of pediatric overuse injuries suggests a pediatric athlete should have at least _____ per week from competitive practices, competitions, and sport-specific training.
    A. 1 to 2 days off
    B. 3 days off
    C. 3 to 5 days off
    D. 2 to 3 days off
    E. ½ to 1 full day off

144. According to the NATA's position statement regarding safe weight loss and maintenance practices in sport and exercise, when determining goal weight, body weight should be assessed relative to what?
    A. Skin-fold measurements
    B. Body mass index
    C. Basal metabolic rate
    D. Bioelectric impedance measurements
    E. Body composition

145. The NATA's position statement on the management of the athlete with type 1 diabetes recommends that each athlete with diabetes have a diabetes care plan. The plan should include all of the following except:
    A. Blood glucose monitoring guidelines
    B. Guidelines for dietary management
    C. Insulin therapy guidelines
    D. Guidelines for hypoglycemia recognition and treatment
    E. Guidelines for hyperglycemia recognition and treatment

146. The NATA's position statement on safe weight loss and maintenance practices in sport and exercise recommends the individual assessing body composition use a valid and reliable body composition assessment technique. These include all of the following except:
    A. Hydrodensitometry
    B. Air displacement plethysmography
    C. Skin-fold measurements
    D. Bioelectric impedance
    E. Doppler measurements

147. According to the consensus statement between the Inter-Association Task Force for Preseason Secondary School Athletics and the NATA's Secondary School Athletic Trainer's Committee, *Preseason Heat Acclimatization Guidelines for Secondary School Athletics*, a 1-hour maximum walk through is permitted during days 1 through 5 of the heat acclimatization period. How long should the recovery period be between the practice and walk through (or visa versa)?
    A. ½ hour
    B. 1 hour
    C. 2 hours
    D. 3 hours
    E. 24 hours

148. According to the NATA's position statement on anabolic-androgenic steroids, an athletic trainer can offer specific support to an athlete suspected of abusing anabolic-androgenic steroids (AAS) through all of the following means except:
    A. Building trust with athletes, coaches, and clients through consistent, year-round, evidence-based educational meetings and inservice sessions .
    B. Avoiding unfounded scare tactics and hype concerning the negative consequences of AAS
    C. Being alert for excessive discussion about and focus on supplements and nutrition practices or self-education about AAS (ie, types, stacks, and cycles)
    D. Remaining attentive because AAS abusers are typically secretive and good at not getting caught; a passed drug screen does not prove AAS nonuse
    E. By supporting the athlete's self-esteem; it is important to compliment his or her physical appearance and strength gains as changes become evident

149. According to the NATA's position statement on anabolic-androgenic steroids, "stacking" of anabolic-androgenic steroids (AAS) is defined as:
    A. Simultaneously administering multiple AAS
    B. Methodically increasing doses within a specific period of time
    C. Alternating 2 types of AAS
    D. Increasing then decreasing dosages over a 48-hour period
    E. Starting with the lowest dosage possible of a given AAS and increasing each subsequent dose by ½ strength

150. Which of the following types of programs appear to be effective anabolic-androgenic steroid (AAS) abuse deterrents for adolescent student-athletes?
    A. Sex-specific, sport-centered, and coach-facilitated educational programs that promote performance-enhancing alternatives (ie, sport nutrition and strength training)
    B. Co-educational, sport-centered, and coach-facilitated educational programs
    C. Gender-specific, community-based, and parent-supported programs
    D. Gender-specific and school- and parent-educational programs focused on behavior altering strategies
    E. Educational programs focused on specific physical and cognitive consequences of AAS abuse

151. According to the NATA's position statement on lightning safety for athletics and recreation, aspects of an emergency action plan specific to lightning safety include all of the following except:
    A. Promote lightning safety slogans
    B. Establish a chain of command
    C. Use a reliable means of monitoring the weather
    D. Identify locations safe from the lightning hazard
    E. Make sure all emergency vehicles are grounded during inclement weather

152. How far from the nose should the facemask of a football helmet be located?
    A. 1 inch
    B. 2 finger widths
    C. 3 finger widths
    D. 0.75 inch
    E. 3 inches

153. Thermomoldable plastics, such as Orthoplast or Aquaplast, may be indicated for many different situations. Which of the following conditions might benefit from the use of this type of material?
    A. Genu recurvatum
    B. Thoracic outlet syndrome
    C. Quadriceps contusion
    D. Anterior cruciate sprain
    E. Genu varum

154. All of the following are ways of reducing risk of injury except:
    A. Assess activity areas for safety
    B. Frequent handwashing
    C. Proper equipment maintenance
    D. Documentation of treatments
    E. All of the above

Clinical Evaluation and Diagnosis

1. A positive Thompson's sign is indicative of what problem?
    A. Tight hip flexor
    B. Tight iliotibial band
    C. Ruptured anterior tibialis tendon
    D. Ruptured posterior tibialis tendon
    E. Ruptured Achilles tendon

2. Which of the following is a simple movement to check the integrity of the radial nerve?
    A. Elbow flexion
    B. Wrist extension
    C. Forearm supination
    D. Thumb-to-little finger opposition
    E. Shoulder flexion

3. A grade I ankle inversion sprain involves which structure?
   A. Tibiofibular ligament
   B. Posterior talofibular ligament
   C. Calcaneofibular ligament
   D. Anterior talofibular ligament
   E. Spring ligament

4. You are covering a football game when 2 players collide. You notice that one player grabs his neck and shakes his arm. When you examine him, he complains of lateral neck discomfort and a feeling of "numbness" or "burning" down his arm. His arm is hanging limp by his side. In a few minutes, the symptoms subside. What do you suspect?
   A. Carpal tunnel syndrome
   B. Long thoracic nerve injury
   C. A "burner" or pinched nerve syndrome
   D. Dorsal scapular nerve injury
   E. Thoracic outlet syndrome

5. Which test, if positive, is indicative of a torn posterior cruciate ligament?
   A. Sag sign
   B. Anterior drawer sign
   C. McMurray's sign
   D. Ober's sign
   E. Lachman's sign

6. At what point should the athletic trainer's initial evaluation of an injury begin?
   A. At the moment the injury is witnessed
   B. Once the patient has been stabilized in the athletic training facility
   C. Once the athletic trainer receives a medical referral from a doctor
   D. After the patient is seen by the team doctor
   E. B and D

7. Panner's disease is an osteochondrosis of which of the following?
   A. Capitellum
   B. Tibial tubercle
   C. Olecranon
   D. First ray of the foot
   E. Talus

8. What quick test can be performed to check if nerve root L5 is intact?
   A. Have the patient flex his or her hip while standing
   B. Have the patient walk on his or her toes
   C. Have the patient extend his or her great toe
   D. Have the patient extend his or her hip
   E. Have the patient flex his or her knee

9. A positive Phalen's sign is suspect of what problem?
   A. Tarsal tunnel syndrome
   B. Long thoracic nerve injury
   C. Thoracic outlet syndrome
   D. Suprascapular entrapment syndrome
   E. Carpal tunnel syndrome

10. Trendelenburg's test is a method used to evaluate the competence of what structures?
    A. Hip flexors
    B. Peroneal muscles
    C. Hip abductors
    D. Erector spinae
    E. Abdominals

11. What evaluative test is used to examine the integrity of the lateral collateral ligament of the knee?
    A. Pivot shift test
    B. Valgus stress test
    C. Lachman's test
    D. Varus stress test
    E. None of the above

12. What does a positive drop-arm sign indicate?
    A. Posterior shoulder subluxation
    B. Torn rotator cuff muscle
    C. Axillary nerve injury
    D. A labral tear
    E. Humeral head fracture

13. If there is inflammation at the site of the medial epicondyle of the elbow, which of the following would be positive?
    A. Tennis elbow test
    B. Golfer's elbow test
    C. Tinel's sign
    D. Finkelstein's test
    E. Allen's test

14. All of the following are signs of an injury except:
    A. Change in skin color or texture
    B. Change in body temperature
    C. Change in blood pressure
    D. Complaint of headaches
    E. Change in respiratory rate

15. Information gained during the palpation phase of the athletic trainer's initial assessment might include all of the following except:
    A. Presence of crepitus
    B. Sensory function
    C. Presence of a deformity
    D. Degree of functional movement
    E. A and B

16. During an upper quarter screen, checking the strength of thumb extension correlates to what nerve root?
    A. T1
    B. T3
    C. C5
    D. C4
    E. C8

17. A positive clunk test is indicative of what pathology?
    A. Unstable ankle
    B. Olecranon fracture
    C. Meniscus tear of the knee
    D. Glenoid labrum tear
    E. Anterior cruciate ligament tear

18. A baseball player comes to see the athletic trainer and is complaining of diffuse pain, clicking, and a sensation of "slipping" of his right shoulder when throwing. What pathology might the athletic trainer suspect with this type of presentation?
    A. Torn rotator cuff
    B. Thrower's exostosis
    C. Acromioclavicular joint pathology
    D. Labral pathology
    E. Bicipital tendinitis

19. Two major symptoms of a spontaneous pneumothorax include _____ and _____.
    A. Bradycardia, cyanosis
    B. Sudden chest pain, dyspnea
    C. Apnea with rales, rhonchi
    D. Left shoulder pain, cyanosis
    E. Diaphoresis, bradycardia

20. The _____ pulse and _____ pulse should be palpated after an acute traumatic injury to the knee area to make sure the peripheral circulation to the involved limb is adequate.
    A. Posterior tibial, dorsalis pedis
    B. Anterior tibial, plantar
    C. Saphenous, dorsalis pedis
    D. Femoral, posterior tibial
    E. Femoral, popliteal

21. Foot drop may be indicative of what pathology?
    A. Plantar nerve injury
    B. Shin splints
    C. Osteochondritis dissecans
    D. Achilles tendinitis
    E. Peroneal nerve injury

22. A type V Salter-Harris fracture involves what kind of fracture through the physeal plate?
    A. The epiphysis and metaphysis separate without fragmentation
    B. A crush injury to the epiphysis
    C. The epiphysis and metaphysis separate with fragmentation
    D. The epiphysis, metaphysis, and physis all separate from each other
    E. The metaphysis is separated with fragmentation

23. A patient you have just evaluated for a possible head injury has a noticeable facial droop on the left side of his face. Which cranial nerve(s) is involved?
    A. I
    B. IV, V
    C. VII
    D. III, IX
    E. II, VI

24. During your examination of a patient who has been complaining of weakness when using the rowing machine in the weight room, you notice his right latissimus dorsi muscle appears atrophied. Which nerve is affected?
    A. Trigeminal
    B. Thoracodorsal
    C. Dorsal scapular
    D. Thoracic spinal
    E. None of the above

25. A second-degree burn will have which of the following characteristics?
    A. A raised, reddened appearance
    B. A white, mottled appearance
    C. A blackened, hard appearance
    D. A reddened area with blisters
    E. Blanched, shiny appearance

26. The athlete may have difficulty performing what actions if the medial and lateral pectoral nerves are injured?
    A. Flexion, adduction, and internal rotation of the upper arm
    B. Shoulder shrugs
    C. Abduction and external rotation of the upper arm
    D. Extension, internal rotation, and adduction of the upper arm
    E. Flexion, abduction, and external rotation of the upper arm

27. A gymnast reports to the athletic trainer with a complaint of low back pain, which has been present for approximately 1 week. After being sent to the doctor for evaluation, a "Scottie dog" defect is seen on x-ray. This finding confirms which condition?
    A. Fractured transverse process of a vertebra
    B. Fractured demifacet of a vertebra
    C. Spondylolisthesis
    D. Spondylolysis
    E. A and B

28. A patient is poked in the eye with a finger and comes to the athletic trainer for evaluation. The patient is having significant difficulty opening his eye. Which of the following muscles might have sustained an injury?
    A. Levator capitis inferioris
    B. Splenius capitis
    C. Levator palpebrae superioris
    D. Levator palpebrae orbitis
    E. Scalenes

29. A patient is brought to the athletic training facility after being struck in the back of the head with a bat by accident. The patient is complaining of blurred vision. Which lobe of the brain has been affected?
    A. Frontal
    B. Parietal
    C. Temporal
    D. Occipital
    E. Cerebellum

30. What internal organ is diseased if the patient presents with jaundice?
    A. Spleen
    B. Pancreas
    C. Gallbladder
    D. Kidney
    E. Liver

31. Which 2 structures are injured with a Bankart lesion?
    A. Anterior capsule of the shoulder and the glenoid labrum
    B. The inferior capsule of the shoulder and glenoid fossa
    C. The articular surface of the humeral head and glenoid labrum
    D. The surgical neck of the humerus and the coracoacromial ligament
    E. The acromioclavicular joint and glenoid fossa

32. A patient has a wrist injury that is limiting his ability to supinate his forearm. In what plane of motion does supination and pronation of the forearm take place (in the anatomical position)?
    A. Frontal
    B. Horizontal
    C. Sagittal
    D. Vertical
    E. A and C

33. What is the sensation that a patient might experience just prior to an epileptic seizure called?
    A. An aura
    B. A hallucination
    C. A delusion
    D. Pre-epileptic vertigo
    E. A premonition

34. The inflammatory process includes all of the following signs and symptoms except:
    A. Redness
    B. Pain
    C. Warmth
    D. Swelling
    E. Numbness

35. Changes in blood pressure may occur as a result of many factors. Two of these factors may include _____ and _____.
    A. Exercise, change in posture
    B. Change in posture, respiratory rate
    C. Level of consciousness, body size
    D. Respiratory rate, pH levels of the blood
    E. Change in mood, respiratory rate

36. Type 1 diabetes is characterized by an impaired capacity to secrete insulin due to a beta cell defect. This type of diabetes is commonly seen in what type of individual?
    A. Obese, geriatric
    B. Lean, insulin dependent
    C. Noninsulin dependent, obese
    D. Noninsulin dependent, juvenile
    E. None of the above

37. All of the following are true about infectious mononucleosis except:
    A. The attack rate is highest between 15 to 25 year olds
    B. The virus is excreted in saliva
    C. The primary symptom is low back pain
    D. It is caused by transmission of the Epstein-Barr virus
    E. It causes splenomegaly in over half of all cases

38. Which of the following organisms is one of the most common causes of vaginitis in women?
    A. AIDS
    B. Genital herpes
    C. Chlamydia trachomatis
    D. Candida
    E. Gonorrhea

39. All of the following are risk factors for osteoporosis except:
    A. Early menopause
    B. High consumption of alcohol, cigarettes, and caffeine
    C. Sedentary lifestyle
    D. Obesity
    E. Lack of folic acid in the diet

40. A patient with an infection or serious disease, such as leukemia, might demonstrate an abnormally raised white blood cell count. What is the normal leukocyte count?
    A. 200,000 to 400,000/cu mm
    B. 500 to 1500/cu mm
    C. 4000 to 10,000/cu mm
    D. 1000 to 40,000/cu mm
    E. 250 to 500/cu mm

41. What is the primary target of the AIDS virus in the body?
    A. Neutrophils
    B. Basophils
    C. T-helper lymphocytes
    D. Phagocytes
    E. Red blood cells

42. EIA stands for what clinical entity?
    A. Exercise-induced arrhythmia
    B. Exercise-induced asthma
    C. Exercise-induced allergy
    D. Exercise-induced aneurysm
    E. Exercise-induced angina

43. What type of gait deviation might the athletic trainer see with a patient who has sustained an ankle injury and has decreased range of motion in dorsiflexion?
    A. Lateral trunk bending
    B. Trendelenburg gait
    C. Hip hiking
    D. Wide walking base
    E. Extension lag

44. A soccer player has fractured his right lower leg, been placed in a cast, and given crutches. The addition of crutches does what to his center of gravity?
    A. Moves it to the left
    B. Moves it to the midabdominal area
    C. Moves it to the right
    D. There is no effect on the center of gravity
    E. Enlarges the base of support

45. You notice one of your gymnasts has lost a significant amount of weight over the past month. She is always concerned about her image when she discusses her performance with you. What might you suspect as the problem?
    A. Drug dependence
    B. Depression
    C. Narcissism
    D. Bipolar disease
    E. Anorexia nervosa

46. A patient who sustains a severe or career-ending injury may go through a progression of emotional reactions, which are frequently seen with an individual who has experienced a significant loss. All of the following are included in this series of reactions except:
    A. Bargaining
    B. Anger
    C. Acceptance
    D. Denial
    E. Guilt

47. All of the following are symptoms of an overtrained patient except:
    A. Emotional liability
    B. Loss of appetite
    C. Reduced concentration
    D. Excessive motivation
    E. Fatigue

48. Which of the following signs/symptoms are present in a depressed patient?
    A. Decreased appetite
    B. Insomnia
    C. Fatigue
    D. Feeling of hopelessness
    E. All of the above

49. The athletic trainer notices one of the baseball players routinely cleans his cleats after every game and practice so no dirt is visible and checks his equipment bag multiple times to assure himself his "lucky towel" is with him. This is an example of what type of behavior?
    A. Schizophrenic
    B. Anxiety
    C. Obsessive-compulsive
    D. Passive-aggressive
    E. A and B

50. All of the following are possible factors regarding why a patient might be injury prone except:
    A. Bad luck
    B. Problems at home
    C. Joint hypermobility
    D. Poor endurance
    E. Poor coordination

51. Results of severe fluid restriction during weight loss attempts by a wrestler may include which of the following?
    A. Higher resting heart rate
    B. Increased renal flow
    C. Increased stroke volume
    D. Higher O$_2$ consumption
    E. Lower resting heart rate

52. What is wrong with an athlete eating a 12- to 16-ounce steak, baked potato, scrambled eggs, and coffee with sugar 4 hours prior to an event?
    A. Coffee with sugar may take as long as 3 hours to metabolize
    B. The intestinal tract will be full at the time of competition because it is a large meal
    C. The athlete may be hungry 8 hours later after he or she competes
    D. Nothing; the pre-event meal should be at least 500 calories or more
    E. Nothing; the athlete should eat whatever makes him or her feel comfortable

53. What happens when a patient consumes a simple sugar prior to an event?
    A. May cause a sudden decrease in blood glucose because of a sudden increase in insulin production
    B. May lead to a sudden increase in blood glucose because of a decrease in insulin production
    C. May lead to increased blood levels of electrolytes
    D. May lead to hyperlipidemia
    E. May cause a sudden increase in bilirubin levels

54. Which of the following is not a good source of vitamin C?
    A. Broccoli
    B. Strawberries
    C. Oranges
    D. Nuts
    E. Spinach

55. A patient informs the athletic trainer that he is taking tetracycline for a respiratory infection. Tetracycline will bind with which of the following 2 minerals to form a nonabsorbable complex (and therefore should not be taken before meals)?
    A. Potassium and zinc
    B. Sodium and magnesium
    C. Iron and calcium
    D. Iron and phosphorus
    E. Folic acid and niacin

56. Body fat percentage should not go below ___ in females because the internal organs lose a protective layer of fat.
    A. 20%
    B. 25%
    C. 17%
    D. 12%
    E. 8%

57. A loss of water equaling what percent of body weight will begin to threaten athletic performances?
    A. 10% to 20%
    B. 0.5% to 1%
    C. 1% to 2%
    D. 1% to 1.5%
    E. 2% to 3%

58. Which of the following medications is not an NSAID?
    A. Aspirin
    B. Motrin
    C. Tylenol
    D. Celebrex
    E. Aleve

59. Which of the following medications is not an antihistamine drug?
    A. Dimetapp
    B. Ultram
    C. Benadryl
    D. Claritin
    E. Allegra

60. A patient comes to your office complaining of intense itching and burning pain between his toes, and he cannot find anything to help alleviate the symptoms. The area is reddened with some white flakes. What might you recommend?
    A. Neosporin ointment
    B. Tinactin spray
    C. Silvadene cream
    D. Eucerin cream
    E. Hydrocortisone

61. An athlete collides with a teammate during an ice hockey game and sustains a blow to the jaw with a hockey stick. He is holding his lower face with his hands and is in intense pain. All of the following procedures will assist the athletic trainer in determining if there is a fracture of the jaw except:
    A. Have the athlete bite and observe for a malocclusion
    B. Palpate the jaw for a hematoma
    C. Ask the athlete to open and close his mouth, noting asymmetry with movement
    D. Palpate for jaw deformity when it is at rest, open, and closed
    E. See if the athlete can retract his jaw and observe for difficulty with movement

62. A patient sustains a blunt trauma injury to the upper right quadrant of the abdomen. What structure might be injured in this area?
    A. Liver
    B. Gallbladder
    C. Spleen
    D. Pancreas
    E. Kidney

63. During a return to play progression for a concussion, what is the typical time frame between stages?
    A. 12 hours
    B. 1 hour
    C. At least 24 hours
    D. 1 month
    E. None of the above

64. "Cauliflower ear" is an injury to which structure of the ear?
    A. Tympanic membrane
    B. External auditory canal
    C. Pinna
    D. Eustachian tube
    E. Internal auditory canal

65. What may proteinuria indicate?
    A. Pancreatitis
    B. Possible gallstones
    C. Renal or urinary tract pathology
    D. Diabetes
    E. Crohn's disease

66. What would be the most appropriate type of roentgenogram for a possible tibial stress fracture?
    A. X-ray
    B. PET scan
    C. MRI
    D. CT scan
    E. Bone scan

67. Which of the following is one of the most common eye injuries sustained in athletics?
    A. Detached iris
    B. Detached retina
    C. Zygomatic fracture
    D. Corneal abrasion
    E. Hypertrophic retina

68. All of the following parameters should be assessed when checking the neurovascular status of an injured limb except:
    A. Sensation
    B. The pulse distal to the injury
    C. Motor function
    D. Joint range of motion
    E. Atrophic changes

69. A baseball player has been stung by a bee. This player has a history of a severe allergy to bee stings. A couple of minutes after being stung, the area becomes red and raised and begins to itch. The athlete begins to complain that his tongue feels thick, and he starts to have difficulty breathing. What type of shock is he beginning to develop?
    A. Neurogenic
    B. Metabolic
    C. Hypovolemic
    D. Respiratory
    E. Anaphylactic

70. After an acute musculoskeletal injury, such as a shoulder dislocation, the body releases a natural opiate-like substance that provides temporary pain relief. What is this substance called?
    A. Prostaglandins
    B. Substance P
    C. Endorphins
    D. Insulin
    E. Histamines

71. What is the typical mechanism of injury for an anterior shoulder dislocation?
    A. Shoulder abduction with internal rotation
    B. Maximal shoulder extension
    C. Shoulder abduction with external rotation
    D. Shoulder adduction with internal rotation
    E. Shoulder flexion with internal rotation

72. Which of the symptoms below are seen with acute mountain sickness?
    I. Insomnia
    II. Vomiting
    III. Shortness of breath with exertion
    IV. Headache
    V. Fatigue
    A. II, III, IV
    B. I, III, IV, V
    C. I, II, IV, V
    D. I, II, III, V
    E. II, III, IV

73. Which muscle grade denotes active muscle movement in a gravity-eliminated position?
    A. -3/5
    B. +3/5
    C. 5/5
    D. 1/5
    E. 2/5

74. All of the following are useful in evaluating low back pathology except:
    A. Valsalva's maneuver
    B. Bilateral straight leg test
    C. Scouring test
    D. Lasègue's test
    E. Slump test

75. What is the best position for the patient to be in to muscle test the piriformis?
    A. Sitting
    B. Prone
    C. Supine
    D. Side-lying
    E. Standing

76. What is the average range of motion of elbow flexion?
    A. 0 to 90 degrees
    B. 0 to 135 degrees
    C. 0 to 115 degrees
    D. 0 to 100 degrees
    E. 0 to 180 degrees

77. What is the proper method to manually muscle test the biceps femoris muscle?
    A. Sitting, resisting knee extension
    B. Lying prone, resisting knee flexion with the tibia in external rotation
    C. Sitting, resisting hip flexion
    D. Lying prone, resisting knee flexion with the tibia in internal rotation
    E. Sitting, resisting elbow flexion

78. What is a quick method of testing the motor ability of the sacroiliac nerve root?
    A. Have the patient walk on his or her toes
    B. Manually resist ankle inversion
    C. Manually resist great toe extension
    D. Assess the patient's ability to squat
    E. Resisted ankle eversion

79. To test the function of the rhomboid major muscle, the athletic trainer should ask the patient to perform what movement?
    A. Scapular retraction
    B. Shoulder internal rotation
    C. Scapular protraction
    D. Shoulder shrug
    E. Shoulder external rotation

80. Which muscle supinates the forearm and flexes the shoulder?
    A. Brachialis
    B. Coracobrachialis
    C. Biceps brachii
    D. Flexor pollicis longus
    E. Pronator quadratus

81. All of the following movements occur in the sagittal plane except:
    A. Hip abduction
    B. Shoulder flexion
    C. Knee extension
    D. Hip flexion
    E. Elbow flexion

82. Which muscle flexes both the foot and the knee?
    A. Biceps femoris
    B. Flexor digitorum
    C. Posterior tibialis
    D. Anterior tibialis
    E. Gastrocnemius

83. The flexor pollicis longus is responsible for which of the following action(s)?
    A. Great toe flexion
    B. Thumb flexion
    C. Thumb flexion and adduction
    D. Thumb flexion and abduction
    E. None of the above

84. Asking the patient to move his or her eyes from side to side and up and down tests the integrity of which cranial nerve?
    A. II
    B. V
    C. I
    D. III
    E. VIII

85. The rectus femoris muscle _____ and _____ when it contracts.
    A. Flexes the hip, externally rotates the hip
    B. Extends the hip, flexes the knee
    C. Flexes the knee, plantar flexes the ankle
    D. Flexes the hip, extends the knee
    E. Extends the hip, extends the knee

86. Which of the following muscles is not involved in internal rotation of the hip?
    A. Adductor magnus
    B. Gluteus maximus
    C. Gracilis
    D. Tensor fasciae latae
    E. Gluteus minimus

87. Which of the following cervical nerve roots represent the sensory dermatomes of the hand?
    I. C5
    II. C6
    III. C7
    IV. C8
    V. T1
    A. I, II, III
    B. II, III IV
    C. III, IV, V
    D. I, III, IV
    E. I, III, V

88. Which of the following muscles does not adduct the shoulder?
    A. Pectoralis major
    B. Teres major
    C. Subscapularis
    D. Latissimus dorsi
    E. Serratus anterior

89. Which of the following muscles does not extend the trunk?
    A. Semispinalis (thoracic)
    B. Erector spinae
    C. Quadratus lumborum
    D. Multifidi
    E. Gluteus maximus

90. The supinator muscle is innervated by which of the following nerves?
    A. Musculocutaneous nerve
    B. Axillary nerve
    C. Radial nerve
    D. Median nerve
    E. A and D

91. Following multiple ankle sprains over the course of the year, the athletic trainer detects some weakness of the invertors and evertors of a patient's ankle. Which of the following muscles does not invert the ankle?
    A. Tibialis posterior
    B. Extensor digitorum longus
    C. Flexor digitorum longus
    D. Flexor hallucis longus
    E. C and D

92. During digestion, food passes through the small intestine as it is being broken down into smaller components. Which area of the small intestine does it pass through first?
    A. Ileum
    B. Esophagus
    C. Jejunum
    D. Cecum
    E. Duodenum

93. What nerve passes through the carpal tunnel?
    A. Musculocutaneous
    B. Radial
    C. Median
    D. Ulnar
    E. Cubital

94. Which of the following structures is not part of the pelvis?
    A. Coccyx
    B. Pubic symphysis
    C. Ileum
    D. Innominate bones
    E. Sacrum

95. Which nerves innervate the hip adductor musculature?
    A. Femoral, superior gluteal
    B. Femoral, tibial
    C. Femoral, obturator
    D. Femoral, obturator, inferior gluteal
    E. Tibial, obturator

96. Which of the following muscles abducts the little finger of the hand?
    A. Interossei
    B. Abductor digiti minimi
    C. Lumbricals
    D. Abductor digitorum brevis
    E. Adductor digiti minimi

97. Which of the following muscles does not extend and laterally flex the neck?
    A. Splenius capitis
    B. Splenius cervicis
    C. Levator scapulae
    D. Sternocleidomastoid
    E. Multifidus

98. Which of these muscles are innervated by the tibial nerve?
    I. Gastrocnemius
    II. Flexor hallucis longus
    III. Extensor hallucis longus
    IV. Tibialis anterior
    V. Biceps femoris
    A. I, II, III, IV
    B. II, III, V
    C. I, II, V
    D. I, III, IV, V
    E. I, II, III

99. All of the following are controlled by the cranial nerves except:
    A. Vision
    B. Smell
    C. Tongue movement
    D. Cervical flexion
    E. Hearing

100. What position is the "recommended" position for manually muscle testing the gluteus medius muscle?
    A. Side-lying, with the affected limb on top
    B. Supine
    C. Prone
    D. Sitting
    E. Standing

101. What is the average range of motion of knee flexion?
    A. 0 to 180 degrees
    B. 0 to 120 degrees
    C. 0 to 100 degrees
    D. 0 to 155 degrees
    E. 0 to 135 degrees

102. True leg-length discrepancy is measured between which 2 points?
    A. The posterior inferior iliac spine to the medial malleolus
    B. The umbilicus to the midpatella
    C. The umbilicus to the lateral malleolus
    D. The anterior superior iliac spine to the medial malleolus
    E. The anterior superior iliac spine to Gerdy's tubercle

103. In what position should the patient be to manually muscle test the hip flexors, and where should the athletic trainer's force be directed during testing?
    A. Prone, with the force directed down onto the posterior thigh
    B. Side-lying, with the force directed down onto the side of the thigh
    C. Sitting, with the force directed down onto the anterior aspect of the thigh
    D. Sitting, with the force directed down onto the medial aspect of the thigh
    E. None of the above

104. What position should the patient's shoulder be in to manually muscle test the deltoids?
    A. Abducted to 0 degrees and externally rotated to 45 degrees
    B. Abducted to 90 degrees
    C. Flexed with the palm down
    D. Extended with the palm up
    E. Extended with the palm down

105. What is an excessive lateral curvature of the vertebral column called?
    A. Kyphosis
    B. Spondylolysis
    C. Scoliosis
    D. Lordosis
    E. Ankylosing spondylolysis

106. During your evaluation of a patient's shoulder, you notice his left scapula is "winging." What does this indicate?
    A. Rhomboid weakness
    B. Deltoid weakness
    C. Serratus anterior weakness
    D. Upper trapezius weakness
    E. Long thoracic nerve entrapment

107. The maximal rate at which oxygen is consumed and utilized while exercising is known as the maximal oxygen consumption, or VO_2 max. What is the normal range of VO_2 max for an average college athlete?
    A. 80 to 100 mL/kg/min
    B. 45 to 60 mL/kg/min
    C. 70 to 80 mL/kg/min
    D. 45 to 60 dL/g/min
    E. 25 to 40 mL/kg/min

108. Which of the following is an indirect method of monitoring oxygen consumption?
    A. Measuring respiratory rate
    B. Measuring vital capacity
    C. Drawing blood gases during testing
    D. Measuring tidal volume
    E. Measuring heart rate

109. During exercise, the body's oxygen stores are greatly diminished. The recovery O_2 is used for all of the following except:
    A. Replacing O_2 dissolved in tissue fluids
    B. Returning muscle myoglobin to resting values
    C. Increasing venous oxyhemoglobin to pre-exercise levels
    D. Returning the catecholamine level in the blood to normal
    E. A and B

110. Submaximal exercise tests, which evaluate physical working capacity by measuring heart rate increases with exercise, include all of the following except:
    A. Progressive pulse rate test
    B. Harvard step test
    C. Cooper 12-minute run-walk test
    D. The Saltin-Astrand VO_2 debt test
    E. None of the above

111. A _____ is a device used to measure joint range of motion.
    A. Goniometer
    B. Dynamometer
    C. Caliper
    D. Flexometer
    E. Sphygmomanometer

112. Tenderness and pain with induration and swelling of the pretibial musculature following overexertion is indicative of which syndrome?
    A. Chondromalacia
    B. Pes anserinus bursitis
    C. Periostitis
    D. Nerve compression syndrome
    E. Tarsal tunnel syndrome

113. Speed's test is an evaluative test for which of the following problems?
    A. Thoracic outlet syndrome
    B. Supraspinatus tendinitis
    C. Bicipital tendinitis
    D. Ruptured biceps tendon
    E. Rupture of the brachialis muscle

114. Signs and symptoms of Sever's disease include which of the following?
    A. Point tenderness with palpation of the hamate bone
    B. Point tenderness and swelling at the base of the fifth metatarsal
    C. Pain with active ankle inversion
    D. Pain between the first and second metatarsal shafts with toe flexion
    E. Point tenderness at or just anterior to the insertion of the Achilles tendon along the posterior border of the calcaneous

115. If the calcaneofibular ligament of the ankle is torn, which of the following would be positive?
    A. Talar tilt test
    B. Anterior drawer sign
    C. Distraction test
    D. Clunk test
    E. Hawkins-Kennedy test

116. When taking a history during a physical examination of a patient, all of the following information is pertinent except:
    A. The mechanism of the injury
    B. If a "pop" or "snap" was heard or felt
    C. If the patient is on medication
    D. Whether the patient has medical insurance or not
    E. History of previous injury

117. What problem might the athletic trainer see if the L4 nerve root was compressed?
    A. Hip flexor weakness
    B. Plantar flexion weakness
    C. Knee extension weakness
    D. Dorsiflexion weakness
    E. Drop foot

118. With the patient sitting, the scapula stabilized, and the shoulder maximally flexed, the patient complains of pain and appears apprehensive. This is a positive _____ test.
    A. Yergason's
    B. Speed's
    C. Neer's
    D. Compression
    E. Hawkins-Kennedy

119. If a palpable "clunk" or shift at approximately 20 to 30 degrees of knee flexion is found during a pivot-shift test, this may be indicative of what?
    A. Anterolateral rotary instability of the knee
    B. Anteromedial rotary instability of the knee
    C. Posterolateral rotary instability of the knee
    D. Posteromedial rotary instability of the knee
    E. Posterior instability of the knee

120. "Spearing" in football is a dangerous technique. Football coaches have discontinued this practice when teaching tackling techniques because it may cause severe head and neck injuries. What is the resulting force on the cervical spine when a football player spears an opponent?
    A. Sudden neck extension
    B. Sudden neck hyperflexion with rotation
    C. Sudden neck lateral flexion
    D. Sudden neck rotation
    E. Sudden vertebral axial distraction

121. What is the most common mechanism of injury for an anterior shoulder dislocation?
    A. Adduction and external rotation
    B. Abduction and internal rotation
    C. Adduction and internal rotation
    D. Abduction and external rotation
    E. Abduction and extension

122. Which of the following conditions often contributes to shoulder impingement?
    A. Acute bicipital tendinitis
    B. Suprascapular nerve entrapment
    C. Adhesive capsulitis
    D. Glenohumeral instability
    E. Serratus anterior weakness

123. A patient has just been diagnosed with plantar fasciitis. All of the following would be appropriate measures to provide support/relief to the affected area except:
    A. An orthotic for arch support
    B. Low dye taping
    C. Metatarsal pad
    D. A heel cup
    E. Stretching program

124. A patient has been diagnosed with bulimia and has a known history of laxative abuse. Complications of chronic laxative use include which of the following?
    A. Electrolyte imbalance and dehydration
    B. Hyperactivity
    C. Hematemesis
    D. Chronic nasal congestion
    E. All of the above

125. A patient comes to the athletic training facility after being kicked in the lower leg by an opponent during a football game. He is complaining of decreased sensation in the L4 dermatome. What is this change in sensation called?
    A. Paresthesia
    B. Hypoesthesia
    C. Hyperesthesia
    D. Referred pain
    E. Anesthesia

126. _____ and _____ are 2 signs of diabetic coma.
    A. Drowsiness, acetone-smelling breath
    B. Seizures, pale/clammy skin
    C. Seizures, a bounding pulse
    D. Flushed skin, giddiness
    E. Pale skin, weak pulse

127. Which of the following tests is used to detect a possible meniscal tear in the knee?
    A. Faber's test
    B. Allen's test
    C. Jerk test
    D. Lachman's test
    E. McMurray's test

128. A patient reports to the athletic trainer with the presence of lesions on his upper lip and mouth area that look like blisters with a crusted yellow appearance and a red, weeping base. What is the probable cause of these lesions?
    A. Impetigo
    B. HIV
    C. Shingles
    D. A fungal infection
    E. Hives

129. A patient is brought to the athletic training facility after sustaining a hard kick to the abdominal area. Which of the following symptoms is not a sign of a significant abdominal injury?
    A. Slow, deep respirations
    B. Increased heart rate, decreased blood pressure
    C. Ashen-colored skin
    D. Rapid, shallow respirations
    E. Rebound tenderness

130. A football quarterback is sacked during a game. He comes off the field holding his throwing arm and complains of chest and anterior shoulder pain. After evaluating the athlete, the athletic trainer suspects a torn pectoralis major muscle. Which of the following physical findings will be seen if the athletic trainer is correct?
    A. Ecchymosis around the xyphoid process
    B. Palpable defect in the posterior axilla
    C. Weakness in abduction and external rotation
    D. Weakness in adduction, flexion, and internal rotation of the affected arm
    E. Weakness in adduction and external rotation

131. While training in a high-altitude climate (eg, 9000 to 10,000 feet), a rock climber experiences acute dyspnea, cough, headache, and weakness. What is the probable cause of these symptoms?
    A. Asthma
    B. Pleurisy
    C. Bronchitis
    D. Pulmonary edema
    E. Pneumonia

132. A second-degree medial collateral ligament sprain is characterized by all of the following except:
    A. Pain along the medial joint line
    B. No gross knee instability, but mild ligamentous laxity is noted in full knee extension during valgus stress testing
    C. Difficulty in actively flexing and extending the knee
    D. Immediate, severe pain following the feeling of a "pop" in the knee; the pain quickly subsides and the athlete is left feeling a dull ache in the knee joint
    E. A and B

133. What is the usual mechanism of injury for a Colles' fracture?
    A. A fall on a closed fist
    B. A fall on a bent elbow
    C. A fall on an outstretched arm and hand
    D. A twisting movement of the knee when the lower leg is planted
    E. Direct trauma to the forearm

134. Allen's test is used to test what?
    A. The integrity of the vertebral arteries
    B. The integrity of the radial and ulnar arteries of the hand
    C. For carpal tunnel syndrome
    D. For tarsal tunnel nerve entrapment
    E. Integrity of the ulnar nerve

135. Which of the carpal bones is most commonly dislocated?
    A. Scaphoid
    B. Lunate
    C. Cuboid
    D. Hamate
    E. Triquetral

136. What type of force typically causes injury to the medial collateral ligament, medial meniscus, and anterior cruciate ligament of the knee?
    A. A valgus force with the tibia in external rotation
    B. A varus force with the knee in full extension
    C. A valgus force with the femur in external rotation
    D. A valgus force with the knee in recurvatum
    E. A valgus force with the knee in full flexion

137. An athlete sustains a neck injury during an ice hockey game and is complaining of numbness and tingling along the ulnar border of his forearm and fourth and fifth fingers. Which of the following roentgenograms would be most appropriate in detecting nerve root compression?
    A. Electromyography or nerve root conduction velocity test
    B. CT scan or MRI
    C. Myelography
    D. Sonography
    E. Plain film radiograph

138. Which of the following is an example of a papule?
    A. A freckle
    B. A wart
    C. A hive
    D. A friction blister
    E. A fungus

139. When testing for paresthesia of the C5 nerve root, where should the athletic trainer perform pinprick testing?
    A. Base of the neck
    B. At the nipple line
    C. The medial aspect of the arm
    D. The lateral aspect of the forearm
    E. The lateral aspect of the upper arm over the middle deltoid

140. What is the proper position to manually muscle test the anterior deltoid?
    A. Shoulder in full internal rotation with the palm facing the floor, the force directed downward
    B. Shoulder at 90 degrees of abduction, full external rotation, and supination with the force directed downward
    C. Resistance to the first 30 degrees of abduction
    D. Arm at 90 degrees of flexion, palm facing downward, and the force is in the downward direction
    E. Shoulder at 45 degrees of abduction

141. What is one of the most common symptoms of a lumbar discogenic injury?
    A. Dull, localized backache
    B. Localized swelling with muscle guarding
    C. Inability to backward bend
    D. Sharp, radiating pain down the back of the leg
    E. Pain with only forward flexion

142. When a patient reports to the athletic trainer complaining of lateral hip pain, all of the following conditions might be the source of pain except:
    A. Trochanteric bursitis
    B. Strain of the glutcus mcdius
    C. Lumbar discogenic disease
    D. Avulsion of the ischial tuberosity
    E. Strain of the tensor fasciae latae

143. All of the following injuries might be associated with a "popping" sensation of the knee joint except:
    A. Anterior cruciate ligament injury
    B. Torn meniscus
    C. Subluxed patclla
    D. Iliotibial band friction syndrome
    E. B and C

144. The contact phase of the running gait is divided into which components?
    A. Forward swing and foot strike
    B. Foot strike, midsupport, and take-off
    C. Follow-through, forward swing, and foot descent
    D. Midsupport, take-off, and foot descent
    E. Foot strike, follow-through, and foot descent

145. Foot pronation results in _____ of the tibia during midsupport in the running gait.
    A. External rotation
    B. Internal rotation
    C. Abduction
    D. Adduction
    E. Retroversion

146. A wrestler comes into the athletic training facility after sustaining a major elbow injury. There is intense pain, and the area is grossly swollen. The athlete is unable to straighten his elbow, and the forearm appears shortened. The athletic trainer suspects an acute dislocation. Which 2 areas would the athletic trainer check for possible vascular impairment?
    A. Ulnar and radial pulses
    B. Radial pulse and color of the nailbeds after compression
    C. Brachial and radial pulses
    D. Arterial and venous circulation
    E. Axilla and anticubital fossa

147. An athlete sustains a blow to the head with a temporary loss of consciousness. He appears to have a lucid period in which he seems to be normal for a period of a couple of hours and then becomes significantly lethargic. What type of medical emergency would the athletic trainer suspect?
    A. Ruptured intervertebral disc at level C3,4
    B. Extradural hemorrhage
    C. Basilar fracture
    D. Subdural hemorrhage
    E. Contrecoup fracture

148. When evaluating a patient for Sinding-Larsen-Johansson disease, the athletic trainer should be sure to do the following:
    A. Abduct, extend, and externally rotate the shoulder while palpating the brachial pulse
    B. Palpate for effusion over Gerdy's tubercle
    C. Perform Thompson's test
    D. Check the level of the sacroiliac joints
    E. Palpate the inferior patellar pole with the patient's knee extended and the patellar tendon relaxed

149. A tennis player comes to the athletic trainer complaining of medial thigh pain. He is limping and has pain with resisted hip adduction and hip flexion. There is diffuse tenderness and ecchymosis along the proximal aspect of the medial thigh. What is the probable cause of the pain?
    A. Hip flexor rupture
    B. Groin strain
    C. Medial hamstring strain
    D. Popliteal strain
    E. Patellar tendon rupture

150. A lacrosse player comes limping into the athletic training facility with assistance from a coach. He is holding his leg in slight hip and knee flexion. There is a large bulge in the proximal thigh. During the exam, the athletic trainer requests the athlete to extend his knee as he sits on the edge of a taping table. He is able to partially straighten his leg, although there is pain down the anterior thigh area with the attempt to move it. What does the athletic trainer suspect is wrong?
    A. Biceps femoris rupture
    B. Femoral nerve injury
    C. Ruptured rectus femoris muscle
    D. Obturator nerve injury
    E. Iliopsoas rupture

151. A basketball player reports to the athletic training facility complaining of a "burning" pain along the lateral aspect of his right knee during and after running. No edema or ecchymosis is found during the exam, but he is tender to palpation of the affected area. Which of the following special tests might be positive?
    A. Lachman's test
    B. Patellar apprehension test
    C. Ober's test
    D. Sag sign
    E. Faber's test

152. A patient presents with loss of strength at the L3 and L4 nerve root levels. What muscle should the athletic trainer test to confirm an injury at this level?
    A. Gluteus minimus
    B. Flexor hallucis longus
    C. Gluteus maximus
    D. Adductor magnus
    E. Quadriceps

153. The athletic trainer asks a patient to shrug his shoulders after a neck and shoulder injury. He has difficulty performing this movement, even though it is not painful. What nerve is injured?
    A. Spinal accessory
    B. Dorsal scapular
    C. Long thoracic
    D. Suprascapular
    E. Thoracoscapular

154. How is the strength of the pes anserinus musculature manually muscle tested?
    A. Resistance to knee flexion and internal rotation of the lower leg
    B. Resistance to knee extension and hip adduction
    C. Resistance to knee flexion and external rotation of the lower leg
    D. Resistance to knee extension and internal rotation of the lower leg
    E. Resistance to knee flexion and ankle inversion

155. During a track meet, you notice one of the runners appears somewhat disoriented. During your assessment of this athlete, you find he is complaining of being lightheaded, his skin is cool and clammy, he is sweating profusely, and his radial pulse is rapid. You take a rectal temperature and find it is mildly elevated (102°F). You suspect the athlete is suffering from which of the following problems?
    A. Heat cramps
    B. Prickly heat
    C. Heat stroke
    D. Heat exhaustion
    E. Hematuria

156. One of your female gymnasts has been complaining of feeling generally fatigued on a constant basis. After being examined by the team physician, he orders a complete blood count. This blood test assesses all of the following except:
    A. Red blood cell count
    B. White blood cell count
    C. Plasma volume
    D. Hemoglobin levels
    E. Platelet count

157. While elevating a patient's shoulder, you note that the patient is unable to abduct through the full range of motion against gravity. When performing a manual muscle test, this finding would be assigned which of the following muscle grades?
    A. +2/5
    B. 3/5
    C. -4/5
    D. 1/5
    E. -3/5

158. You evaluate a basketball player who has sustained a finger injury while attempting to catch a ball. During your examination, you observe that the athlete is unable to extend the distal phalanx and the tip of his finger is positioned in approximately 30 degrees of flexion. You determine the athlete has a mallet finger. This injury is caused by which of the following?
    A. Tenosynovitis of the abductor pollicis longus
    B. A subungual hematoma
    C. A sprain of the extensor pollicis brevis
    D. An avulsion of the extensor tendon from its insertion
    E. Dupuytren's contracture

159. During your examination of a football player who has sustained a low back injury during a tackle, you find that he is reporting dulled sensation along the dorsum of his right foot, he has difficulty walking on his heels, and his patellar tendon reflex is diminished. You suspect which of the following nerve root(s) is affected?
    A. L3
    B. L4
    C. L2
    D. S1 to S3
    E. L5

160. When evaluating the inert structures of a joint, passive range of motion is used to determine all of the following except:
    A. The patient's willingness to move
    B. Limitations of joint motion
    C. Joint stability
    D. Muscle elasticity
    E. Soft tissue elasticity

161. Sickle-cell anemia may cause rhabdomyolysis in the athlete. Which of the following is a cardinal sign of rhabdomyolysis?
    A. Bleeding from the ear
    B. The presence of myoglobin in the urine
    C. Yellowing of the nailbeds of the fingers and toes
    D. Yellowing of the conjuctiva of the eyes
    E. Dyspnea

162. What are the 3 most commonly affected organ systems in Marfan syndrome?
    A. Skeletal, auditory, sensory
    B. Dermatological, auditory, neurological
    C. Neurological, cardiovascular, gastrointestinal
    D. Skeletal, ocular, cardiovascular
    E. Neurological, cardiovascular, ocular

163. Which of the following conditions is also known as Graves' disease?
    A. Hyperthyroidism
    B. Hypothyroidism
    C. Hirsutism
    D. Hyperparathyroidism
    E. Polymyositis

164. A patient reports having had a recent upper respiratory infection 2 weeks ago and is now having rapidly evolving bilateral muscle weakness of unknown origin. He is afebrile. What should the athletic trainer suspect?
    A. Systemic lupus erythematosus
    B. Autonomic dysreflexia
    C. Guillain-Barré syndrome
    D. Acute myelogenous lymphoma
    E. Lyme disease

165. Which of the following are common complications of hepatitis C?
    A. Cirrhosis and liver cancer
    B. Bile duct constricture and gastroesophageal reflux disease
    C. Cirrhosis and colon cancer
    D. Ascites and pancreatic cancer
    E. Gastritis

166. What is the incubation period for HIV and human papillomavirus?
    A. 4 to 7 days
    B. 1 to 6 months
    C. 2 to 14 days
    D. 1 to 13 weeks
    E. 1 to 6 weeks

167. Which of the following diseases is the most commonly inherited disorder among White Americans?
    A. Cystic fibrosis
    B. Tay-Sachs disease
    C. Down syndrome
    D. Sickle-cell anemia
    E. Hemophilia

168. Which of the following structures is affected in an individual who has been diagnosed with amyotrophic lateral sclerosis (also known as Lou Gehrig disease)?
    A. Epidermis
    B. Motor neuron
    C. Axon
    D. Neuromuscular junction
    E. Prefrontal cortex of the brain

169. A young gymnast sustains a fracture/dislocation of the right talus and is immobilized in nonweightbearing for 6 weeks. After the cast is removed, she begins to complain of skin hypersensitivity, pain that is disproportional to the injury, and a significant resistance to move her ankle or toes. The athletic trainer recognizes this to be the initial symptoms of which of the following disorders?
    A. Cauda equina
    B. Post fracture syndrome
    C. Myasthenia gravis
    D. Reflex sympathetic dystrophy
    E. Muscular dystrophy

170. Which of the following is the underlying cause of multiple sclerosis?
    A. Hyperactivity of the synapses within the brain
    B. Inflammation of the middle cerebral artery
    C. A genetic disorder
    D. Low levels of dopamine production
    E. Demyelination of the neurons of the central nervous system

171. Mumps is a contagious viral disease that is primarily manifested by:
    A. Parotitis
    B. Splenomegaly
    C. Retinopathy
    D. Maculopapular rash
    E. Pancreatitis

172. What is spina bifida occulta?
    A. Complete herniation of the spinal cord and meninges through a defect in the neural tube
    B. Complete herniation of the meninges through a defect in the neural tube
    C. Partial herniation of the spinal cord and meninges through a defect in the neural tube
    D. Partial herniation of the meninges through a defect in the neural tube
    E. The incomplete formation of the posterior vertebral arch without herniation of the meninges or spinal cord

173. The biceps brachii tendon reflex correlates to what spinal level?
    A. C2
    B. C4
    C. C5
    D. C6
    E. C7

174. The patellar tendon reflex correlates to what spinal level?
    A. L1
    B. L2-4
    C. L5
    D. L5-S1
    E. S1

175. A soccer player sustains a mild head injury during a game. The athletic trainer administers a Romberg's test on the sideline, assessing which of the following?
    A. Disorder of the medulla
    B. Function of the cerebral cortex
    C. Function of the temporal lobe of the brain
    D. Cerebellum or basal ganglia dysfunction
    E. Disorder of the parietal lobe of the brain

176. How is cranial nerve VIII tested?
    A. Having the patient identify an odor
    B. Using a Snellen chart
    C. Crumpling paper near the ear
    D. Resisting a shoulder shrug
    E. Having the patient stick out his or her tongue

177. How is cranial nerve XI tested?
    A. Having the patient identify an odor
    B. Using a Snellen chart
    C. Having the patient smile
    D. Resisting a shoulder shrug
    E. Checking pupil reaction to light

178. How is cranial nerve IX tested?
    A. Having the patient identify an odor
    B. Using a Snellen chart
    C. Having the patient stick out his or her tongue
    D. Having the patient swallow
    E. By touching the patient's cheek lightly with a finger

179. Changes in cognition and behavior and disorientation after a traumatic head injury are indicative of dysfunction of which part of the brain?
    A. Basal ganglia
    B. Pons
    C. Cerebellum
    D. Occipital lobe
    E. Cerebrum

180. The adrenal glands release all of the following hormones except:
    A. Aldosterone
    B. Cortisol
    C. Epinephrine
    D. Norepinephrine
    E. Growth hormone

181. One of the hormones that the pancreas produces is glucagon. What is the function of this hormone?
    A. It stimulates the increase of glucose transport out of the blood and into cells
    B. It facilitates a build-up of glucose in the liver
    C. It stimulates an increase in metabolism
    D. It facilitates the breakdown of fat in the pancreas
    E. It stimulates the release of glucose from the liver into the blood

182. Mast cells release which of the following chemicals to initiate the inflammatory response?
    A. Bradykinins
    B. Antigens
    C. Lysosomes
    D. Histamine
    E. Antibodies

183. Lysosomes function to do which of the following during the inflammatory process?
    A. Increase vascular permeability
    B. Cease the inflammatory process
    C. Cause platelets to adhere to the collagen matrix
    D. Act as a catalyst in the formation of bradykinins
    E. Contain enzymes that digest material brought into the cytoplasm of the cells during phagocytosis

184. During the inflammatory response, leukocytes are drawn to the site of injury by chemical mediators. This process is known as which of the following?
    A. Margination
    B. Coaxing
    C. Chemotaxis
    D. Emigration
    E. Integration

185. What is one of the greatest concerns and primary life-threatening effect of rhabdomyolysis?
    A. Renal failure
    B. Heart failure
    C. High blood glucose levels
    D. Heart arrhythmias
    E. Blunt trauma to the abdomen

186. After a severe head injury, an individual may posture as follows: extension of the lower limbs and flexion of the elbows, wrists, and fingers. This condition is known as what?
    A. Decortication
    B. Decerebration
    C. Decellebration
    D. Dystonia
    E. Dyskinesia

187. If a patient whom an athletic trainer is working with has a history of asthma, what daily test should he or she use to monitor the patient's condition?
    A. Metered-dose inhaler
    B. Peak flow meter
    C. Ventilator
    D. Breatholizer
    E. Volume spirometer

188. A leading cause of hypothyroidism is Hashimoto's thyroiditis, which is an autoimmune disorder. What is the primary symptom of this disease?
    A. Depression
    B. "Butterfly" rash
    C. Atrophic skin
    D. Deviated trachea
    E. Goiter

189. Wolff-Parkinson-White syndrome is characterized by which of the following?
    A. A depressed QT interval
    B. A short PR interval and prolonged QRS complex
    C. A long PR interval and shortened QRS complex
    D. An elevated QT interval
    E. Very late depolarization of the heart

190. Which of the following diagnostic tests is considered the "gold standard" for detecting signs of hypertrophic cardiomyopathy?
    A. CT scan
    B. Echocardiogram
    C. Genetic testing
    D. Electrocardiogram
    E. Cardiac stress testing

191. Which of the following signs is tested for when a deep vein thrombosis is suspected after a traumatic incident occurs involving the lower leg?
    A. Babinski's sign
    B. Thompson's sign
    C. Homan's sign
    D. Battle's sign
    E. Ballotment sign

192. What is the hallmark sign of peripheral arterial disease?
    A. Numbness of the hands and feet
    B. Pallor of the hands and feet
    C. Hyperlipidemia
    D. Intermittent claudication
    E. Pain and cramping of the lower extremities while in sitting

193. All of the following are symptoms of caffeine withdrawal except:
    A. Diaphoresis
    B. Fatigue
    C. Headache
    D. Irritability
    E. Runny nose

194. When the athletic trainer places his or her thumb over the patient's distal bicep tendon and strikes the thumb with the reflex hammer, which nerve level is being evaluated?
    A. C8
    B. C7
    C. C6
    D. C5
    E. C4

195. The athletic trainer performs a cervical distraction test on a patient. A positive finding is observed. This is indicative of which of the following?
    A. Tumor
    B. Soft tissue inflammation
    C. Traction injury to the brachial plexus
    D. Cervical disc herniation
    E. A nerve root compression or facet dysfunction

196. Which dermatome correlates to the T7 nerve root?
    A. Axilla
    B. Nipple line
    C. Xyphoid process, costal margin
    D. Umbilicus
    E. Anterior superior iliac spine

197. Which of the following tests is appropriate to perform if the athletic trainer suspects the patient has meningitis?
    A. Brudzinski-Kernig test
    B. Milgram's test
    C. Beevor's test
    D. Halstead's maneuver
    E. Bowstring test

Immediate and Emergency Care

1. All of the following drugs may be used with phonophoresis during the acute phase of treatment except:
    A. Dexamethasone
    B. Hydrocortisone 1%
    C. Lidocaine
    D. Naproxen
    E. Hydrocortisone 10%

2. One of your athletes has been diagnosed with psoriasis. All of the following medications are appropriate for treatment of this condition except:
    A. Aristocort
    B. Keflex
    C. Zoloft
    D. Betadine
    E. Benadryl

3. Which of the following is not a medication that is delivered via a metered-dose inhaler for exercise-induced asthma?
    A. Proventil
    B. Alupent
    C. Atrovent
    D. Ventolin
    E. Butisol

4. What medication is often used for anxiety or panic attacks?
    A. Zantac
    B. Xanax
    C. Thorazine
    D. Prozac
    E. Lyrica

5. What is the primary mode of action of penicillin?
    A. Increases the number of T-lymphocytes in the bloodstream
    B. Inhibits the metabolism of the bacteria
    C. Prevents bacterial reproduction
    D. Breaks down the cell wall of the bacteria
    E. Prevents viral reproduction

6. Which of the following is considered a medical emergency?
    A. Acute compartment syndrome
    B. Navicular fracture
    C. Bulimia
    D. Mitral valve prolapse
    E. Cellulitis

7. All of the following treatments would be inappropriate for an acute quadriceps contusion except:
    A. Light massage
    B. Pulsed ultrasound
    C. Ice massage followed by gentle stretch
    D. Ice pack with compression wrap with the knee in flexion
    E. Heat pack and massage

8. Deep frostbite is a medical emergency. What would the proper course of treatment be for this problem?
   A. Very slow, careful rewarming of the body part with warm water
   B. Firm, sustained pressure of the hand on the affected body part
   C. Rapid rewarming of the affected body part with warm water
   D. Quick friction in order to increase local circulation
   E. None of the above

9. During which of the circumstances below should an athlete be immediately referred to a dentist?
   I. The tooth is knocked out
   II. When a tooth is displaced 2 mm or more
   III. When a crown is fractured and the tooth is still alive
   IV. When a filling is knocked out or fractured and the athlete is sensitive to hot or cold food
   V. When an artificial plate is broken during competition
   A. I, II, III
   B. I, II, III, V
   C. I, V
   D. II, III, IV
   E. I, III, IV

10. A male patient sustains a direct blow to the genital area. How can the athletic trainer immediately decrease the pain?
    A. Use an ice pack to the area with the patient in supine, knees in extension
    B. Use direct pressure on the testes
    C. Have the patient lie supine with his knees bent to his chest to decrease the strain on the scrotum and apply ice to the affected area
    D. Have the patient lie on his side with his knees extended
    E. Place a moist heat pack over the area

11. When performing 2-person adult CPR, what is the correct compression-to-breath ratio?
    A. 5:2
    B. 30:2
    C. 15:1
    D. 5:1
    E. 2:5

12. Shock after a severe injury can result from _____ or _____.
    A. Pain, increased blood pressure
    B. Decreased heart rate, infection
    C. Hemorrhage, hypothermia
    D. Hemorrhage, stagnation of blood
    E. Increased heart rate, pain

13. A patient who had been diagnosed with infectious mononucleosis has just been cleared by the team doctor to return to full activity. How long should the patient remain out of contact participation from the time of onset to the time of full recovery?
    A. 2 weeks
    B. At least 3 weeks
    C. 6 months
    D. A maximum of 6 weeks
    E. A minimum of 2 months

14. A rugby player sustains a confirmed head injury during a game and is removed from the game. All of the following are symptoms/signs of increasing intracerebral pressure that the athletic trainer should monitor except:
    A. Nausea and vomiting
    B. Pupil irregularity
    C. Increase in systolic blood pressure with decrease in diastolic blood pressure
    D. Romberg's sign
    E. Changes in cognition

15. If an athlete is unconscious from a blow to the head, he or she should be assumed to have a neck injury in addition to a possible head injury. If the airway appears to be impaired, all of the following would be appropriate steps in management except:
    A. Cut the facemask with an appropriate tool and move it out of the way
    B. Leave the helmet on
    C. Stabilize the head and neck
    D. Do a finger sweep of the mouth to remove any debris and clear the airway
    E. Activate EMS

16. During the foreign body airway obstruction maneuver, the athletic trainer should grasp one fist with the other hand and place the thumb side of the fist where?
    A. On the abdomen between the xyphoid process and the umbilicus
    B. On the manubrium
    C. On the abdomen between the umbilicus and the symphysis pubis
    D. Between the scapula
    E. On the left side of the sternum

17. An athlete is brought into the athletic training facility with a 2.5-inch nail embedded in his foot. All of the following actions are appropriate in the treatment of this injury except:
    A. Immediately remove the nail from the foot
    B. Keep the athlete calm
    C. Pack the nail and foot as they are in a large dressing to help control the bleeding and stabilize the object
    D. Transport the athlete to the hospital with the nail still embedded in the foot
    E. Verify that the athlete's tetanus shot is current

18. Which of the measures below are appropriate steps in the management of an athlete who is experiencing a seizure?
    I. Keep spectators out of the way
    II. Protect the athlete's head and body from injury
    III. Turn the athlete on his or her side
    IV. If the athlete is in status epilepticus or it is a first seizure, immediately seek further medical support
    V. Try to keep the athlete's mouth open by any means to prevent airway obstruction
    VI. Call the athlete's next of kin to inform him or her of the problem and of the care given
    A. II, IV, V, VI
    B. I, II, III, IV
    C. II, III, IV, VI
    D. I, II, IV, V
    E. III, IV, V, VI

19. It is critical that CPR be administered as soon as possible during a life-threatening situation. In what amount of time is brain damage likely to occur if the brain is deprived of oxygen?
    A. 2 to 4 minutes
    B. 10 to 12 minutes
    C. 4 to 6 minutes
    D. 10 minutes
    E. After 15 minutes

20. During CPR, it is most convenient and efficient to monitor the athlete's circulation by palpating the carotid artery. Where is the pulse located?
    A. In the groove between the larynx and the sternocleidomastoid muscle
    B. Between the mastoid process and pharynx
    C. At the base of the neck superior to the manubrium
    D. 2 inches below the base of the earlobe on the side of the neck
    E. Antecubital fossa of the elbow

21. During CPR, the adult sternum must be compressed to what depth for compression to be effective?
    A. 0.5 to 1 inch
    B. 1 to 1.5 inches
    C. 2 to 2.4 inches
    D. 2 to 3 inches
    E. As deep as you can

22. Which type of heat injury is considered a medical emergency?
    A. Dehydration
    B. Heat cramps
    C. Heat stroke
    D. Heat exhaustion
    E. All of the above except A

23. Which of the following signs and symptoms are characteristic of a tension pneumothorax?
    I. Tracheal deviation
    II. Distended neck veins
    III. Unilateral absence of breath sounds
    IV. Dizziness
    V. Cyanosis
    A. II, III, IV
    B. I, IV, V
    C. I, III, IV, V
    D. I, II, III, V
    E. I, III, IV

24. An athlete has been kicked in the low back area during a soccer game. He is complaining of significant flank pain, is having difficulty voiding, and there is blood in his urine. What should the athletic trainer suspect is injured?
    A. The spleen
    B. The large intestine
    C. The lumbar fascia
    D. The testicles
    E. The kidney

25. When evaluating an unconscious athlete, what should the athletic trainer do first?
    A. Check for sources of bleeding
    B. Take vital signs
    C. Check for normal extremity movement
    D. Take the athlete's pulse rate
    E. Check that the athlete's airway is open and he or she is breathing normally

26. What is the most common and devastating mechanism of injury seen in neck injuries sustained during football?
    A. Cervical hyperextension
    B. Forceful cervical lateral flexion
    C. Cervical hyperflexion and rotation
    D. Cervical hyperflexion and axial compression
    E. Cervical hyperextension and lateral compression

27. Where would the athlete complain of pain with acute appendicitis?
    A. Lower right quadrant of the abdomen
    B. Right lateral hip area
    C. Inner right thigh
    D. Anterior right thigh area
    E. Lower back

28. What is the prudent method of transporting an athlete with a suspected spinal injury?
    A. Do not move the athlete until a doctor is present
    B. Use a stretcher
    C. Fireman's carry
    D. Use a spine board with medical assistance
    E. Use a wheelchair

29. When fitting an athlete for crutches, the elbow should be bent to approximately what angle?
    A. 90 degrees
    B. 10 degrees
    C. 45 degrees
    D. 0 degrees
    E. 30 degrees

30. Under what condition can CPR be stopped?
    A. If a rib is fractured during the effort
    B. The athlete vomits
    C. The athlete aspirates
    D. Not until the athlete trainer is exhausted, spontaneous respirations and pulse have returned, or a physician or another party continues CPR in place of the athletic trainer
    E. A and C

31. After an athlete has suffered a ruptured spleen, he or she may experience pain that radiates down the left shoulder and approximately one-third of the way down the upper left arm. What is this pain called?
    A. Visceral pain
    B. Radicular pain
    C. Kehr's sign
    D. Angina
    E. Radiation

32. What is the appropriate treatment for an athlete who has sustained a rib fracture?
    A. Use of a rib belt
    B. There is no specific treatment
    C. Total bedrest
    D. Use of a pillow to splint the ribs when coughing
    E. C and D

33. All of the following are basic functions of athletic taping and bandaging except:
    A. To support an injured body part
    B. To protect wounds from infection
    C. To enhance the athlete's skill
    D. To hold protective equipment in place
    E. B and D

34. Taping continuously around a limb may cause what problem?
    A. Ineffective support
    B. Difficulty in tape removal
    C. Compromised circulation
    D. There is no problem with this method
    E. Blisters

35. What is the compression-to-breath ratio during one-person adult CPR?
    A. 5:1
    B. 30:2
    C. 15:1
    D. 5:2
    F. 2:15

36. An athlete reports to the athletic trainer with a deep laceration to his thigh. The cut is approximately 1/8-inch deep, 1-inch long, and bleeding moderately. What would be the proper steps for the athletic trainer to take to treat this wound?
    A. Use a pressure bandage to control the bleeding, keep the wound clean and free of debris, use butterfly strips for temporary closure, and apply ice and compression to the area
    B. Use a pressure bandage to control the bleeding, keep the wound clean, suture the laceration, and cover with a sterile dressing
    C. Wipe the area clean with soap and water, use an antibiotic ointment to minimize infection, suture the wound, and cover it with a sterile dressing
    D. Wipe the area clean with soap and water, apply a large adhesive bandage, and apply ice to the area
    E. None of the above

37. An athlete comes to the athletic trainer holding a tooth that has just been knocked out of his mouth. What would be the proper steps for the athletic trainer to take to allow for a successful reimplantation?
    A. Try to put it back in place and use a topical ointment for pain
    B. Put the tooth in a jar of water and tell the athlete to store it in a refrigerator until he can see a dentist
    C. There is nothing the athletic trainer can do because the tooth is dead
    D. Place the tooth in a cloth soaked with saline or water and get the athlete to a dentist within 30 minutes
    E. None of the above

38. During an emergency, all of the following information should be given over the telephone by the athletic trainer to emergency personnel except:
    A. The type of emergency
    B. The current status of the athlete
    C. Where the athlete is currently located
    D. The type of treatment currently being given to the athlete
    E. The name of the next of kin

39. An athlete has a suspected fracture involving the knee. Which of the following areas should be splinted?
    A. The ankle and lower leg areas
    B. The knee and thigh
    C. The ankle, knee, and thigh
    D. The lower limb joints and one side of the trunk
    E. The hip and ankle

40. Which of the following cells release histamine and serotonin during the cellular response phase of tissue healing?
    A. Macrophages
    B. Erythrocytes
    C. Granulocytes
    D. Leukocytes
    E. Mast cells and platelets

41. The acute phase of an injury lasts approximately 3 to 4 days. What occurs at the time of initial trauma?
    A. Phagocytosis, followed by vasoconstriction and diapedesis
    B. Transitory vasodilatation, inflammation, and phagocytosis
    C. Transitory vasoconstriction, followed by vasodilatation and increased permeability
    D. Vasoconstriction, increased permeability, and granulation
    E. All of the above

42. Where do primitive stem cells mature into red and white blood cells and platelets?
    A. Liver
    B. Spleen
    C. Gallbladder
    D. Bone marrow
    E. Epididymis

43. An athlete has just been injured on the basketball court, and the athletic trainer begins administering first aid. During the initial contact, the athletic trainer notices the athlete is hyperactive, argumentative, and sarcastic in his responses to questions. All of the following actions by the athletic trainer are inappropriate except:
    A. Telling the athlete he or she is a wimp and that it is "not that bad"
    B. Being abrupt and telling the athlete to snap out of it
    C. Allowing the athlete to express his emotions as they occur
    D. Calling the referee over to calm the athlete
    E. Walking away to prevent an argument

44. The athletic trainer notices an athlete is prone to abnormal bruising. After discussing the problem with the team doctor, he recommends which of the following vitamins?
    A. E
    B. D
    C. C
    D. Niacin
    E. K

45. An acronym used for the immediate care of an acute musculoskeletal injury is which of the following?
    A. RICE
    B. NSAID
    C. REST
    D. STAT
    E. HOPS

46. A drug that is used to increase the effect of another, such as aspirin when used in combination with codeine, is known as what?
    A. Synergistic
    B. Cumulative
    C. Paradoxical
    D. Potentiating
    E. Titrating

47. Which of the following is not the proper action for an athlete to take if lightning is observed during a game?
    A. Avoid standing near metal bleachers on the field
    B. Stand near a telephone pole
    C. Assume a crouched position in a ditch
    D. Take cover in an automobile if he or she cannot get indoors
    E. A and C

48. One of your cross-country runners has an ongoing problem with tinea pedis. Which of the following actions should you take to assist this athlete in minimizing the problem?
    A. Use talcum powder daily and keep his or her feet dry after showering
    B. Use Kwell shampoo twice a day or as directed by a physician
    C. Remove the infected toenail to prevent the infection from spreading
    D. Make sure the athlete uses sunblock with an SPF of 15 or higher
    E. None of the above

49. A patient comes to the athletic training facility with what appears to be a tick embedded in his lower leg. The athletic trainer should instruct the patient not to do which of the following?
    A. Keep the area clean and free of other debris
    B. Pull the tick off with tweezers
    C. Cover the tick with mineral oil
    D. Put fingernail polish remover onto the tick's body
    E. All of the above

50. What is a major side effect of the NSAID group?
    A. Vertigo
    B. Tinnitus
    C. Drowsiness
    D. Blurred vision
    E. Gastrointestinal upset

51. Your patient is on a medication for a *Staphylococcus aureus* infection. Which of the following adverse reactions might you expect with antibiotic treatment?
    A. Palpitations
    B. Abdominal cramping
    C. Dry mouth
    D. Headache
    E. Dry skin

52. What is the normal dosage for one tablet of aspirin?
    A. 200 mg
    B. 400 mg
    C. 500 mg
    D. 375 mg
    E. 325 mg

53. All of the following are possible side effects of oral contraceptives except:
    A. Nausea and vomiting
    B. Shortness of breath
    C. Fluid retention
    D. Amenorrhea
    E. Feeling sluggish

54. Anabolic steroids are often abused by athletes. Which of the following results may occur in the female athlete after ingesting testosterone?
    A. Decreased libido
    B. Gynecomastia
    C. Hirsutism
    D. Increased body fat
    E. All of the above

55. What is the best way to prevent otitis externa?
    A. Avoid contact activities for 7 to 10 days
    B. Use ear plugs during activity
    C. Dry the external auditory canal after swimming
    D. Wear adequate protective devices for the ear
    E. All of the above

56. Under which of the following conditions should an athletic helmet be removed after an injury?
    A. If the athlete requests it be removed
    B. If, after a reasonable period of time, the facemask cannot be removed to gain access to the airway
    C. The chief EMT requests that it be removed
    D. If the helmet causes immobilization of the head or jaw
    E. The helmet should never be removed

57. Which of the following tools has the Inter-Association Task Force recommended not be used as the primary tool for loop-strap removal on a football helmet after an injury?
    A. FM Extractor
    B. The Trainer's Angel
    C. A flathead screwdriver
    D. The anvil pruner
    E. B and D

58. A predisposing condition such as spinal stenosis may mean an athlete is more likely to:
    A. Experience vertigo after an injury to the head
    B. Demonstrate nystagmus after an injury to the head
    C. Develop "glove and stocking" symptoms after a neck injury
    D. Develop paralysis after a fracture-dislocation
    E. Develop lower extremity neuropathies

59. Spinal immobilization is best achieved with the full-body splint. All of the following are examples of full-body immobilization equipment except:
    A. The standard rigid spine board
    B. Vacuum mattress
    C. A Stryker frame
    D. Scoop stretcher
    E. Miller full-body splint

60. After an acute injury, chemical mediators are given off by various cells. Which of the following chemicals is the first to appear?
    A. Serotonin
    B. Heparin
    C. Prostaglandins
    D. Histamine
    E. Thrombin

61. Which of the following means "the abnormal development of tissue"?
    A. Atrophy
    B. Dysplasia
    C. Metaplasia
    D. Hyperplasia
    E. Hypertrophy

62. _____ and _____ are 2 conditions that will interfere with fracture healing.
    A. Poor blood supply, poor immobilization
    B. Infection, callus formation
    C. Granulation, callus formation
    D. Hematoma formation, the influx of endosteal cells
    E. Increased blood supply, callus formation

63. One of your patients has just been stung by a bee. He appears to be showing signs of anaphylaxis. Which of the following medications would be appropriate to administer to stop the reaction?
    A. Epinephrine
    B. Heparin
    C. An antitussive
    D. A histamine-2 blocker
    E. None of the above

64. _____ and _____ are both examples of histamine-2 blockers.
    A. Xanax, Tegretol
    B. Benadryl, Seldane
    C. Proventil, Ventolin
    D. Tagamet, Zantac
    E. Benadryl, Tagamet

65. Which of the following drugs must the athletic trainer determine the athlete is not allergic to prior to administering a NSAID?
    A. Famotidine
    B. Acetaminophen
    C. Sulfa
    D. Sudafed
    E. Aspirin

66. When transporting an athlete off the field by manual conveyance, it is most convenient to do this with how many athletic trainers?
    A. 8
    B. 4
    C. 1
    D. 3
    E. 2

67. What is the average respiratory rate for a healthy adult (18 years of age or older)?
    A. 30 to 80 breaths/min
    B. 20 to 30 breaths/min
    C. 12 to 15 breaths/min
    D. 5 to 10 breaths/min
    E. 40 to 50 breaths/min

68. Where should the bell of a stethoscope be placed when taking blood pressure?
    A. Over the brachial artery
    B. Over the brachial vein
    C. Over the popliteal fossa
    D. Over the radial artery
    E. Over the ulnar artery

69. Orthostatic syncope is caused by which of the following conditions?
    A. Increased intracranial pressure
    B. Sudden peripheral vasodilatation
    C. Poisoning
    D. An acute reduction in cardiac output
    E. All of the above

70. Which type of food should the athletic trainer recommend the patient avoid if gallbladder pathology is suspected?
    A. Foods low in carbohydrates
    B. Foods high in protein
    C. Fatty foods
    D. Foods high in vitamin K
    E. All of the above

71. A patient who has a seizure should be referred to a physician under which of the following conditions?
    A. After a seizure that lasts more than 5 minutes
    B. There is no history of previous seizures
    C. If the seizure does not fit into the patient's pattern of previous seizures
    D. All of the above
    E. None of the above

72. Your team physician sends a prescription to you for your athlete that reads "whirlpool treatments TID." What does TID mean?
    A. Twice a day
    B. Every 3 hours
    C. Four times a day
    D. Three times a week
    E. Three times a day

73. If necessary, the removal of the helmet and shoulder pads from an athlete with a suspected spinal cord injury should be coordinated to avoid which of the following?
    A. Cervical hyperextension
    B. Airway obstruction
    C. Cervical hyperflexion
    D. Thoracic rotation
    E. Thoracic compression

74. The Inter-Association Task Force recommends that no fewer than _____ persons lift athletes suspected of having a spinal cord injury.
    A. Four plus
    B. Two plus
    C. Three plus
    D. Ten plus
    E. Eight plus

75. Which of the following instruments is used to visually examine the ear canal and tympanic membrane?
    A. Ophthalmoscope
    B. Laryngoscope
    C. Arthroscope
    D. Endoscope
    E. Otoscope

76. What is the primary reason an athletic trainer would perform pulmonary auscultation?
    A. To check for a systolic bruit
    B. To identify potential abnormal breath sounds
    C. To diagnose cardiothoracic pathology
    D. To diagnose pulmonary pathology
    E. All of the above

77. One of your female patients presents with dysuria, a sense of urgency to urinate, decreased urine volume, nocturia, low back pain, and pyuria. What do you suspect this patient has?
    A. Pyoperitonitis
    B. Dermatitis
    C. Prostatitis
    D. Vaginitis
    E. Cystitis

78. One of your athletes presents with rhinorrhea, rhinitis, a sore throat, nonproductive cough, low grade fever, headache, chills, and malaise. What action(s) should the athletic trainer take?
    A. Do not allow the athlete to work out for 10 to 14 days and refer him or her to a physician
    B. Transport the athlete to the nearest emergency facility
    C. Limit the athlete's activities until the fever resolves and resume full activity as the symptoms resolve
    D. Begin the athlete on a course of antipyretics and analgesics
    E. Call the team physician for advice

79. All of the following symptoms should alert the athletic trainer to serious pathology that requires immediate referral to a physician except:
    A. Itchy skin, especially when it involves areas on the feet and toes
    B. Painful urination
    C. Unexpected weight loss
    D. Night pain
    E. Palpable lump in the breast or axilla

80. For which of the following injuries would the use of a hard-shell pad be appropriate?
    A. Cover a large skin infection
    B. A toe injury
    C. A painful contusion
    D. Plantar fasciitis
    E. None of the above

81. When choosing a prophylactic knee brace, the brace should meet all of the following criteria except:
    A. It should always be custom molded to avoid a poorly fitting brace
    B. It should not interfere with normal knee function
    C. It should not increase injuries to the lower extremity
    D. It should be cost effective and durable
    E. B and D

82. When recommending a running sneaker the athletic trainer should recommend a sole that has what major qualities?
    A. Shock absorbing with a wide last
    B. Durable and noncompressive
    C. Shock absorbing and durable
    D. Durable with a rigid midsole
    E. None of the above

83. Which of the following materials can the athletic trainer use to construct a custom protective or supportive device?
    A. Felt
    B. Gauze padding
    C. Cotton
    D. Foam
    E. All of the above

84. An AED is used for what purpose?
    A. To provide immobilization of the lumbar spine and pelvis after a spinal injury
    B. To treat arrhythmias of the heart
    C. To treat hypovolemic shock
    D. To assess the athlete's level of consciousness after a head injury
    E. To defibrillate the heart when an unconscious victim has no pulse

85. When resolving a conflict, there are many approaches that an athletic trainer can take to successfully manage a difficult situation. Of the following conflict resolution methods, which one is least likely to successfully resolve a problem?
    A. Compromise
    B. Collaboration
    C. Negotiation
    D. Avoidance
    E. A and B

86. One of your patients presents with abnormal pain that he describes as burning. He states that it becomes worse when he lies in supine or consumes caffeine, spicy foods, or alcohol. What might you suspect is the problem?
    A. Kidney stone
    B. Ruptured spleen
    C. Bowel obstruction
    D. Hernia
    E. Esophageal reflux or peptic ulcer

87. One of your patients presents with a sudden onset of chest pain, dyspnea, hemoptysis, and cyanosis. What do you suspect is the problem?
    A. Pneumothorax
    B. Lung cancer
    C. Endocarditis
    D. Pulmonary infection
    E. Acute appendicitis

88. One of your athletes presents with diarrhea, vomiting, and abdominal cramping 1 to 6 hours after eating at a local restaurant. What do you suspect is the problem?
    A. Kidney stone
    B. Bowel obstruction
    C. Viral gastroenteritis
    D. Dysentery
    E. Food poisoning

89. How long should the abdomen be auscultated before the athletic trainer decides if the bowel sounds are absent?
    A. 30 to 60 seconds
    B. 2 to 3 minutes
    C. 60 to 90 seconds
    D. At least 5 minutes per region
    E. None of the above

90. One of your patients begins to complain of intense itching of the skin under the cold pack that you applied to his shoulder 5 minutes ago. When you remove the pack you notice that hives have developed on the area that has been cooled. What is the patient experiencing?
    A. Paroxysmal cold hemoglobinuria
    B. Hypothermia
    C. Cold urticaria
    D. Raynaud's disease
    E. Frostbite

91. When treating an athlete who presents with undifferentiated somatoform disorder, the athletic trainer should do all of the following except:
    A. Provide care for a bona fide injury
    B. Develop a sound relationship with the athlete to gain his or her trust
    C. Avoid doing more harm by dismissing the athlete as a "symptom magnifier"
    D. Provide the athlete with psychological counseling focused on having the athlete recognize and acknowledge the source of his or her anger
    E. All of the above

92. When using iontophoresis, the athletic trainer should be aware of possible _____ and _____ as a result of ion flux during treatment.
    A. Vertigo, light-headedness
    B. Sensation changes, increased swelling
    C. Skin irritation, chemical burns
    D. Vasodilatation, skin mottling
    E. Allergic reaction, increased swelling

93. Why is it important that an athlete with an abdominal injury never be given anything to eat or drink?
    A. It increases the risks of surgery if an operative procedure becomes necessary
    B. It will increase the athlete's blood glucose
    C. It will cause blood to be shunted to the viscera, causing hypovolemic shock
    D. It will cause metabolic acidosis
    E. None of the above

94. One of your diabetic athletes appears confused and is dizzy, apprehensive, and diaphoretic. How should this athlete be treated?
    A. This athlete is in diabetic ketoacidosis and should be given an immediate insulin injection
    B. This athlete should be treated for insulin shock and should be transported to the nearest hospital if he or she does not respond to sugar within 2 to 3 minutes
    C. This athlete is hyperthermic and needs to be placed in a cool, dark room until the symptoms pass
    D. The athletic trainer should monitor vital signs every 15 minutes, keep the athlete oriented, and administer insulin by mouth. If there is no change in 5 to 10 minutes, the athlete should be transported to the hospital
    E. None of the above

95. When taking a blood pressure with a sphygmomanometer, at what point is the systolic pressure noted?
    A. The point at which the pulse disappears
    B. The point at which the pulse is first heard
    C. At a point between 150 and 200 mm Hg
    D. When the brachial pulse is first palpated as the cuff is deflated
    E. When the radial pulse is first heard as the cuff deflates

96. The ideal relationship between the athletic trainer and athlete is built on _____ and _____.
    A. Encouragement, effective listening
    B. A positive attitude, a sense of humor
    C. Luck, "good chemistry"
    D. Trust, mutual respect
    E. Trust, a good insurance policy

97. Which of the following is not a good reason to refer an athlete to a psychiatrist or psychologist?
    A. The athlete is showing undue concern over minor injuries, but the concern is brief
    B. His or her psychological stress is intense or persistent
    C. There is any suggestion of suicide
    D. There is a loss of contact with reality
    E. C and D

98. An athlete receives a head injury during a soccer game. While performing the on-field evaluation, the athletic trainer notices that the athlete has a hearing defect after testing for air and bone conduction using a tuning fork. Which cranial nerve is injured?
    A. IX (glossopharyngeal)
    B. VI (abducens)
    C. XII (hypoglossal)
    D. IV (trochlear)
    E. VIII (vestibulocochlear)

99. Which of the following is the proper protocol for administering Tylenol to an adult patient (assuming the patient is not allergic to acetaminophen)?
    A. Initial dose: 2 tablets, 200 mg each, repeat every 6 to 8 hours, PRN
    B. Initial dose: 2 tablets, 225 mg each, repeat every 4 to 6 hours, PRN
    C. Initial dose: 2 tablets, 325 mg each, repeat every 4 to 6 hours, PRN
    D. Initial dose: 2 tablets, 12.5 mg each, repeat every 6 hours, PRN
    E. Initial dose: 3 tablets, 200 mg each, repeat every 8 to 12 hours, PRN

100. Which of the following is the proper protocol for administering Advil to an adult patient (assuming he or she is not allergic to ibuprofen or aspirin and does not have renal or gastrointestinal pathology)?
    A. Initial dose: 1 to 2 tablets, 200 mg each, repeat every 6 hours, PRN. Do not exceed 6 tablets in a 24-hour period without consulting with a physician
    B. Initial dose: 4 tablets, 200 mg each, repeat every 6 hours, PRN
    C. Initial dose: 1 tablet, 400 mg, repeat in 4 to 6 hours with 2 tablets, 100 mg each, PRN
    D. Initial dose: 1 tablet, 600 mg, repeat in 4 to 6 hours, PRN. Do not exceed 4 tablets in a 24-hour period without consulting with a physician
    E. None of the above

101. Which of the following is the proper protocol for administering Pepcid AC to an adult patient (assuming the patient does not have difficulty swallowing or persistent abdominal pain)?
    A. Initial dose: 2 tablets, 5 mg each with milk up to twice a day. Do not administer more than 4 tablets in a 24-hour period
    B. Initial dose: 1 tablet, 10 mg each with water up to twice a day. Do not administer more than 2 tablets in a 24-hour period
    C. Initial dose: 1 tablet, 75 mg with water up to twice a day. Do not administer more than 2 tablets in a 24-hour period
    D. Initial dose: 1 tablet, 5 mg with water up to 4 times a day
    E. None of the above

102. One of your athletes is complaining of constipation related to a dietary change. Which of the following would be the most appropriate recommendation for the athletic trainer to make?
    A. Recommend a diet high in fish oils
    B. Recommend increased fluid intake and increased intake of fruits, bulk vegetables, and cereal
    C. Recommend an increased diet of red meat and legumes
    D. Decrease the intake of green, leafy vegetables, and cereals to decrease bulk
    E. All of the above

103. Which of the following categories of drugs does not have a synergistic effect to cryotherapy?
    A. Nonsteroidal anti-inflammatory analgesics
    B. Skeletal muscle relaxants
    C. Systemic antibiotics
    D. Anti-inflammatory steroids (glucocorticoids)
    E. A and B

104. Which of the following categories of drugs has an antagonistic effect to superficial and deep heat therapy?
    A. Peripheral vasodilators
    B. Skeletal muscle relaxants
    C. Nonsteroidal anti-inflammatory analgesics
    D. Systemic vasoconstrictors
    E. All of the above

105. Which of the following are the 3 most common sites for avulsion fractures and apophysitis in the pelvic region?
    I. Ischial tuberosity and hamstring attachment
    II. Pubic symphysis and the adductor magnus attachment
    III. Anterior inferior iliac spine and the rectus femoris attachment
    IV. Iliac crest and quadratus lumborum attachment
    V. Anterior superior iliac spine where the sartorius attaches
    A. I, III, V
    B. III, IV, V
    C. I, II, IV
    D. I, III, IV
    E. I, II, III

106. What is the possible consequence of a poorly managed shin contusion?
    A. Anterior tibialis tendinitis
    B. A fasciotomy
    C. Osteochondritis dissecans
    D. Osteomyelitis
    E. Extensor digitorum contracture

107. Which of the following is not part of the treatment for plantar fasciitis?
    A. Heel cups
    B. Soft orthotics
    C. Ultrasound
    D. Arch taping
    E. Use of a metatarsal bar

108. All of the following structures should be evaluated before and after a dislocated elbow is reduced except:
    A. The median nerve
    B. The radial nerve
    C. The neurovascular status of the brachial artery
    D. The ulnar nerve
    E. The axillary nerve

109. Which of the following is the appropriate treatment of a Bennett's fracture?
    A. RICE and analgesics followed by immobilization of the metatarsophalangeal joint for 3 weeks
    B. RICE and analgesics followed by immobilization of the carpometacarpal joint; it is structurally unstable and the athlete should be immediately referred to an orthopedic surgeon
    C. RICE and analgesics followed by immobilization of the wrist in slight flexion for 6 weeks
    D. RICE and analgesics followed by a protective splint of the proximal interphalangeal joint for 6 to 8 weeks
    E. None of the above

110. One of your athletes is experiencing an anxiety attack. He is hyperventilating. You talk to him to calm him down and have him slowly rebreathe into a paper bag. What process does rebreathing into a paper bag reverse?
    A. The release of adrenocorticotropic hormone from the pituitary gland
    B. Respiratory acidosis
    C. Metabolic alkalosis
    D. Metabolic acidosis
    E. Respiratory alkalosis

111. Which end feel is an abrupt, firm, springy resistance to motion?
    A. Tissue stretch
    B. Bony block
    C. Capsular restriction
    D. Muscle spasm
    E. Scar tissue adhesions

112. Which of the following is not a component of a primary survey?
    A. Check for sensations of numbness, tingling, or burning
    B. Check surroundings and environment
    C. Check athlete for ABC
    D. Check for severe bleeding
    E. B and D

113. Which of the following should be done for an unconscious patient suffering from insulin shock?
    A. Immediately give the patient an injection of epinephrine so his or her airway will open
    B. Immediately give the patient a glass of orange juice or other high-sugar drink
    C. Immediately transport the patient to an emergency care facility
    D. Immediately give the patient some sugar-free candy in order to counteract the high levels of sugar in his or her body
    E. All of the above

114. When symptoms are experienced distal to the pathology, this is known as what?
    A. Referred symptoms
    B. Physiological symptoms
    C. Radicular symptoms
    D. Psychosomatic symptoms
    E. Contrecoup symptoms

115. Which is not a sign/symptom of postconcussion syndrome?
    A. Dizziness
    B. Restlessness
    C. Behavioral changes
    D. Visual disturbances
    E. All of the above are signs or symptoms of postconcussion syndrome

116. What special test identifies ulnar nerve compression or transmission interference at the elbow?
    A. Finkelstein's test
    B. Tarsal tunnel test
    C. Elbow flexion test
    D. Tinel's sign
    E. Yergason's test

117. All of the following are signs/symptoms of anaphylactic shock except:
    A. Development of rash or hives
    B. Wheezing sounds coming from the chest
    C. An increase in blood pressure
    D. Rapid, weak pulse
    E. A and D

118. Which of the following is not a major type of open wound?
    A. Laceration
    B. Contusion
    C. Abrasion
    D. Avulsion
    E. Incision

119. Which of the following is a condition of rapidly rising internal body temperature that occurs when the body's mechanisms for the release of heat are overwhelmed?
    A. Hyperthermia
    B. Heat exhaustion
    C. Heat stroke
    D. Hypothermia
    E. Raynaud's phenomenon

120. Which pulse should always be assessed with any injury to the lower extremity?
    A. Carotid pulse
    B. Brachial pulse
    C. Axillary pulse
    D. Radial pulse
    E. Dorsal pedal pulse

121. What type of shock is commonly referred to as fainting?
    A. Respiratory shock
    B. Cardiogenic shock
    C. Metabolic shock
    D. Anaphylactic shock
    E. Psychogenic shock

122. When a minor is injured and it is a life-threatening situation, the athletic trainer must try to contact the parents of the child. If the parents of the child cannot be contacted and they did not give consent in writing before the child began participation, the athletic trainer still has the right to give the child emergency care. Which type of consent is this?
    A. Informed
    B. Implied
    C. Complied
    D. Restrictive
    E. None of the above

123. Which of the following is a sign of heat stroke?
    A. Pale, cold, clammy skin
    B. Unequal pupils
    C. Hot and relatively dry skin
    D. Slow pulse
    E. Diaphoresis

124. Which of the following is not a sign of a diabetic coma?
    A. Fast and weak pulse
    B. Deep and sighing respirations
    C. Livid, later pale, skin
    D. Slow and weak pulse
    E. Fruity-smelling breath

125. What are the 2 most common sites to apply direct pressure to control severe bleeding of the upper and lower extremities?
    A. Brachial artery and femoral artery
    B. Popliteal artery and radial artery
    C. Brachial artery and suprascapular artery
    D. Brachial vein and femoral vein
    E. Carotid artery and femoral artery

126. _____ shock is a widely disseminated infection in many areas of the body, with the infection being borne through the blood from one tissue to another.
    A. Cardiogenic
    B. Septic
    C. Psychogenic
    D. Metabolic
    E. Hypovolemic

127. Which of the following is not a sign of hypovolemic shock?
    A. Low blood pressure
    B. Rapid and weak pulse
    C. Shallow and extremely rapid respiration
    D. Slow and weak pulse
    E. Agitation

128. How long can the brain be deprived of oxygen until brain cells begin to die?
    A. 10 to 15 minutes
    B. 1 to 3 minutes
    C. 4 to 6 minutes
    D. 17 to 20 minutes
    E. 12 to 16 minutes

129. Which of the following is a sign of inadequate breathing?
    A. Steady rise and fall of the chest
    B. The sound of air passing through the athlete's nose or mouth
    C. The sensation of the athlete breathing on the side of your face
    D. Noisy respiration, such as wheezing or gurgling
    E. None of the above

130. A football helmet should be removed only under which of the following circumstances?
    A. The injured athlete is not moving
    B. The injured athlete is no longer comfortable and says the helmet is hurting his neck
    C. You cannot gain adequate access to the airway
    D. If the EMTs think it is a great idea
    E. Never remove the helmet

131. What is a common bony process broken during adult CPR?
    A. Olecranon process
    B. The clavicle
    C. Styloid process
    D. Mastoid process
    E. Xyphoid process

132. Profuse sweating, dizziness, and nausea are signs and symptoms of which of the following?
    A. Heat stroke
    B. Heat exhaustion
    C. Hypothermia
    D. Frostbite
    E. Heat cramps

133. Which of the following things would you not want to do for someone who has gone into shock?
    A. Maintain the airway
    B. Keep the athlete calm
    C. Provide care for specific injury
    D. Give food or drink to the athlete
    E. Monitor his or her vital signs

134. An athlete with a skull fracture will have which of the following?
    A. Battle's sign
    B. Raccoon eyes
    C. Tenderness in the hard palate
    D. All of the above
    E. None of the above

135. Where would you place direct pressure on a wound that is bleeding?
    A. Directly on the wound
    B. On the right side of the wound
    C. Above the wound
    D. Below the wound
    E. On the closest artery

136. What is the first thing you should do if you suspect a spinal injury?
    A. Place the athlete on a spine board with assistance
    B. Hold in-line stabilization
    C. Help the athlete to sit up
    D. Have the athlete move his or her head
    E. Have the athlete move his or her legs

137. Which of the following is not included in a rehabilitation program after an injury?
    A. Plyometrics
    B. PNF
    C. Agility drills
    D. Immobilization
    E. Joint mobilizations

138. With ice application during the initial care of an acute injury, all of the following occur except:
    A. Increased metabolism in the area
    B. Inhibition of the hypoxic response
    C. Disruption of the pain/spasm cycle
    D. Reduction of edema
    E. Decreased nerve conduction

139. Which of the following carries impulses toward the central nervous system?
    A. Synaptic connections
    B. Afferent pathways
    C. Efferent pathways
    D. Dendrites
    E. Efferent axons

140. Deep stroking during massage is known as what?
    A. Tapotement
    B. Vibration
    C. Pétrissage
    D. Effleurage
    E. Friction massage

141. To determine if an athlete is breathing, you should do all of the following except:
    A. Place your ear over the athlete's mouth to listen for breath sounds
    B. Observe the chest
    C. Feel for the rise and fall of the chest
    D. Ask the athlete to say his or her name
    E. A and C

142. _____ pupils indicate possible shock, hemorrhage, or cardiac arrest.
    A. Unequal
    B. Constricted
    C. Dilated
    D. Discolored
    E. Closed

143. Which of the following does not occur when an individual is in shock?
    A. Skin is pale and cool
    B. Blood pressure is high
    C. Pulse is rapid
    D. Blood pressure is low
    E. Respiration is shallow

144. Frostbite includes which of the following signs?
    A. Skin appears blotchy white to yellow-gray
    B. Skin is purple
    C. Skin is pale
    D. Skin is warm
    E. All of the above

145. The athletic trainer should do which of the following when dealing with an athlete with heat exhaustion?
    A. Administer cool fluids
    B. Remove unnecessary clothing
    C. Move to a cool place
    D. All of the above
    E. None of the above

146. Transport to a medical facility for a concussion may be necessary for all of the following reasons except:
    A. If the patient is unconscious for a prolonged period of time (> 1 min)
    B. Shows declining mental status during evaluation
    C. Shows declining mental status after evaluation
    D. Demonstrates signs and symptoms of an injury more than a concussion
    E. If the athlete complains of a headache

147. Cranial nerve dysfunction and altered breathing patterns are signs of pathology of what part of the brain?
    A. Frontal lobe
    B. Midbrain and medulla
    C. Cerebellum
    D. Spinal cord
    E. Occipital lobe

148. Commotio cordis is a result of which of the following?
    A. Electrolyte imbalances
    B. Hyperthermia
    C. Blunt trauma to the chest
    D. Infection
    E. Thrombosis

149. Diabetic ketoacidosis may result from which of the following conditions?
    A. Hypoglycemia
    B. Insulin shock
    C. A blood glucose level of 70 to 110 mg/dL
    D. High blood glucose levels
    E. High blood bicarbonate

150. Which of the following conditions has a cardiac etiology as it relates to sudden death in the athlete?
    A. Heat illness
    B. Pulmonary embolism
    C. Exercise-induced anaphylaxis
    D. Substance abuse
    E. Wolff-Parkinson-White syndrome

151. An athlete who is not properly dressed when exercising in the cold weather may be subject to hypothermia. At what core body temperature does shivering cease, skeletal muscle stiffen, and cold diuresis occur?
    A. Below 64°F
    B. Below 95.5°F
    C. Below 90°F
    D. At 93°F
    E. Below 100°F

152. Pulse oximetry is used to measure oxygen saturation. Which of the following is a normal reading?
    A. 95% to 100%
    B. 91% to 94%
    C. 86% to 90%
    D. 81% to 85%
    E. 75% to 80%

153. What is the normal systolic blood pressure range for a child between 6 to 10 years of age?
    A. 60 to 105 mm Hg
    B. 80 to 122 mm Hg
    C. 90 to 140 mm Hg
    D. 90 to 110 mm Hg
    E. 80 to 110 mm Hg

154. When developing an emergency action plan, it is critical that the athletic trainer identify certain aspects of the venue he or she is working in prior to an event. All of the following should be considered except:
    A. Condition of the court or field of play
    B. Location of the emergency exits
    C. Location of emergency equipment
    D. Location of the ambulance or entrance where the ambulance or EMS will arrive
    E. Location of the press box

155. How is the correct size of an oropharyngeal airway measured and selected?
    A. Measure the distance between the tip of the ear to the corner of the mouth
    B. Measure the distance between the tip of the nose to the tip of the ear
    C. Measure the distance between the angle of the mandible to the tip of the nose
    D. Measure the distance between the chin to the tip of the ear
    E. Measure the distance between the external auditory meatus and the corner of the mouth

156. An indication for suctioning includes which of the following?
    A. If the athlete complains of excessive mucus in the mouth
    B. Blood in the mouth from a dislodged tooth
    C. When the athletic trainer notices "frothing at the mouth"
    D. Vomiting in an unresponsive individual
    E. Vomiting in an alert individual

157. Which of the following is considered a medical emergency?
    A. Colles' fracture
    B. Posterior elbow dislocation
    C. Gamekeeper's thumb
    D. Lunate dislocation
    E. Scaphoid fracture

158. Which of the following is not part of the management of turf toe?
    A. Ice
    B. NSAIDs
    C. Rest
    D. Taping to limit motion of the first metatarsophalangeal joint
    E. Taping to limit motion of the distal interphalangeal joint

159. Athletic trainers are qualified to use emergency oxygen systems to care for an ill or injured athlete. All of the following are true regarding emergency oxygen systems except:
    A. They have a pressure-reducing system
    B. It delivers oxygen at a fixed flow rate
    C. It has a container holding medical-grade oxygen
    D. A prescription is required for its use
    E. It delivers oxygen at a flow rate of at least 6 LPM for at least 15 minutes

160. What precautionary measures should be taken prior to transferring and securing an athlete with protective equipment (as in football or ice hockey) to a rigid immobilization device such as a spine board?
    A. Facemask removal and preparation of shoulder pads
    B. Make sure a cervical collar is applied and the athlete is rolled to the side to prevent aspiration of vomit
    C. The helmet and shoulder pads are removed
    D. The facemask is removed and the arms are secured to the chest
    E. Secure the arms across the chest with a strap and remove the helmet

161. What is the first step in treating an abrasion or laceration?
    A. Close the wound with butterfly strips
    B. Wrap the wound with sterile gauze
    C. Check the distal pulses
    D. Control the bleeding with direct pressure
    E. Reduce wound contamination

162. When a bronchodilator is used more often than recommended, it can cause which of the following?
    A. Hypertension
    B. A sudden drop in forced expiratory volume
    C. An increased ejection fraction
    D. Tachycardia
    E. Bradycardia

163. Portable radios and landline telephones are preferred over personal cell phones when communicating in an emergency primarily because of which of the following?
    A. Cell phones are easy to misplace
    B. Personal equipment should not be used in an emergency
    C. Cell phones do not have a secured frequency
    D. The use of cell phones violates HIPAA laws
    E. A cell phone may be unreliable in some areas due to weak cellular signals

164. A capillary refill time of greater than _____ seconds is a sign of inadequate perfusion.
    A. 0.25
    B. 0.50
    C. 1.0
    D. 1.5
    E. 2.0

Treatment and Rehabilitation

1. What does "extension lag" mean?
    A. Ability to only flex the knee
    B. Inability to fully backward bend (lumbar movement)
    C. One leg drags behind the other during gait
    D. Inability to fully extend the knee
    E. Inability to fully extend the hip

2. What is the best method of determining the recovery status of the hand and forearm after a flexor injury?
    A. Use of a KT-1000 arthrometer
    B. Assessing the strength of a handshake
    C. Manual muscle testing of the wrist
    D. Use of a hand dynamometer
    E. Electromyography testing

3. Which of the following is the correct sequence of tissue healing?
    A. Cellular response, regeneration, remodeling
    B. Remodeling, regeneration, cellular response
    C. Rejection, regeneration, resolution
    D. Regeneration, resolution, remodeling
    E. None of the above

4. What amount of time may it take for complete remodeling of tissues to occur after a soft tissue injury?
    A. 1 to 3 months
    B. 6 to 9 months
    C. 4 to 6 weeks
    D. 12 to 24 months
    E. Up to 1 year

5. Where is the primary location for adenosine triphosphate production in skeletal muscle?
    A. Sarcomere
    B. Sarcoplasm
    C. Sarcolemma
    D. Sarcoplasmic reticulum
    E. Mitochondria

6. Sensory receptors located at the musculotendinous junction, which monitor active tension generated by the muscle during a contraction, are called:
    A. Pacinian corpuscles
    B. Ruffini receptors
    C. Golgi tendon organs
    D. Muscle spindles
    E. Contractile sensory receptors

7. Which of the following describes a neurapraxia?
    A. Demyelination of the axon sheath that leads to a conduction block. Usually heals in approximately 1 to 2 weeks
    B. Loss or disruption of the axon and myelin sheath. The epineurium is still intact
    C. An injury to the endoneurium, perineurium, and epineurium with a permanent neurological deficit
    D. A crush injury to a nerve causing damage to the epineurium. The perineurium is intact
    E. None of the above

8. Bone grows via a process of apposition and resorption on its surface. Which of the following cells are responsible for the resorption of bone during its growth or repair?
    A. Osteoblasts
    B. Osteocytes
    C. Osteophils
    D. Osteoclasts
    E. None of the above

9. Why is the repair response so limited in the articular cartilage of a joint after an injury in the adult athlete?
    A. Articular cartilage cells do not undergo mitosis in the mature athlete
    B. Articular cartilage has a poor venous supply
    C. Articular cartilage has a low water content
    D. There are fewer mitochondria present in articular cartilage than in hyaline cartilage
    E. All of the above

10. What are the 4 sensations an athlete will experience with the application of cryotherapy?
    A. Cold, burning, cramping, numbness
    B. Pain, aching, stinging, cold
    C. Aching, burning, pain, numbness
    D. Cold, burning, aching, numbness
    E. Cold, burning, stinging, aching

11. The effects of treating a subacute musculoskeletal injury with a warm whirlpool include all of the following except:
    A. Analgesia
    B. Stimulation of local circulation
    C. Decreased muscle spasm
    D. Increased deep tissue temperature
    E. Decreased joint stiffness

12. Which cells are active after an injury to begin building collagen?
    A. Osteocytes
    B. Osteoblasts
    C. Granulocytes
    D. Osteoclasts
    E. Fibroblasts

13. Heat is dissipated in the body by all of the following except:
    A. Shivering
    B. Convection
    C. The lungs
    D. Sweat evaporation
    E. Vasodilatation

14. External muscular force available for useful work is the result of all of the following factors except:
    A. The velocity of muscular shortening
    B. Whether the muscle is fast or slow twitch
    C. The angle of the pull of the muscle
    D. The length of the muscle
    E. C and D

15. Balance and coordination are critical for athletic performance. Feedback from the muscles as to what they are doing during a particular activity is known as _____. The area of the brain that assists in controlling movement is the _____.
    A. Proprioception, brain stem
    B. Muscle perception, medulla
    C. Kinesthesia, cortex
    D. Proprioception, cerebellum
    E. Kinesthesia, cerebrum

16. What is a stretching exercise that consists of a "stretch and hold" position called?
    A. Static stretch
    B. PNF pattern
    C. Ballistic stretch
    D. Warm-up
    E. B and C

17. If hyperventilation does not adequately increase the oxygen supply in the blood during aerobic exercise, what must occur to meet the gas exchange demands?
    A. Increased cardiac output
    B. Decreased cardiac output
    C. Supplemental iron pills must be provided
    D. The activity must be discontinued
    E. None of the above

18. An injured athlete is led through a therapeutic mental process in which he pictures himself being evaluated by the athletic trainer and assured the injury is not serious. He then pictures himself moving through rehabilitation, recovering nicely, and, finally, returning to his sport fully healed. What is this therapeutic approach to the recovery process called?
    A. Regression
    B. Thought stopping
    C. Biofeedback
    D. Meditation
    E. Visualization

19. What must the athletic trainer establish with the athlete prior to and during the rehabilitation in order for the rehabilitation of an injured athlete to be successful?
    A. A good rapport
    B. A position of dominance
    C. A deadline by which the athlete must return to full-time participation in his or her sport
    D. The understanding that the coach has the final decision in his or her rehabilitation sessions
    E. B and C

20. A basketball player who has sprained her ankle for the second time in 3 months reports to the athletic training facility for her third treatment session. The athletic trainer notices she is demanding and wants to know why the athletic trainer "did not fix her ankle the right way the first time." She becomes somewhat threatening, stating that she will find someone else to help her if she is not successfully helped this time. What would be the best response to an attention-seeking athlete?
    A. Give up and let her seek help elsewhere
    B. Work with the athlete as long as necessary to satisfy her need for attention
    C. Set specific but reasonable time limits with the athlete per treatment session so the athletic trainer is not overtaxed
    D. Encourage the athlete to take a more positive position on her rehabilitation and use humor to divert her attention away from the injury
    E. None of the above

21. If an athlete needs to lose weight for health reasons, how many calories must his or her daily diet be reduced by in order to lose 1 to 2 pounds per week?
    A. 250 to 500 calories/day
    B. 1000 to 2000 calories/week
    C. 1000 to 2000 calories/day
    D. 500 to 1000 calories/day
    E. None of the above

22. Which modality would be best utilized if the desired therapeutic effect is decreased pain, edema, and inflammation?
    A. Moist heat packs
    B. Ultrasound
    C. Diathermy
    D. Fluidotherapy
    E. Ice packs

23. What are heat-producing currents in the body that are formed by a magnetic field that is externally applied in short-wave diathermy called?
    A. Induction currents
    B. Magnetic currents
    C. Eddy currents
    D. Alternating currents
    E. Interferential currents

24. High-voltage pulsed monophasic generators deliver current to deep tissues without damaging superficial tissues and are used for pain modulation. What type of waveform is used with this type of stimulator?
    A. Asymmetrical biphasic spiked pulse
    B. Monophasic squared pulse
    C. Symmetrical biphasic pulses
    D. Monophasic spike delivered in pairs
    E. None of the above

25. A moist heat pack causes all of the following effects except:
    A. Higher superficial tissue temperatures
    B. Increases in muscle tissue temperatures
    C. Sedation
    D. Reduction of muscle spasms
    E. Vasodilatation

26. What physiological effects occur under the cathode of an electrical stimulator?
        I. Vasodilatation
        II. Vasoconstriction
        III. Tissue softening
        IV. Irritation
    A. I, III, IV
    B. II, III, IV
    C. I, II, III
    D. I, II, IV
    E. None of the above

27. All of the following are contraindications for using cryotherapy except:
    A. Raynaud's phenomenon
    B. Inflammation
    C. Vasculitis
    D. Cold urticaria
    E. A and D

28. What would be a functional skill for a patient in an ankle rehabilitation program?
    A. Gastrocnemius flexibility
    B. Single-leg hopping
    C. Lifting tolerance
    D. Anterior tibialis strengthening
    E. All of the above

29. When rehabilitating a musculoskeletal injury, what is the proper progression of treatment?
    A. Range of motion, strength, endurance, proprioception
    B. Pain relief, agility, range of motion, strength
    C. Range of motion, pain relief, endurance, proprioception
    D. Proprioception, range of motion, strength, endurance
    E. Range of motion, endurance, strength, proprioception

30. Which of the following PNF techniques is not a strengthening technique?
    A. Slow reversal
    B. Rhythmic stabilization
    C. Slow-reversal-hold-relax
    D. Rhythmic initiation
    E. All of the above

31. During a lower extremity D1 flexion PNF pattern, what movements are taking place at the hip?
    A. Extension, abduction, internal rotation
    B. Flexion, abduction, internal rotation
    C. Extension, adduction, external rotation
    D. Flexion, adduction, external rotation
    E. Flexion, abduction, external rotation

32. During a D2 extension pattern of the upper extremity, what is the proper timing sequence?
    A. Shoulder extension, forearm pronation, finger flexion
    B. Shoulder flexion, scapular retraction, finger extension
    C. Shoulder abduction, forearm supination, finger extension
    D. Shoulder extension, forearm supination, finger flexion
    E. None of the above

33. According to Maitland's 5 grades of joint motion, which grade would be most appropriate when joint movement is limited by pain and spasm?
    A. I
    B. II
    C. III
    D. IV
    E. V

34. A patient is seen by the athletic trainer 4 weeks post-operatively after shoulder arthroscopy. During the athletic trainer's assessment, it is found that the patient has limited abduction secondary to capsular stiffness. Which of the following joint glides would be appropriate to improve this motion?
    A. Inferior humeral glide
    B. Anterior humeral glide
    C. Posterior humeral glide
    D. Superior humeral glide
    E. All of the above/combined glides

35. Which of the following statements accurately describes isokinetic training?
    A. Generation of a muscular force with no visible joint movement
    B. Generation of a muscular force with visible joint movement that occurs at a constant speed but with variable external resistance
    C. Generation of a muscular force with visible joint movement at a variable speed but with a fixed external resistance
    D. Generation of a muscle force during muscular lengthening
    E. None of the above

36. Which of the following massage techniques is a method of tapotement?
    A. Cupping
    B. Hacking
    C. Pinching
    D. All of the above
    E. None of the above

37. When massage is utilized to induce a sedative effect, which type of massage technique is indicated?
    A. Tapotement
    B. Vibration
    C. Pétrissage
    D. Danish
    E. Effleurage

38. What conditioning component is needed to perceive the position of the foot as it lands on the ground after the swing phase of gait?
    A. Agility
    B. Balance
    C. Proprioception
    D. Kinesthesia
    E. Eccentric stretching

39. Descending hills during running requires what type of muscular contraction by the quadriceps to decelerate the body?
    A. Positive
    B. Concentric
    C. Isokinetic
    D. Isometric
    E. Eccentric

40. What should a postseason conditioning program specifically focus on?
    A. Endurance activities
    B. Strengthening and flexibility exercises
    C. Sport-specific activities
    D. Identifying and improving the areas of conditioning in which the athlete is deficient
    E. All of the above

41. During the acute phase of an ankle injury, the water temperature of a whirlpool should be set at what temperature?
    A. 37°C to 37.7°C
    B. 55°F to 65°F
    C. 30°F to 35°F
    D. 70°F to 80°F
    E. 40°C to 50°C

42. Before returning an athlete to full activity, all of the following criteria should equal those taken from the uninvolved side at the end of the rehabilitation program except:
    A. Strength of each muscle group
    B. Girth measurements at 6 inches above and below the joint line
    C. Proprioception of both extremities
    D. Flexibility of the involved muscle groups
    E. C and D

43. Which of the following components of a rehabilitation program is most often overlooked by the athletic trainer during rehabilitation?
    A. Endurance
    B. Flexibility
    C. Proprioception
    D. Functional testing prior to returning to the sport
    E. Strength

44. What type of exercises may be safely initiated immediately after knee surgery?
    A. Closed-chain eccentric exercises
    B. Isotonic exercises
    C. Isometric exercises
    D. Functional exercises
    E. None of the above

45. When rehabilitating a patient who has been diagnosed with "jumper's knee," which muscle group should eventually be strengthened?
    A. Hamstrings
    B. Quadriceps
    C. Hip adductors
    D. Hip extensors
    E. Triceps surae

46. When treating an athlete with trochanteric bursitis, flexibility should be increased in which of the following muscles?
    A. Gluteus maximus
    B. Tensor fasciae latae
    C. Iliacus
    D. Piriformis
    E. Lumbar

47. A tight Achilles tendon can cause _____ or _____ in order to allow the lower leg to move over the foot during running.
    A. Late heel-off, early heel strike
    B. Early heel-off, excessive supination
    C. Late heel-off, late toe-off
    D. Early heel-off, excessive pronation
    E. Early heel-off, early heel strike

48. Which of the following is not a factor in designing an appropriate treatment program?
    A. The stage of tissue healing
    B. Pain with joint motion
    C. The severity of the injury
    D. How soon the coach feels the athlete should return to play
    E. A and B

49. When rehabilitating a cervical strain, what must the athletic trainer maintain the integrity of?
    A. Shoulder girdle
    B. Lower back
    C. Upper arm
    D. Hand
    E. Kyphosis of the thoracic spine

50. Which of the following sequences contains the appropriate steps in rehabilitating a grade II ankle sprain?
    A. RICE, stretching the Achilles tendon, isometric exercises, proprioceptive exercises, isotonic exercises
    B. RICE, isotonic exercises, hopping exercises, stretching the Achilles tendon, active range of motion exercises
    C. RICE, isotonic exercises, isokinetic exercises, active range of motion exercises
    D. RICE, treadmill ambulation, active range of motion exercises, figure-8 exercises, stretching of the Achilles tendon, foot intrinsic exercises
    E. None of the above

51. When is the best time to begin a rehabilitation program after an injury?
    A. Immediately
    B. After the injured part is "healed"
    C. After the inflammation is under control
    D. Once the pain subsides
    E. All of the above

52. When following the DAPRE technique of progressive resistive exercise, the first set of 10 repetitions is performed with a weight that is _____ of the weight that will be lifted in set 3.
    A. 10%
    B. 25%
    C. 100%
    D. 75%
    E. 50%

53. When rehabilitating a patient with patellofemoral pain syndrome, which muscle groups should be strengthened?
    A. Quadriceps, hamstrings
    B. Hip abductors, hamstrings
    C. Hip adductors, quadriceps
    D. Hip flexors, hip external rotators
    E. Iliotibial band, hip external rotators

54. Which of the following exercises are appropriate in attempting to decrease the symptoms of thoracic outlet syndrome?
    A. Cervical range of motion exercises, anterior shoulder strengthening
    B. Cervical range of motion exercises, cervical isometrics
    C. Anterior chest wall strengthening, cervical isometrics
    D. Stretching the anterior chest wall, strengthening the posterior midthoracic area
    E. None of the above

55. What are the most appropriate exercises for a diagnosis of lumbar spinal stenosis?
    A. Kegel exercises
    B. McKenzie extension exercises
    C. Lumbar stabilization exercises
    D. Postural awareness exercises
    E. Williams' flexion exercises

56. Which of the following exercises does not address proprioception?
    A. Recumbent stationary bicycling
    B. Mini-trampoline exercises
    C. Stork-standing exercises with the eyes open
    D. Treadmill exercises
    E. All of the above

57. When rehabilitating a shoulder, in what area should strengthening exercises be initiated first?
    A. Rotator cuff musculature
    B. Cervical musculature
    C. Scapular musculature
    D. Shoulder abductors, flexors, and internal rotators
    E. A and D

58. When rehabilitating a patient who has undergone an anterior cruciate ligament reconstruction, which of the following muscle groups must be strengthened to support the graft?
    A. Triceps surae
    B. Hip adductors
    C. Quadriceps
    D. Gluteals
    E. Hamstrings

59. Which of the following pieces of equipment is not considered closed kinetic chain?
    A. Treadmill
    B. Leg-press machine
    C. Upper body ergometer
    D. Isokinetic knee extension machine
    E. BAPS board

60. When rehabilitating the lateral epicondylitis, which muscle group needs to be strengthened?
    A. Wrist flexors
    B. Wrist extensors
    C. Elbow flexors
    D. Elbow extensors
    E. Shoulder abductors

61. When rehabilitating a patient with a recent herniated lumbar disc, which of the following exercises are most appropriate?
    A. Williams' flexion exercises
    B. McKenzie extension exercises
    C. Lumbar stabilization exercises
    D. Posterior pelvic tilts and knee-to-chest exercises
    E. PNF stretching exercises

62. A patient needs instruction on how to properly perform an abdominal sit-up. What should the athletic trainer recommend?
    A. Place his hands behind his head, take a deep breath and hold it, and pull his torso up toward his bent knees
    B. Cross his arms across his chest, tuck in his chin, bend his knees, inhale, and then exhale as he pulls his torso up toward his knees
    C. Place his hands behind his head, bend his knees, exhale completely first, and inhale deeply as he pulls his torso up toward his knees
    D. Keeping his arms down by his sides, bend his knees, inhale deeply, and hold it as he pulls his torso up toward his knees
    E. None of the above

63. Knee braces can be classified as either functional, prophylactic, or rehabilitative. Which type of brace might be worn for 1 to 2 weeks after a grade II medial collateral ligament tear?
    A. Functional
    B. Prophylactic
    C. Rehabilitative
    D. Custom fit
    E. No brace is necessary for this injury

64. In terms of specificity of training, which type of exercise would be appropriate during the late phases of rehabilitation of a soccer player?
    A. Stairmaster
    B. Swimming
    C. Stationary bicycle
    D. Leg press
    E. Treadmill exercise

65. Which of the following conditions is not indicated for mechanical traction?
    A. An acute interspinous sprain
    B. Degenerative joint disease
    C. Herniated discs or protrusions
    D. Degenerative disc disease
    E. Muscle spasm

66. Which of the muscle groups listed below are involved during a bench press?
    - I. Anterior deltoid
    - II. Rhomboids
    - III. Triceps
    - IV. Pectoralis major
    - V. Latissimus dorsi
    - VI. Upper trapezius
    - A. I, II, III, IV
    - B. III, IV, V, VI
    - C. I, III, IV, V
    - D. II, III, IV, VI
    - E. I, II, III, V

67. Which of the following muscle groups are involved during a full squat with weights?
    - I. Quadriceps
    - II. Hamstrings
    - III. Erector spinae
    - IV. Middle deltoid
    - V. Gluteus maximus
    - VI. Serratus anterior
    - A. I, II, IV, V
    - B. II, III, IV, V
    - C. I, II, III, V
    - D. II, III, V, VI
    - E. All of the above

68. Which of the following muscles are involved in a seated military press?
    - I. Trapezius
    - II. Latissimus dorsi
    - III. Pectoralis major
    - IV. Serratus anterior
    - V. Posterior deltoid
    - VI. Triceps
    - A. II, III, VI
    - B. I, III, IV, V
    - C. I, IV, V, VI
    - D. I, III, IV, VI
    - E. All of the above

69. Which of the following describes a grade III joint mobilization technique?
    - A. Small amplitude movement at the end range
    - B. Large amplitude movement throughout the full available range of motion of the joint
    - C. Small amplitude movement in the beginning of the range of motion
    - D. Thrusting movement done at the anatomical limits of the joint
    - E. None of the above

70. When rehabilitating a patient, it is important that the area being rehabilitated is stressed with a variety of intensities and durations during conditioning. The body responds to these stresses by adapting to the specific demands imposed on it. What is this principle known as?
    - A. The SAID principle
    - B. The DAPRE principle
    - C. The RICE principle
    - D. The SITS principle
    - E. None of the above

71. Which of the following is not an example of an isotonic device?
    - A. Free weights
    - B. A total gym
    - C. A squat rack
    - D. Wall pulleys
    - E. A wall

72. When stretching during a warm-up routine, which type of stretching should not be encouraged because it may lead to an injury?
    - A. Ballistic
    - B. Active
    - C. Static
    - D. Plyometric
    - E. PNF

73. In which of the following sports would plyometric training be beneficial?
    - A. Rock climbing
    - B. Cross-country
    - C. Volleyball
    - D. Archery
    - E. Swimming

74. Which of the following exercises improves proprioceptive feedback when rehabilitating a lower extremity injury?
    - A. Stationary bicycling
    - B. Single-leg standing on a mini-trampoline
    - C. Using a knee extension machine
    - D. Bilateral calf raises
    - E. All of the above

75. An athlete is recovering from a partial meniscectomy performed 5 days ago. All of the following actions would be appropriate at this time except:
    - A. Achilles stretching
    - B. Four quadrant straight leg raises
    - C. Stationary bicycling with minimal/no resistance
    - D. Eccentric quadriceps strengthening
    - E. Hip flexor strengthening

76. Which of the following exercises should be avoided in the early stages (phase I) of anterior cruciate reconstruction rehabilitation?
    A. Full knee extension exercises
    B. Resisted hip abduction
    C. Toe raises
    D. Hamstring curls
    E. Isometric contraction of the quadriceps

77. Two exercises that are designed to stabilize the lumbar spine during low back rehabilitation include _____ and _____.
    A. Single knee-to-chest exercise, double knee to chest
    B. Hamstring stretching, bridging exercises
    C. Partial sit-ups, active trunk extension in prone
    D. Resisted hip abduction exercise, iliotibial band stretching
    E. Hamstring stretching, piriformis strengthening

78. An athletic trainer working in a sports medicine clinic may have to read a SOAP note. In what section would a finding such as a positive Lachman's test be recorded?
    A. Subjective (S)
    B. Objective (O)
    C. Assessment (A)
    D. Plan (P)
    E. Special tests (S)

79. Bracing for scoliosis of the spine may be effective with all ages except:
    A. 5 year olds
    B. 10 year olds
    C. 18 year olds
    D. 14 year olds
    E. Bracing is not effective at any age

80. Ultrasound is based on the _____ effect.
    A. Resonance
    B. Sounding
    C. Cavitation
    D. Phoresor
    E. Reverse piezoelectric

81. What medium does not transmit ultrasound waves?
    A. Water
    B. Gel
    C. Body lotion
    D. Steroid creams
    E. Air

82. What kind of heating method does a warm whirlpool utilize?
    A. Conduction
    B. Convection
    C. Radiation
    D. Evaporation
    E. All of the above

83. What is the term used in ultrasound to describe the time that sound waves are being emitted during one pulse period?
    A. Ultrasound frequency
    B. Cavitation
    C. Attenuation
    D. Duty cycle
    E. Intensity

84. A moist heat pack offers what type of thermotherapy?
    A. Superficial
    B. Deep
    C. Cutaneous
    D. Surface
    E. None of the above

85. Conventional TENS uses a frequency in the _____ pulses per second range with a phase duration of _____ μseconds.
    A. 50 to 100, 250
    B. 50 to 100, 2 to 50
    C. 2 to 4, >150
    D. >100, 20 to 30
    E. <10, 50

86. What is one of the most serious adverse reactions during iontophoresis treatment?
    A. Galvanic burns
    B. Anaphylactic shock
    C. Dermatitis
    D. Histamine reaction
    E. None of the above

87. Paraffin bath therapy is commonly used on the hands and feet as a method of superficial heating. To keep the paraffin mixture in a molten state, the temperature should be maintained between:
    A. 100°F to 115°F
    B. 80°F to 105°F
    C. 126°F to 130°F
    D. 118°F to 125°F
    E. 140°F to 150°F

88. The therapeutic conversion of electrical energy into high-frequency sound energy above the audible range to create heat in the tissues is the definition of what modality?
    A. Diathermy
    B. Ultrasound
    C. Electric stimulation
    D. TENS
    E. Interferential current

89. Ultrasound waves are reflected by _____ and absorbed by _____.
    A. Bone, skin
    B. Skin, connective tissue
    C. Skin, blood
    D. Bone, muscle
    E. Nerve, muscle

90. Which of the following are contraindications to massage?
    I.   Inflammation
    II. Pregnancy
    III. Hemorrhage
    IV. Infection
    V.   Phlebitis
    A. I, II, III, IV
    B. I, III, IV, V
    C. II, III, IV
    D. II, III, IV, V
    E. All of the above

91. Which of the following is not an indication for diathermy?
    A. To increase local circulation
    B. Reduction of spasms
    C. Pain relief
    D. Cardiac abnormalities
    E. Osteoarthritis

92. Which of the following is not a contraindication or precaution for the use of ultrasound?
    A. Scarring
    B. Acute hemorrhage
    C. Anesthesia
    D. Treating over the endocrine gland
    E. Open wounds

93. Which physical law is applied with the use of an infra-red lamp?
    A. Joule's law
    B. Inverse square law
    C. Wolff's law
    D. Ohm's law
    E. Newton's law

94. _____ and _____ are 2 means that deliver medication via sound waves and electricity.
    A. Ultrasound, iontophoresis
    B. Ultrasound, phonophoresis
    C. Micromassage, phonophoresis
    D. Phonophoresis, iontophoresis
    E. High-volt electric stimulation, iontophoresis

95. What is a primary indication for cervical traction?
    A. Muscle spasm
    B. Hemorrhage
    C. Muscle weakness
    D. Vertigo
    E. None of the above

96. The athletic trainer of a collegiate women's swimming and diving team suspects one of his patients might have a severe eating disorder. After lengthy discussions with both the coach and patient, the athletic trainer decides it would be best for the patient if she is referred for professional help. To which of the following professionals should the patient be initially referred?
    A. An endocrinologist
    B. A chiropractor
    C. A registered dietitian
    D. A registered nurse
    E. A psychologist

97. One of your male patients notices a tingling sensation in his urethra followed by a discharge of greenish-yellow pus from his penis. He is also complaining of pain during urination. You suspect which sexually transmitted disease and recommend which of the following actions?
    A. Syphilis; have the patient take Zovirax for 7 to 10 days
    B. Trichomoniasis; have the patient drink acidic fluids, call his family physician, and have the patient refrain from all sexual contact
    C. Genital candidiasis; have the patient apply a fungicide to his penis
    D. Gonorrhea; refer the patient to a physician and have him refrain from all sexual contact
    E. Genital herpes; have the patient take Diflucan

98. During the rehabilitation of a knee injury, the athletic trainer decides the use of neuromuscular stimulation is indicated. As the athletic trainer is applying the electrodes to the patient's thigh, the patient says he has never had electric stimulation and is scared of electricity. Which of the following would be an appropriate response by the athletic trainer?
    A. Tell him he is being childish
    B. Demonstrate how it works
    C. Teach him about the general principles of electric stimulation
    D. Tell a joke about electricity to relax him
    E. Do not use an electrotherapeutic modality on the patient

99. A cross-country runner comes to you because he would like to begin a strength-training program for general body development. He informs you that he "has never really lifted weights before." How would you instruct him regarding his breathing pattern during a lift?
    A. Have the athlete inhale deeply at the beginning of the lift and then forcefully exhale at the end of the lift
    B. Have the athlete hold his breath during the lift
    C. Have the athlete inhale during the lift and hold his breath at the end of the lift
    D. Have the athlete breathe in, blow out, and breathe in again at the end of the lift
    E. Breathe normally

100. What should the athletic trainer do when teaching a patient how to properly use crutches?
    A. Make sure the patient's weight is fully supported on his or her hands and armpits
    B. Caution the patient not to lean on the crutches so that his or her weight is on the crutches' axillary pads
    C. Teach him or her how to use a cane first
    D. Teach the patient a 4-point gait
    E. Teach the patient a 5-point gait

101. You suspect one of your soccer players is experiencing "training staleness." Which of the following should you assess when developing a counseling approach with the patient?
    A. The level of the patient's ability to play the sport
    B. The relationship between the patient and his family
    C. The patient's training schedule and diet
    D. The patient's competition schedule
    E. The relationship between the patient and coach

102. When rehabilitating an athlete following a ligamentous wrist injury, once the ligament has healed enough where active motion can be initiated, it is important to educate the athlete to exercise only:
    A. Isometrically
    B. In water
    C. While using a prophylactic brace
    D. First thing in the morning
    E. In a pain-free range

103. One of your patients has been diagnosed with Sinding-Larsen-Johansson disease. Which of the following is not appropriate when advising the patient in regard to minimizing his symptoms?
    A. To increase the strength of the vastus medialis obliquus muscle with isotonic quadriceps strengthening exercises
    B. Use ice packs frequently to minimize pain and swelling
    C. Avoid stressful activities, such as running, for approximately 6 months
    D. Avoid deep squatting
    E. All of the above

104. When counseling a patient about the proper way to self-administer a medication, it is important that the athletic trainer make the patient aware of what 2 factors?
    A. Any side effects and, in detail, how the drug works on the body
    B. If the drug may be addictive and how long the effects will last
    C. If the drug may cause depression and, in detail, how the drug works on the body
    D. When to take the medication and what foods/drugs not to mix with it
    E. B and C

105. An athlete experiences a catastrophic injury in which she is permanently unable to return to playing the only sport with which she is familiar. What would be the athletic trainer's appropriate response when discussing the injury with the athlete?
    A. Tell her it is not appropriate to deny her condition and that it is best to accept her limitations
    B. Tell her it is OK for her to feel a variety of emotions and to openly express her needs and concerns
    C. Tell her to speak to her coach about her future in athletics
    D. Tell her to seek psychological counseling until she is no longer angry about her injury
    E. Tell her it happens all of the time and eventually she will get used to her situation

106. When advising a patient about his year-long strength-training program, the athletic trainer should have the patient limit his heavy lifting workouts to which periods?
    A. In-season and postseason
    B. Preseason and in-season
    C. Postseason and off-season
    D. Off-season and preseason
    E. None of the above

107. A swimmer reports to the athletic training facility complaining of symptoms related to Scheuermann's disease. Which type of exercises are beneficial in trying to diminish the symptoms during the early stages of the disease?
    A. Cervical range of motion exercises
    B. Extension and postural exercises
    C. Williams' flexion exercises
    D. Hughston exercises
    E. Deep breathing exercises

108. When rehabilitating an athlete following a lumbar strain, the athletic trainer should emphasize the significance of having the athlete improve the flexibility of all of the following structures except:
    A. The abdominals
    B. The iliopsoas
    C. The paraspinals
    D. The hamstrings
    E. The hip extensors

109. One of your basketball players often complains about localized lumbar "backaches." After performing your evaluation on this patient, it appears his primary problem is postural. All of the following are actions that the patient can take to prevent low back pain except:
    A. When standing for long periods of time, rest one foot on a stool if it is available
    B. Avoid sleeping in side-lying position with the knees slightly bent
    C. Carry objects at waist level when possible
    D. Sit on chairs with a firm seat and straight back
    E. Keep his abdominals strong

110. Which of the following individuals should the athletic trainer advise and consult with when developing a reconditioning program for a patient following a musculoskeletal injury while playing football?
    A. The team physician
    B. The school nurse
    C. The head football coach
    D. The patient's parents if he is a minor
    E. The team strength and conditioning coach

111. _____ and _____ are important qualities that an athletic trainer must possess when counseling a patient during a time of distress.
    A. Honesty, respect
    B. Sympathy, pity
    C. Confidence, logic
    D. Objectivity, decisiveness
    E. Logic, detachment

112. If the patient complains of a burning sensation during an ultrasound treatment, all of the following may be the source of the problem except:
    A. The intensity is too high
    B. Not enough ultrasound medium is being used
    C. Too much ultrasound gel is being used
    D. The movement of the transducer head is too slow
    E. B and D

113. Pain occurring at a site distant to damaged tissue that does not follow the course of a peripheral nerve describes what type of pain?
    A. Muscular
    B. Referred
    C. Radicular
    D. Visceral
    E. Parasympathetic

114. Which of the following is not a contraindication to the use of diathermy?
    A. Acute inflammation and joint effusion
    B. Muscle spasm
    C. Pregnancy
    D. Open wounds
    E. C and D

115. What occurs during a joint mobilization technique when a convex surface moves on a concave surface?
    A. Roll and glide occur in opposite directions
    B. Glide and spin occur in opposite directions
    C. A shearing force occurs at the joint surface
    D. Roll and glide occur in the same direction
    E. Straight glide in same direction

116. Contraindications to cervical traction include all of the following except:
    A. A positive vertebral artery test
    B. A positive alar ligament test
    C. Disc herniation
    D. Increased radicular symptoms with treatment
    E. Nystagmus

117. Which of the following is a manual technique in which an injured patient's muscles are actively contracted against a counterforce in a specific position?
    A. Myofascial release
    B. Muscle energy techniques
    C. Joint mobilization
    D. Strain-counterstrain
    E. Multi-angle isokinetics

118. Delayed-onset muscle soreness normally occurs how long after a strenuous exercise session?
    A. 1 hour after exercise
    B. 12 hours after exercise
    C. 24 to 72 hours after exercise
    D. 4 to 6 hours after exercise
    E. Immediately after exercise

119. Physiologic adaptations of the respiratory system during aerobic endurance training include all of the following except:
    A. Reduced submaximal heart rate
    B. Enhanced oxygen exchange within the lungs
    C. Decreased submaximal pulmonary ventilation
    D. Improved circulation throughout the lungs
    E. B and D

120. Which of the following muscles are involved in a seated row exercise?
    I. Latissimus dorsi
    II. Teres minor
    III. Teres major
    IV. Middle trapezius
    V. Rhomboids
    VI. Pectoralis major
    A. I, III, IV, VI
    B. II, III, IV, V
    C. I, IV, V, VI
    D. I, III, IV, V
    E. I, II, III, IV

121. Which of the following muscles are the primary muscles involved when performing a resisted wrist curl (palms up)?
    I. Flexor digitorum longus
    II. Flexor digiti minimi
    III. Adductor pollicis
    IV. Flexor carpi radialis
    V. Flexor carpi ulnaris
    VI. Brachialis
    A. I, II, IV
    B. I, IV, V, VI
    C. II, III, IV, VI
    D. IV, V
    E. III, IV, V

122. Which of the following structures is responsible for relaying information regarding muscle dynamics to the conscious and subconscious parts of the central nervous system?
    A. Muscle spindle
    B. Proprioceptors
    C. Golgi tendon organs
    D. Type III muscle fibers
    E. Brain stem

123. Which of the following is the most effective motivator for compliance to rehabilitation of an athletic injury?
    A. Coercion
    B. Bribery
    C. Fear
    D. Collaboration
    E. Goal setting

124. Which of the following types of exercise can produce a spike in systolic blood pressure that can result in a potentially life-threatening cardiovascular accident?
    A. Isometric
    B. Plyometric
    C. Isotonic
    D. Eccentric
    E. Isokinetic

125. Which of the following is an example of muscle spindle activity?
    A. Nystagmus
    B. Babinski's reflex
    C. Knee-jerk reflex
    D. Moro's reflex
    E. None of the above

126. When the length of a muscle prevents full range of motion at the joint or joints over which the muscle crosses, it is known as what?
    A. Adhesive capsulitis
    B. Passive insufficiency
    C. Hypomobility
    D. Muscle contracture
    E. None of the above

127. All of the following principles must be considered before the athletic trainer begins an activity designed to improve balance except:
    A. Multiple planes of motion must be stressed
    B. The activities must progress to sport-specific activities
    C. The activity should incorporate a unisensory approach
    D. The exercises must be safe but challenging
    E. A and B

128. Which of the following positions must be avoided when rehabilitating an athlete who has posterior instability of the glenohumeral joint?
    A. Abduction with external rotation
    B. Full forward flexion
    C. Internal rotation with horizontal adduction and flexion
    D. Internal rotation with shoulder extension
    E. A and B

129. When developing a functional progression for an athlete who is undergoing a rehabilitation program, all of the following factors need to be considered except:
    A. The physician's expectations for the athlete's return to activity
    B. The athlete's expectations for his or her return to activity
    C. The severity of the athlete's disability
    D. The length of the rehabilitation program
    E. The athlete's position in the sport

130. Upper extremity closed kinetic chain exercises are used primarily for strengthening and improving proprioception of which of the following structures?
    A. Muscles that stabilize the shoulder girdle
    B. Ligaments that stabilize the glenohumeral joint
    C. Tendons that support the joints of the cervical spine, shoulder, and elbow
    D. The articular surfaces of the glenohumeral and acromioclavicular joints
    E. The articular surfaces of the acetabulum and femoral head

131. Hans Selye's phenomenon of the general adaptation syndrome, which occurs when an individual responds to a stressful situation, includes which 3 stages of the stress response?
    A. Fright, flight, exhaustion
    B. The alarm stage, resistance stage, exhaustion
    C. The alarm stage, flight stage, acceptance stage
    D. Anger stage, bargaining stage, acceptance stage
    E. The alarm stage, flight, exhaustion

132. What is the temperature range of an ice bath?
    A. 35°F to 50°F
    B. 70°F to 75°F
    C. 65°F to 70°F
    D. 50°F to 60°F
    E. 60°F to 80°F

133. Which of the following actions may help to decrease skin-electrode resistance when performing an electrotherapy treatment?
    A. Moisten the electrodes with water
    B. Cool the skin first with an ice pack
    C. Place the electrodes on skin that has excessive hair
    D. Use a plastic-meshed cloth electrode
    E. Apply body lotion on the skin

134. Which of the following acoustical interfaces is most reflective of ultrasound energy?
    A. Water–soft tissue
    B. Soft tissue–fat
    C. Soft tissue–bone
    D. Soft tissue–air
    E. None of the above

135. Which of the following electrode placement techniques is most commonly used when treating an individual with "brief-intense" TENS?
    A. Direct placement
    B. Dermatome placement
    C. Stimulation point placement
    D. Continuous placement
    E. Bracket method

136. It is important to set specific short- and long-term goals when developing a treatment program. Goals serve all of the following purposes except:
    A. Insure full reimbursement from a third-party payer
    B. Identify outcomes
    C. Measure the effectiveness of the treatment protocol
    D. Establish timeliness of the treatment program
    E. Allows the athlete to be a part of the treatment

137. When using shortwave diathermy, which of the following objects should not be located within the treatment area?
    A. Towels
    B. Wooden treatment tables (metal-free)
    C. A container of ultrasound gel
    D. Swiss balls and Theraband
    E. Metal stools

138. _____ and _____ are 2 medications that can be combined when utilizing iontophoresis.
    A. Acetic acid, lidocaine
    B. Dexamethasone, lidocaine
    C. Dexamethasone, epinephrine
    D. Hydrocortisone, Medrol
    E. Antibiotic creams, lidocaine

139. How often should an ultrasound unit be calibrated to ensure the safe application of ultrasound?
  A. Every 3 months
  B. Every month
  C. Every other year
  D. Every 5 years
  E. At least once per year

140. A patient presents to the athletic training facility complaining of a "sore spot" on the back of his neck. It appears as a dark red, hard area, which later develops as a lesion discharging yellowish-red pus from numerous areas. The athletic trainer suspects the patient has what type of infection?
  A. Viral
  B. Fungal
  C. Systemic
  D. Parasitic
  E. Bacterial

141. Herpes simplex labialis is caused by which of the following?
  A. Virus
  B. Fungus
  C. Bacteria
  D. Parasite
  E. None of the above

142. Pediculosis is most effectively treated with which of the following?
  A. Mouthwash
  B. An antibiotic
  C. Time
  D. An antifungal
  E. A parasiticide

143. Which of the following may occur as a result of a puncture wound that has not been properly treated?
  A. A tetanus infection
  B. A streptococcus infection
  C. A spirochete infection
  D. A staphylococcus infection
  E. Dissemination of the wound

144. How quickly may the adaptations in skeletal muscle reverse if strength training is discontinued or interrupted during rehabilitation?
  A. 24 hours
  B. 36 hours
  C. 48 hours
  D. 1 week
  E. 4 weeks

145. Circuit training is an effective training technique if the athletic trainer desires to improve _____ and _____.
  A. Agility, endurance
  B. Strength, flexibility
  C. Agility, proprioception
  D. Power, endurance
  E. Strength, power

146. The athletic trainer should look for all of the following features when purchasing a stationary bicycle except:
  A. A comfortable seat
  B. An easily modified workload
  C. Good construction
  D. An on-board computer for easy programming
  E. Adjustable to fit all athletes

147. All of the following are contraindications for the use of aquatic therapy except:
  A. An excessive fear of the water
  B. An open wound
  C. An athlete who is unable to tread water
  D. Urinary tract infection
  E. A skin infection

148. Which of the following medications is not a medication that could predispose an athlete to heat illness?
  A. Decongestants
  B. Antihistamines
  C. Diuretics
  D. NSAIDs
  E. Beta-adrenergic blockers

149. How long does it take for a patient's heartrate to plateau at a given level during a cardiorespiratory training session?
  A. 10 minutes
  B. 30 seconds
  C. 45 seconds
  D. 5 minutes
  E. 2 to 3 minutes

150. What is the efferent response to sensory information called?
  A. Kinesthesia
  B. Neuromuscular control
  C. Proprioception
  D. Coordination
  E. Parathesia

151. What type of fracture fails to heal spontaneously within a normal time frame?
    A. Malunion
    B. Oblique
    C. Osteogenesis
    D. Nonunion
    E. Spiral

152. Which is not a thermal effect of ultrasound?
    A. Increased blood flow
    B. Secretion of chemotactics
    C. Reduction of muscle spasm
    D. Edema reduction
    E. Muscular heating

153. Which of the following modalities results in the movement of ions into the body through the use of an electrical current?
    A. Iontophoresis
    B. Pulsed diathermy
    C. Phonophoresis
    D. Direct coupling
    E. Ultrasound

154. _____ is a method of massage that involves the lifting and kneading of the skin, subcutaneous tissue, and muscle with the fingers or hand.
    A. Friction
    B. Tapotement
    C. Effleurage
    D. Rolfing
    E. Pétrissage

155. Which of the following is a cardinal sign of inflammation?
    A. Cyanosis
    B. Loss of function
    C. Cold skin
    D. Numbness
    E. None of the above

156. What is a vascular reaction to cold that results in a white, red, or blue discoloration of the extremities?
    A. Neurapraxia
    B. Analgesia
    C. Raynaud's phenomenon
    D. Hypothermia
    E. Cyanosis

157. All of the following are indications for the use of a warm whirlpool except:
    A. Cleaning large, open wounds
    B. Relieving pain
    C. Initial edema reduction
    D. Increasing range of motion
    E. Reflexation

158. The most common form of hyperthyroidism identified by tremors, weakness, difficulty in swallowing/speaking, and facial/eye tics is known as:
    A. Graves' disease
    B. Legg-Calvé-Perthes disease
    C. Paget's disease
    D. Reye's syndrome
    E. Sarcoidosis

159. What is air hunger marked by labored or difficult breathing called?
    A. Dysuria
    B. Dystrophy
    C. Diaphoresis
    D. Dysphagia
    E. Dyspnea

160. A stretch injury to a nerve resulting in transient symptoms of paresthesia and weakness is known as what?
    A. Neurotmesis
    B. Neurapraxia
    C. Neurofibromatosis
    D. Nerve gliding
    E. Myopraxia

161. All of the following muscles form the pes anserinus muscle group except:
    A. Semimembranosus
    B. Semitendinosus
    C. Gracilis
    D. Sartorius
    E. B and D

162. What is the internal reaction or resistance of tissue to an external load called?
    A. Mechanical failure
    B. Strain
    C. Stress
    D. Yield point
    E. Threshold

163. An involuntary muscle contraction characterized by alternate contraction and relaxation in rapid succession is known as which of the following?
    A. Tonic contraction
    B. Alternating contraction
    C. Eccentric contraction
    D. Clonic contraction
    E. Phasic contraction

164. Which of the following is a term that refers to a group of techniques used for the purpose of relieving soft tissue from the abnormal grip of tight fascia?
    A. Glides
    B. Traction
    C. Myofascial release
    D. Therapeutic massage
    E. Joint mobilization

165. The rate at which a drug disappears from the body through metabolism, excretion, or both is known as which of the following?
    A. Biotransformation
    B. Half-life
    C. Efficacy
    D. Bioavailability
    E. Expiration rate

166. A type of training that employs a series of stations that consist of various combinations of weight training, flexibility, calisthenics, and brief aerobic exercise is known as which of the following?
    A. Isokinetic training
    B. Circuit training
    C. Plyometrics
    D. Progressive resistance exercises
    E. Specificity training

167. Diaphoresis is also known as which of the following?
    A. Rapid heart beat
    B. Body odor
    C. Bad breath
    D. Slow heart beat
    E. Sweating

168. Joint mechanoreceptors are found in all of the following structures except:
    A. Ligaments
    B. The brain
    C. Menisci
    D. Fat pads
    E. Musculotendinous junction

169. Cognitive function may be affected by all of the following conditions except:
    A. Dehydration
    B. Malnutrition
    C. Abnormal body temperature
    D. Depression
    E. Medication

170. Polydipsia is also known as which of the following?
    A. Excessive urination
    B. Excessive hunger
    C. Excessive blood glucose
    D. Low urine pH
    E. Excessive thirst

171. The progression for strengthening exercises is usually in what order?
    A. Isometric, isokinetic, isotonic, plyometric
    B. Isokinetic, isometric, plyometric, isotonic
    C. Isotonic, plyometric, isokinetic, isometric
    D. Isometric, isotonic, isokinetic, plyometric
    E. Plyometric, isometric, isotonic, isokinetic

172. Isotonic external rotation of the glenohumeral joint during shoulder rehabilitation focuses on what muscles?
    A. Infraspinatus
    B. Teres minor
    C. Posterior deltoid
    D. All of the above
    E. None of the above

173. Injury or disease of the pancreas creates pain in which quadrant of the abdomen?
    A. Lower right
    B. Upper right
    C. Upper left
    D. Lower left
    E. Central

174. Where is a Morton's neuroma most commonly located?
    A. Between the first and second metacarpals
    B. Between the third and fourth metatarsals
    C. Between the second and third metacarpals
    D. Between the second and third metatarsals
    E. Plantar surface of the heel

175. An excessive valgus force to the knee may result in an injury to which ligament?
    A. Lateral collateral ligament
    B. Medial collateral ligament
    C. Anterior cruciate ligament
    D. Posterior cruciate ligament
    E. Arcuate ligament

176. The female athletic triad describes the simultaneous presence of which of the following?
    A. An eating disorder, amenorrhea, and osteoporosis
    B. Depression, premenstrual syndrome, and osteoporosis
    C. A medial collateral and anterior cruciate ligament sprain with meniscus tear
    D. Menstrual cramping, overeating, and premenstrual syndrome
    E. Dysmenorrhea, eating disorder, and osteoporosis

177. All of the following are tests for glenohumeral instability except:
    A. Clunk test
    B. Anterior apprehension
    C. Anterior glide
    D. Load and shift
    E. Neer's test

178. Which of the following involves the use of ice or a cold spray before performing a stretch?
    A. Cryokinetics
    B. Cryostretch
    C. Cold therapy stretching
    D. Dynamic stretching
    E. Cryogenics

179. Indications for ultrasound include all of the following except:
    A. Bursitis
    B. Fasciitis
    C. Acute hemorrhage
    D. Plantar warts
    E. Tendinitis

180. Which of the following are braces used after rehabilitation?
    A. Functional
    B. Prophylactic
    C. Patellofemoral
    D. Rehabilitative
    E. Postoperative

181. _____ is a type of electrotherapy used to re-educate muscle.
    A. Interferential
    B. Russian
    C. Iontophoresis
    D. Premodulated
    E. Low intensity

182. What is a protective spasm of the muscular abdominal wall called?
    A. Gas pains
    B. Rigidity
    C. Myositis
    D. Splinting
    E. Very painful

183. What does the production of black, tar-like stools indicate?
    A. Upper gastrointestinal bleeding
    B. Infection
    C. Lower gastrointestinal bleeding
    D. A diet that is too high in iron
    E. Colon cancer

184. Which of the following devices is more effective in decreasing skin temperature during a cryotherapy treatment?
    A. A microwaveable pack
    B. A chemical spray
    C. A cold towel
    D. An ice pack
    E. A fan

185. A dry, nonproductive cough is most often caused by which of the following?
    A. Lung infection
    B. Bronchitis
    C. Allergies
    D. Pneumothorax
    E. Cancer

186. A dynamic program of prescribed exercise for preventing or reversing the destructive effects of inactivity while returning an individual to his or her former level of competition is known as what?
    A. Pilates
    B. Rehabilitation
    C. A DAPRE program
    D. Cardiovascular program
    E. Yoga

187. What is an upward force experienced by a body in a fluid that acts in the opposite direction of gravity and is responsible for the feeling of weightlessness in water?
    A. Specific gravity
    B. Viscosity
    C. Hydrostatic pressure
    D. Buoyancy
    E. None of the above

188. Electrical stimulating currents are classified into 3 categories. Which of the following is not one of these categories?
    A. Interferential current
    B. Direct current
    C. Pulsed current
    D. Alternating current
    E. Galvanic current

189. All of the following are contraindications for electrical stimulation electrode placement except:
    A. Stimulation across the heart
    B. Stimulation over an acute thrombophlebitis
    C. Control of labor pain by stimulation of the lower back
    D. Stimulation over the temples
    E. Directly over the spine

190. "Like charges repel while unlike charges attract each other." This is known as what law?
    A. Ohm's
    B. Coulomb's
    C. Murphy's
    D. Wolff's
    E. Horner's

191. All of the following are indications of ice massage application except:
    A. Subacute injuries
    B. Contusions
    C. Anesthetized skin
    D. Muscle spasm
    E. Overuse injuries

192. Which of the following types of electrical stimulators is considered "subsensory"?
    A. Interferential stimulator
    B. Low-intensity stimulator
    C. TENS
    D. Diathermy
    E. High-intensity stimulator

193. Which of the following is defined as an uninterrupted direct current?
    A. Interferential current
    B. Microcurrent
    C. Galvanic current
    D. Pulsed current
    E. None of the above

194. The amount of power generated by an ultrasound unit is defined as what?
    A. Frequency
    B. Duty cycle
    C. Duration
    D. Intensity
    E. An ohm

195. When using fluidotherapy, the treatment temperature range is normally set at which of the following temperatures?
    A. 60°F to 70°F
    B. 85°F to 100°F
    C. 100°F to 113°F
    D. 75°F to 96°F
    E. 40°F to 60°F

196. The D2 flexion pattern of the hip works which group of muscles?
    A. Abductors, flexors, internal rotators
    B. Abductors, flexors, external rotators
    C. Adductors, flexors, internal rotators
    D. Adductors, extensors, external rotators
    E. The abductors and flexors only

197. Strengthening of which muscle is vital in the throwing athlete?
    A. Lower trapezius
    B. Pectineus
    C. Serratus posterior
    D. Obliques
    E. Rhomboids

198. Treatment for facet dysfunction consists of all of the following except:
    A. Facet joint mobilization
    B. Passive rotation
    C. Pelvic rock exercises
    D. McKenzie extension exercises
    E. Abdominal strengthening

199. Which muscle does not need to be strengthened after a rotator cuff repair?
    A. Supraspinatus
    B. Biceps
    C. Teres minor
    D. Sternocleidomastoid
    E. Triceps

200. When a muscle is stretched to a point where a mild discomfort is felt and the limb is held in one position, it is known as what type of stretch?
    A. Ballistic
    B. PNF
    C. Static
    D. Dynamic
    E. None of the above

201. What is a form of exercise that helps develop eccentric control during dynamic movements?
    A. Isometric
    B. PNF
    C. Hydraulic training
    D. Isokinetics
    E. Plyometric

202. A patient presents with an acute injury of the foot and has an antalgic gait pattern. Which of the following should you do first?
    A. Have the patient run half speed on a treadmill for cardiorespiratory health
    B. Give the patient crutches
    C. Instruct the patient in a heel-to-toe gait pattern
    D. Observe/palpate the injured area for gross deformity and point tenderness
    E. Have the patient wear an open toe shoe

203. The athletic trainer should perform which of the following tests for posterior cruciate ligament laxity?
    A. Apley distraction test
    B. Jerk test
    C. Apley compression test
    D. Pivot shift test
    E. Posterior drawer test

204. When palpating the knee joint after an injury, the athletic trainer should be sure to palpate which of the following structures?
    A. Anterior superior iliac spine
    B. The navicular
    C. Medial condyle of the femur
    D. The tibial crest
    E. Dorsalis pedis

205. A patient presents with insidious pain along the posterior aspect of the thigh. Which of the following steps should be performed first by the athletic trainer?
    A. Palpate the muscle bellies of the posterior thigh
    B. Ask how and when the pain started
    C. Manual muscle test the hamstring muscles
    D. Perform a functional test
    E. Assess sensation of the hip

206. Articular cartilage has limited ability to heal because of which of the following reasons?
    A. Constant movement of the joint does not allow for healing
    B. Cartilage has limited or no direct blood supply
    C. The high incidence of aseptic necrosis
    D. Poor results with NSAID treatment
    E. None of the above

207. Which of the following is the least occurring type of shoulder subluxation/dislocation?
    A. Superior
    B. Inferior
    C. Anterior
    D. Posterior
    E. C and D

208. Treatment of "snapping hip" syndrome includes all of the following except:
    A. Ice and NSAIDs
    B. Biomechanical correction
    C. Flexibility exercises
    D. Excision of the greater tuberosity in severe cases
    E. Instruction in proper training techniques

209. Treatment for cystic fibrosis includes which of the following?
    A. Nutritional counseling/modification, pulmonary therapies to clear secretions, antibiotics
    B. Regular exercise, nutritional counseling/modifications, expectorants
    C. Bed rest, daily suction to clear secretions, antihistamines
    D. Bed rest, daily suction to clear secretions, antibiotics and expectorants
    E. Bronchodilators, antihistamines and expectorants

210. Which of the following modalities should be used sparingly, if at all, with a patient who has been diagnosed with multiple sclerosis?
    A. Cold whirlpool
    B. Interferential current
    C. TENS
    D. Ice packs
    E. Moist heat packs

211. Although no cure exists for myasthenia gravis, medical treatment to minimize the symptoms include which of the following?
    A. Medications that act on the neuromuscular junction
    B. Cold laser
    C. Skeletal muscle relaxants
    D. Radiation
    E. Antipyretic drugs

212. What types of medications are most commonly used in the treatment of epilepsy?
    A. Tranquilizers and sedatives
    B. COX-2 inhibitors
    C. Beta-blockers
    D. Vasopressors
    E. Psychogenic drugs

213. Which of the following is the only NSAID used topically in the United States?
    A. Salicylate
    B. Ibuprofen
    C. Meloxicam
    D. Celebrex
    E. Naproxen NA

214. The term dexamethasone is the _____ name of this medication
    A. Secondary
    B. Brand
    C. Generic
    D. FDA approved
    E. Trade

215. Which of the following pairs are chemically identical?
    A. Diazepam, Skelaxin
    B. Cimetidine, Tagamet
    C. Triacetin, Tinactin
    D. Tetracaine, Lanacane
    E. Ibuprofen, Naprosyn

216. Which of the following is the trade or brand name of the drug hydrocodone?
    A. Darvocet-N 100
    B. Percocet
    C. Demerol
    D. Codeine
    E. Vicodin

217. Which of the following is a common adverse effect of an opioid analgesic?
    A. Constipation
    B. Headache
    C. Stomach upset
    D. Diarrhea
    E. Anxiety

218. The "half-life" of a drug refers to which of the following?
    A. The amount of time it takes for a drug to lose half its potency while it is in storage
    B. Half the amount of time it takes for a drug to reach its therapeutic level in the bloodstream
    C. The time required for the amount of the drug in the blood to be increased by one-half
    D. The time required for half the therapeutic drug level to be excreted in the urine
    E. The time required for the amount of drug in the blood to be reduced by one-half

219. All of the following are routes of drug administration except:
    A. Oral
    B. Topical
    C. Parenteral
    D. Sublingual
    E. Pressurization

220. When rehabilitating an athlete, goal setting influences performance by increasing confidence levels and reducing anxiety. Which of the following is not a specific type of goal that is found in the goal-setting literature?
    A. Subjective goals
    B. General objective outcome goals
    C. Specific objective/performance goals
    D. Process goals
    E. Reward-based goals

221. Which of the following medications has antipyretic properties?
    A. Tylenol
    B. Aspirin
    C. Benadryl
    D. Codeine
    E. A and B

222. Which of the following proton pump inhibitors is an over-the-counter medication?
    A. Nexium
    B. Prilosec
    C. Prevacid
    D. Protonix
    E. Aciphex

223. At what concentrations is topical hydrocortisone available over the counter?
    A. 1% and 5%
    B. 0.25% and 1%
    C. 1.5% and 2%
    D. 10% and 15%
    E. 2% and 5%

224. The use of a reusable cold pack may significantly increase the possibility of frostbite because of which of the following?
    A. The chemicals in the packs are caustic to the skin
    B. Wet toweling significantly drops the skin temperature
    C. Reusable cold packs cause anesthesia after 10 minutes
    D. It decreases the cellular metabolic rate
    E. It may lower the skin temperature below the freezing point

225. Although ice bags are the most commonly used modality in the treatment of acute injuries, a drawback of this modality may be which of the following?
    A. They leak easily
    B. They take longer to cool the skin than reusable ice packs
    C. Ice machines are expensive and their cost may be too prohibitive
    D. Ice takes a long time to make on a regular basis
    E. Ice machines tend to be unreliable

226. Massage can be used as an effective modality to control pain because it activates which of the following?
    A. Central nervous system and chemosensitive receptors
    B. Parasympathetic nervous system and mechanosensitive receptors
    C. Parasympathetic nervous system and the pacinian receptors
    D. Autonomic nervous system and the pacinian receptors
    E. Autonomic nervous system and chemosensitive receptors

227. Contraindications for joint mobilization include all of the following except:
    A. Acute inflammation
    B. Osteoporosis
    C. Malignancy
    D. Infection
    E. Joint hypomobility

228. During rehabilitation, closed-chain exercises are recommended because they do all of the following except:
    A. Stimulate proprioceptors
    B. Increase joint stability
    C. Isolate a specific muscle group for strengthening
    D. Reduce shear forces
    E. Increase muscle co-contraction

229. "Rehabilitation" includes all of the following components except:
    A. Assessment of level of function/dysfunction
    B. Organization and interpretation of results of the initial evaluation
    C. Formulation of patient problems
    D. Establishment of long- and short-term goals
    E. Diagnosis of the patient's condition

230. High-voltage pulsed stimulation may be used as an adjunct treatment in controlling acute and chronic pain through which 2 mechanisms?
    A. Gate control and opiate release mechanisms
    B. Gate control and histamine release mechanisms
    C. Analgesia production and counterirritation
    D. Edema control and spasm reduction
    E. Stimulation of both motor and sensory nerves

231. When using massage to reduce edema in an extremity, the athletic trainer should begin the technique _____ and move _____.
    A. Medially, laterally
    B. Proximally, distally
    C. Distally, proximally
    D. Deeply, superficially
    E. Superficially, deeply

232. The condition intertrigo is treated by which of the following?
    A. Application of a topical astringent
    B. Application of a topical antibiotic
    C. There is no known treatment for intertrigo
    D. Application of a warm compress
    E. Application of a cold compress, cleaning the area with mild soap and water, followed by the application of a soothing ointment

233. When using ultrasound under water, a rubber-type basin should be used. Which of the following is the reason this technique should not be performed in a metal basin or whirlpool?
    A. Cavitation may occur
    B. The ultrasound transmission is significantly increased
    C. Minerals in the water block the transmission of the ultrasound energy
    D. Ultrasound energy is reflected off metal and may damage the transducer head
    E. Ultrasound energy is reflected off metal, increasing the intensity in various areas near the metal

Organizational and Professional Health and Well-Being

1. All of the following forms are critical parts of the patient's permanent medical record and should be completed before the patient is permitted to participate in the first team practice except:
    A. Permission-to-treat form
    B. Preparticipation physical examination form
    C. Release form for patients subjected to high risk
    D. Coach's injury report form
    E. Medical history form

2. How would you define a policy?
    A. A specific plan for members of an organization to follow
    B. A broad statement of an intended action
    C. An organizational plan that provides program direction for 1 or 2 years
    D. A mission statement of an organization
    E. A vision statement of an organization

3. What general topics should be addressed in an athletic training program policies and procedures manual?
    A. Who the athletic training program will serve
    B. Facility use and maintenance
    C. Risk management plans
    D. Chains of command and supervision
    E. All of the above

4. Maintaining up-to-date records is extremely important. How often should the athletic trainer document?
    A. Monthly
    B. Weekly
    C. Daily
    D. Every 6 months
    E. Every 2 weeks

5. An athletic trainer can release a patient's medical records to which of the following?
    A. Professional athletic team organizations
    B. Insurance companies
    C. The media
    D. No organization or individual without the consent of the patient or legal guardian
    E. B and C

6. A high school athlete is pitching during a baseball game and is hit in the head with a line drive. He is seriously injured. The assistant coach is also the athlete's father. In this situation, who is legally responsible for the athlete's immediate care?
    A. The head coach
    B. The assistant coach/parent
    C. The athletic trainer
    D. The high school at which the event is taking place
    E. All of the above

7. _____ is a form of record keeping that allows the athletic trainer to list the athlete's injury information, the actions taken by the athletic trainer, and the response of the athlete to the athletic trainer's treatment in column form.
    A. SOAP notes
    B. Focus charting
    C. Charting by exception
    D. Computerized documentation
    E. WOTS UP

8. You have been given the opportunity to assist in hiring a new team physician. What type of agreement should be drawn up between the school and the physician?
    A. School emergency systems agreement
    B. A noncompete agreement
    C. A medical consent agreement
    D. A physician's letter of agreement
    E. Liability contract agreement

9. Which of the following best describes an athletic trainer in a nontraditional athletic training setting?
    A. Controller
    B. Organizer
    C. Director
    D. Planner
    E. Manager

10. What guidelines does the athletic trainer have to follow regarding maintaining proper hygiene and sanitation in the athletic training facility?
    A. JCAHO
    B. AMA
    C. CARF
    D. OSHA
    E. CAATE

11. Which of the following organizations establishes standards of quality for organizations that provide rehabilitative services?
    A. TJC
    B. AMA
    C. APTA
    D. OSHA
    E. CARF

12. All of the following are components of a well-written SOAP note except:
    A. It is legible, clear, and concise
    B. It contains many objective measurements
    C. Progress is expressed in functional terms
    D. It is written with the intent to mislead an insurance company
    E. It describes a clear plan of treatment

13. Which of the following documents would be most likely subpoenaed during a civil litigation suit against an athletic trainer?
    A. Equipment inventory
    B. Treatment log
    C. Budget reports
    D. Sporting event schedules
    E. Proof of athletic trainer credentials and certifications

14. Fixed payments made on a monthly basis to a managed care provider are known as what type of reimbursement?
    A. Point-of-service plan
    B. Fee for service
    C. Third-party reimbursement
    D. Capitation
    E. Managed care option

15. Which of the following forms should the athletic trainer fill out to gain the quickest reimbursement from an insurance company?
    A. HCFA-1500 form
    B. CPT 1-A form
    C. UCR form
    D. An incident report form
    E. None of the above

16. The athletic trainer may use any of the following to treat an injured or ill patient except:
    A. Prescription drug
    B. Hydrotherapy
    C. Cryotherapy
    D. Electrotherapy
    E. Massage

17. Maintaining accurate medical records is the responsibility of which of the following individuals in the high school setting?
    I. Athletic trainer
    II. Athletic director
    III. Principal
    IV. School nurse
    V. Team physician
    A. I, II, III
    B. II, IV, V
    C. III, IV, V
    D. I, IV, V
    E. All of the above

18. What type of analysis would be considered a useful tool in the strategic planning of an existing athletic training program?
    A. The HCFA analysis
    B. The strengths/weaknesses analysis
    C. The WOTS UP analysis
    D. The Samson analysis
    E. Flow chart analysis

19. What is the primary care physician who is appointed by an insurance company to oversee the medical care given to a patient and assigns any specialty and ancillary services called?
    A. The gatekeeper
    B. The participating provider
    C. The third-party administrator
    D. The policyholder
    E. None of the above

20. The _____ is a charge that represents the maximum amount that an insurance company will pay a provider.
    A. HCFA
    B. NCR
    C. ADA
    D. CPT
    E. UCR

21. The _____ is a nongovernmental, nonprofit organization that gathers injury data from a number of sources including educational institutions.
    A. NSC
    B. NOCSAE
    C. ACSM
    D. OSHA
    E. ISS

22. Which organization must certify facemasks that are used in ice hockey helmets?
    A. CSA
    B. HECC
    C. NOCSAE
    D. ASTM
    E. NCAA

23. _____ supplies include such items as adhesive tape, gauze pads, and bandages.
    A. Permanent
    B. Capital
    C. Nonexpendable
    D. Nonfixed
    E. Expendable

24. _____, _____, and _____ must be taken into consideration when developing a risk management plan.
    A. Security, liability, competence
    B. Security, fire safety, management of emergency injuries
    C. Insurance procedures, policies/procedures, materials
    D. Licensing, certifications, administrative policy
    E. Employees, liability, security

25. Large purchases for an educational institution are usually done through a process known as what?
    A. Direct purchase
    B. Indirect purchase
    C. Soliciting
    D. Bid process
    E. None of the above

26. Which of the following best describes a copayment?
    A. An occasional payment made by a policyholder to an insurance company
    B. The amount owed yearly by the policyholder before the insurance company will begin to pay for services
    C. The amount of money that both an employee and employer share when paying for medical benefits
    D. A percentage of the total amount the policyholder is required to pay for medical services rendered
    E. The amount of money that a provider offers as a discount for services

27. You are in the position to hire an assistant athletic trainer. You have a specific person in mind, but your athletic director implies he is not comfortable with this person's gender. Which level of the law mandates the hiring and firing of employees?
    A. State
    B. Local
    C. City
    D. District
    E. Federal

28. Which piece of information is not part of the athletic trainer's daily documentation?
    A. Treatment technique
    B. Playing status
    C. Daily injury log
    D. Patient's insurance information
    E. Rehabilitation progression

29. All of the following are important steps in avoiding legal problems when administering care to the patient except:
    A. Keeping accurate records
    B. Staying familiar with the health history of the patient
    C. Following orders of the team physician
    D. Allowing the coach to decide when the patient should return to play after injury
    E. B and C

30. Which of the following is not a responsibility of the athletic trainer?
    A. Counsel and advise the athlete about health care
    B. Diagnose and treat illnesses
    C. Administer first aid as necessary
    D. Supervise proper equipment fitting
    E. Organize and set up preparticipation physical exams

31. Which of the following is not characteristic of a managed care organization?
    A. They require provider accountability
    B. They promote the use of a physician as a gatekeeper
    C. They are based on a fee-for-service model
    D. They utilize various strategies
    E. They utilize specific providers

32. All of the following are reasons why an insurance claim might be denied except:
    A. Lack of patient progress
    B. The duration of care is considered excessive
    C. Improper coding
    D. The goals are based on functional outcomes
    E. Treating beyond the approved number of visits

33. What is the series of codes used by insurance agencies and providers alike to identify a patient's diagnosis for reimbursement purposes called?
    A. International Classification of Diseases or ICD-10 codes
    B. Interclinician Codes of Diagnoses or ICD-5 codes
    C. Third-party payer codes
    D. International Procedure and Diagnoses or IPD-10 codes
    E. None of the above

34. All of the following are reasons why good documentation skills are an absolute necessity for the athletic trainer except:
    A. To protect the legal rights of the patient and athletic trainer
    B. To improve the communication between the athletic trainer and other health care providers
    C. To enhance the care given by the athletic trainer and to determine when release from the athletic trainer's immediate care is appropriate
    D. To improve the athletic trainer's position for financial gain through reimbursement by the insurance company
    E. To keep an accurate log of treatment as a means of evaluating successful outcomes

35. You are part of a planning committee that has been given the responsibility of designing the new athletic training facility at your school. You have been through the initial process of conducting a needs assessment and selecting an architect/contractor. You now are meeting with the architect to begin the development of the schematic drawings that will be submitted for approval. _____ and _____ are 2 major elements that must be addressed in these schematic drawings.
    A. Plumbing, electrical layouts
    B. Space needs, traffic patterns
    C. Field access, escape routes
    D. Aesthetics, large equipment positioning
    E. Color, furniture location

36. When acquiring capital equipment for your athletic training facility, a decision must be made regarding leasing or purchasing the equipment. What might be a possible advantage in leasing the equipment?
    A. Less risk that the equipment will become obsolete
    B. Lower overall cost
    C. Outright ownership of the equipment
    D. Purchased equipment has little resale value
    E. All of the above

37. As the director of a free-standing sports medicine clinic, it is important to keep accurate records of an employee's personnel record. All of the following should be included in this file except:
    A. Performance evaluation records
    B. Salary and promotion records
    C. Time-off request sheets
    D. Employee contracts
    E. B and D

38. In athletic training, database software has been primarily used to perform what function?
    A. Write letters and produce forms
    B. Perform simple calculations and integrate text with graphics
    C. Store and retrieve information regarding athletic injury and treatment
    D. Merge lists and develop spreadsheets
    E. All of the above

39. Which of the following describes an insurance "rider?"
    A. A supplementary clause to an insurance contract that covers the cost of conditions that extend beyond those associated with the standard policy
    B. The usual fee charged by a health care provider for a particular service
    C. A policy that pays for medical expenses only after all of the athlete's other medical insurance policies have reached their limit
    D. A universally accepted insurance claim form used by hospitals
    E. None of the above

40. All of the following are methods of enhancing a budget plan except:
    A. Keep an accurate inventory on all disposable and nondisposable supplies
    B. Figure out how much of your disposable supplies have been used and estimate how much more will be needed to finish out the fiscal year
    C. Consult with a certified public accountant or professional financial advisor and follow his or her direction regarding the development of a budget plan
    D. Consult with several vendors to get an estimate of how much prices will rise in the upcoming year
    E. Determine how many athletes will be receiving care

41. When developing an emergency plan, all of the following should be established except:
    A. The athletic trainer and coaches should have the appropriate keys to important gates and locks
    B. There should be a phone accessible for immediate use
    C. The athletic trainer should be familiar with the community emergency medical system
    D. Making sure there is a student athletic trainer available to accompany an injured athlete to the hospital if necessary
    E. A and C

42. Which of the following is a prudent action that the athletic trainer should take prior to an emergency arising?
    A. The athletic trainer should arrange a meeting between him- or herself, the local rescue squad, team physician, and any other individual involved in handling an injured athlete at least once per year to establish and practice procedures that will be used in the event of an emergency
    B. Make sure all of the golf carts are fully charged and ready to roll
    C. Make sure the athletic director and school nurse are on campus
    D. Know all of the emergency routes of the campus and have directions to the nearest hospital
    E. B and D

43. Which of the following is the biggest budgetary obstacle that many high school athletic trainers must face?
    A. Lack of a room and special facilities/equipment necessary to operate an adequate athletic training program
    B. Lack of athletic tape and wraps, athletic training kits, and a table
    C. Location of the athletic training facility
    D. Lack of an athletic training student program, which would provide the certified athletic trainer with free help
    E. Lack of a budget plan

44. There are different models of supervision that may be used by a head athletic trainer when managing an athletic training staff. Two of these models are known as _____ and _____ supervision.
    A. Monarchical, sovereign
    B. Clinical, directional
    C. Transitional, directional
    D. Inspection-production, administrative
    E. Clinical, developmental

45. Which of the following is not one of the 3 phases of the needs assessment as it is related to budget planning?
    A. Exploration
    B. Information gathering
    C. Negotiation
    D. Decision making
    E. A and B

46. What is the process in which health care practitioners are reimbursed by a policyholder's insurance?
    A. Primary-party reimbursement
    B. Secondary-party reimbursement
    C. Third-party reimbursement
    D. Tertiary-party reimbursement
    E. Direct reimbursement

47. Which of the following is a growing concept in the insurance industry stressing cost control through coordination of medical services?
    A. A primary care provider
    B. Health maintenance organization
    C. Exclusive provider organization
    D. Preferred provider organization
    E. Managed care

48. Which of the following is not an error when planning the design of a sports medicine facility?
    A. Concentrating on function rather than style
    B. The use of wood for the main flooring material
    C. Having the adaptive access on the other side of the building
    D. Non-ground fault interrupter receptacles placed within the hydrotherapy area
    E. Having only one entrance and exit

49. Which of the following is not a type of insurance policy that is offered to organizations seeking to purchase insurance for athletic teams?
    A. Accident insurance
    B. Indemnity policy
    C. Basic medical coverage
    D. Group insurance
    E. Capitation

50. What is one of the most important steps an athletic trainer needs to take when starting a new high school athletic training program?
    A. Make an emergency plan
    B. Make sure there is enough tape and first-aid kits
    C. Have uniforms made for the athletic training staff so they may be identified by the coaches
    D. Meet with the school's booster clubs to begin fundraising
    E. Network with local physical therapists

51. Which of the following is a priority when developing a sports medicine center for the local community?
    A. An area for massage therapy
    B. A mission statement
    C. An open house
    D. An educational seminar for coaches
    E. All of the above

52. The codes that were established by the AMA for health care providers to receive third-party reimbursement are CPT codes. What does CPT mean?
    A. Current Procedural Treatments
    B. Current Provider Terminology
    C. Consensus Procedural Treatments
    D. Current Provider Treatments
    E. Current Procedural Terminology

53. What is a type of organizational culture characterized by autonomy in decision making and problem solving?
    A. Organizational culture
    B. Collegial culture
    C. Personalistic culture
    D. Informal culture
    E. Independent culture

54. All of the following are basic steps in the purchasing process except:
    A. Request a quotation
    B. Negotiation
    C. Purchase order
    D. Bid requests
    E. Quality control

55. An ICD-10 code identifies which of the following?
    A. The cost of a medical procedure
    B. Who the provider is
    C. The prognosis of the injury
    D. A diagnosis
    E. A treatment procedure

56. When developing preparticipation physical examination forms, it is important to make sure all patients have all of the following included in their medical folders except:
    A. Treatment consent form signed by their parents if the patient is 18 years of age or older
    B. History of any previous conditions documented
    C. Documentation of medications being taken
    D. Assumption-of-risk forms
    E. C and D

57. Who should be involved in making the decisions about transporting an injured athlete?
    A. Athletic trainer
    B. Team physician
    C. Paramedics
    D. Emergency medical technicians
    E. All of the above

58. What is the state law that gives an individual the length of time (in years) to file a claim?
    A. Foreseeable harm
    B. Liability negligence
    C. Statute of limitations
    D. Tort
    E. Statute of suitability

59. If a patient who is covered by an HMO insurance policy needs to see a specialist, who must make the referral in most cases?
    A. Athletic trainer
    B. Specialist
    C. Primary care physician
    D. Patient
    E. None of the above

60. According to program management theory, which of the following is defined as a decision-making process in which a course of action is determined in order to bring about a future state of affairs?
    A. Vision statement
    B. Mission statement
    C. Planning
    D. Program evaluation
    E. Implementation evaluation

61. Which of the following describes a person or organization that supports a program but has a history of untrusting behavior (these people tend to be manipulative in their dealings)?
    A. Opponents
    B. Challengers
    C. Allies
    D. Adversaries
    E. Bedfellows

62. The process by which something is done in a sports medicine program is defined as a(n) _____ .
    A. Procedure
    B. Policy
    C. Agreement
    D. Chain of command
    E. Protocol

63. What are cost-based providers contracted by the federal government and charged with reviewing Medicare claims made by hospitals called?
    A. An intermediary
    B. An insurance "carrier"
    C. A joint review board
    D. An insurance network
    E. Business manager

64. What is the potential to influence the behavior of a superior called?
    A. Superior power
    B. Position power
    C. Counter power
    D. Subordination power
    E. Personal power

65. Which of the following is not a type of budget?
    A. Fixed budgeting
    B. Variable budgeting
    C. Laissez-faire budgeting
    D. Lump-sum budgeting
    E. Line-item budgeting

66. Primary coverage is defined as which of the following?
    A. "Self-pay" insurance
    B. A coverage that begins to pay for covered expenses after the deductible has been met
    C. Protection for an individual against future loss of earnings because of injury
    D. The invoiced cost of an insurance policy
    E. Third-party payment

67. Medical records are defined as which of the following?
    A. Cumulative documentation of a person's medical history and health care interventions
    B. Widely accepted principles that are intended to guide the professional activities of the health care practitioner
    C. The act of recording health care assessments or treatment on cassette tapes or directly into a computer for later transcription
    D. A method of recording details of an athlete's assessment and treatment using a detailed prose-based format
    E. All of the above

68. Which of the following is not part of a SOAP note?
    A. Subjective information
    B. Objective information
    C. Assessment
    D. Participation level
    E. Plan

69. All of the following are ways athletic trainers can help keep insurance premiums to a minimum except:
    A. Insist that the athletes purchase their own personal insurance
    B. Adopt and communicate policies that increase the institution's financial obligations to those injuries that are covered by the school's insurance policy
    C. Spread the risk among all concerned parties
    D. Pass the cost or some fraction of the cost to the athlete
    E. Have the team physician see athletes in the athletic training facility

70. Which of the following is a contract between a policyholder and an insurance company to reimburse a percentage of the cost of the policyholder's medical bills?
    A. An insurance claim
    B. Point-of-service insurance
    C. A promissory note
    D. Medical insurance
    E. Treatment agreement

71. All of the following are exceptions to the rule of confidentiality except:
    A. When the media desires information regarding the athlete's health status
    B. When there is clear and imminent danger to the athlete
    C. When there is clear and imminent danger to other persons
    D. When legal requirements demand that confidential information be released
    E. C and D

72. Athletic training equipment can be either leased or bought. Which of the following is an advantage to leasing equipment?
    A. Higher overall cost
    B. No ownership
    C. Lower initial cost
    D. Higher effective interest rate than traditional financing
    E. None of the above

73. Which of the following is a type of organizational culture characterized by consensus, teamwork, and participatory decision making?
    A. Transformational
    B. Personalistic
    C. Formulistic
    D. Organizational
    E. Collegial

74. Which of the following is the most common order for steps in recruiting and hiring sports medicine personnel?
    A. Request for position, application collection, position request approval
    B. Application collection, position vacancy notice, offer of contract
    C. Request for position, telephone interviews, hiring
    D. Hiring, offer of contract, request for position
    E. Application collection, interview, request for position

75. Which of the following is a method that allocates a fixed amount of money for an entire program without specifying how the money will be spent?
    A. Lump-sum budgeting
    B. Request for quotation
    C. Lump-sum bidding
    D. Line-item budgeting
    E. Need-based budgeting

76. Which type of budgeting model requires justification for every budget line item without reference to previous spending patterns?
    A. Fixed
    B. Variable
    C. Zero-based
    D. Performance
    E. Need-based

77. What is a type of tort in which an athletic trainer fails to act as a reasonably prudent athletic trainer would act under the same circumstances?
    A. Breach of contract
    B. Omission
    C. Abandonment
    D. Negligence
    E. Foreseeable harm

78. Which of the following standards are performance evaluation standards intended to help foster practicality in the employee appraisal process?
    A. Accuracy standards
    B. Feasibility standards
    C. Utility standards
    D. Proprietary standards
    E. Quality standards

79. You were just given permission to hire a new staff athletic trainer. What order should these components follow when conducting staff selection activities?
    I. Retention
    II. Hiring
    III. Promotion
    IV. Performance evaluation
    V. Demotion
    A. III, V, IV, II, I
    B. II, III, I, IV, V
    C. I, II, III, IV, V
    D. IV, I, V, III, II
    E. I, II, IV, V, III

80. Which one of these is not a step for recruiting and hiring sports medicine personnel?
    A. Placing a position vacancy notice in the NATA Career Center
    B. Interviewing
    C. Creating program goals
    D. Hiring a head athletic trainer
    E. All of the above

81. An "operational plan" is a plan that defines organizational activities in the short-term and should be no longer than which of the following?
    A. 10 years
    B. 15 years
    C. 25 years
    D. 7 years
    E. 2 years

82. The equal employment operating chief works with employees who have filed what type(s) of complaint?
    A. Discrimination
    B. Sexual harassment
    C. Racism
    D. All of the above
    E. None of the above

83. A patient with a disability should not be discriminated against, but he or she must have documentation that supports his or her condition. How can he or she justify the disability?
    A. He or she tells you about the condition
    B. He or she has a record of such impairment with medical documentation
    C. He or she has trouble performing in class or in the sport
    D. All of the above
    E. None of the above

84. You are beginning to lay the foundation for your new athletic training facility at North High School. In order to expedite the process and cut down on the amount of individuals you must deal with, you have decided to use one of the following construction process models. Which of the following uses only one firm to both design and construct the new building?
    A. Lump-sum bidding model
    B. Construction development model
    C. Design/build model
    D. Contractor supply model
    E. None of the above

85. Which of the following would help an athletic trainer determine space needs when planning to build a sports medicine center?
    A. Enlisting the help of a doctor who is in private practice
    B. Developing a traffic pattern chart
    C. Buying the equipment first and then determining space needs
    D. Performing site visits at various gyms to get ideas
    E. All of the above

86. Which of the following methods for funding public sector sports medicine facilities utilizes an institution's assets in cash and investments not normally used for operational purposes?
    A. Capital campaign
    B. Tax-exempt bonds
    C. An endowment
    D. Commercial loans
    E. Unrestricted loans

87. Which of the following is covered in a "rider" in an athletic accident insurance policy?
    A. Acute traumatic injuries
    B. Chronic overuse injuries
    C. Long-term permanent disabilities
    D. All of the above
    E. None of the above

88. What is a deductible?
    A. An out-of-pocket expense before the insurance policy begins paying
    B. The amount of coverage provided by an insurance company
    C. The monthly premium for insurance coverage
    D. The amount of money you will pay for each medical visit
    E. The maximum amount of money the insurance company will pay minus your co-pay

89. What is a type of athletic insurance that pays for covered medical expenses only after all other insurance policies have reached their limits?
    A. Self
    B. Primary coverage
    C. Secondary coverage
    D. Catastrophic
    E. Liability coverage

90. What organization publishes CPT codes on an annual basis?
    A. AMA
    B. NATA
    C. CAATE
    D. BOC
    E. None of the above

91. What would be included in the capital expenses of an athletic training program?
    A. Staff salaries
    B. Equipment under $500
    C. Athletic training supplies
    D. Buildings and room construction
    E. All of the above

92. A properly organized athletic training facility should have separate, designated areas for all of the following except:
    A. Modality area
    B. Hydrotherapy area
    C. Storage facilities
    D. Changing room for the athletes
    E. Physician treatment

93. Which of the following are factors that influence space requirements when designing a sports medicine facility?
    A. Number of clients to be served
    B. Types of clients to be served
    C. Amount and type of equipment needed
    D. Projected growth of the program
    E. All of the above

94. How high should the electrical outlets be placed above the floor in the athletic training facility?
    A. 2 to 3 feet
    B. 4 to 5 feet
    C. 6 feet
    D. 1 to 2 feet
    E. None of the above

95. Which of the following could present a problem for the athletic trainer when using a computer to store medical records?
    A. Maintaining security
    B. Retrieving specific information
    C. Loading files
    D. Using email
    E. All of the above

96. How many hours of evidence-based practice continuing education is a certified athletic trainer required to get every 2 years?
    A. 25
    B. 50
    C. 80
    D. 10
    E. 20

97. The BOC *Standards of Professional Practice* consists of 2 sections. What are the 2 sections?
    A. Code of Ethics and Professional Responsibility
    B. Practice Standards
    C. Code of Professional Responsibility
    D. A and B
    E. B and C

98. Which organization has identified the domains of athletic training as defined by the Role Delineation Study?
    A. AMA
    B. APTA
    C. BOC
    D. NATA Ethics Committee
    E. CAATE

99. Which of the following pieces of information are important for the athletic trainer to keep on record in the athletic training facility?
    A. Injury reports
    B. Injury evaluations and progress notes
    C. Daily treatment logs
    D. All of the above
    E. None of the above

100. Which type of budget allocates a fixed amount of money for specific program functions and activities?
    A. Lump-sum budgeting
    B. Fixed budgeting
    C. Need-based budgeting
    D. Variable budgeting
    E. Line-item budget

101. Which of the following is the most restrictive form of regulation for the profession of athletic training?
    A. Exemption
    B. Certification
    C. Registration
    D. Licensure
    E. Reciprocity

102. To be a successful athletic trainer, an individual must possess all of the following personal qualities except:
    A. The ability to adapt to a changing environment
    B. A good sense of humor
    C. An interest in making money
    D. Empathy
    E. B and D

103. Which of the following best describes the function of the school nurse in the sports medicine program of a high school?
    A. As a liaison between the athletic director and the athletic trainer
    B. The direct supervisor of the "health" services
    C. As the "first assistant" to the team physician
    D. As a liaison between the athletic trainer and the school health services
    E. All of the above

104. Which of the following organizations was established in 1950 and created a code of ethics and standards for the profession of athletic training?
    A. AOSSM
    B. ACSM
    C. APTA
    D. NATA
    E. NASM

105. You find out that a certified athletic trainer in your conference is selling a protein shake to his athletes on a regular basis for personal profit. Which of the following codes is the individual violating?
    A. APTA *Code of Honor*
    B. NASM *Code of Ethics*
    C. NCAA *Code of Honor*
    D. ACSM *Code of Medicine*
    E. NATA *Code of Ethics*

106. When explaining to a parent the difference between an athletic trainer and a physical therapist, the expertise of a physical therapist might best be described by which of the following?
    A. Expertise in the rehabilitation of the handicapped individual
    B. Those health care professionals trained in the rehabilitation of orthopedic injuries
    C. Those individuals trained in the rehabilitation of a diverse population
    D. Expertise in the rehabilitation of athletic, geriatric, and neurologically impaired populations
    E. None of the above

107. Over the past 6 months, you notice one of the athletic trainers on your staff exhibiting some behaviors that are out of character for that individual. You recognize these behaviors as signs of "burnout." Which of the following are signs of job burnout?
    I. Insomnia
    II. Angry behavior
    III. Manic behavior
    IV. Self-preoccupation
    V. Attentiveness
    VI. Daily feelings of exhaustion
    A. I, II, IV, VI
    B. I, III, IV, V
    C. II, III, V, VI
    D. II, III, IV, VI
    E. All of the above

108. Which of the following is not among the best means by which an athletic trainer may educate the general public and other health care workers regarding the profession of athletic training?
    A. Organizing professional seminars and conferences
    B. Providing high-quality care to the physically active individual
    C. Publishing articles in professional journals and participating in research
    D. Developing television advertisements
    E. A and C

109. What is the most important thing an athletic trainer should do when taking a history from an athlete after an injury has occurred or when a problem arises?
    A. Be an active listener
    B. Make sure the athlete "gets to the point"
    C. Find out when the injury occurred
    D. Be sure to ask plenty of leading questions
    E. Ask what type of insurance policy he or she has

110. When assisting the general public in understanding the term *sports medicine*, the definition should include which of the following descriptors?
    A. Strength training
    B. Physician
    C. Rehabilitation
    D. Fitness
    E. Multidisciplinary

111. Which of the following qualities is needed in order to be an effective educator in an athletic training program?
    A. Competence in classroom teaching methods
    B. Competence in speech writing and communication skills
    C. A background in sociology
    D. Competence in computer language and audiovisual technology
    E. All of the above

112. Torts are legal wrongs committed against a person or his or her property. Such wrongs may be a direct result of _____ or _____.
    A. Negligence, commission
    B. Negligence, liability
    C. Omission, commission
    D. Omission, negligence
    E. Commission, liability

113. Athletic trainers should carry what type of insurance?
    A. Catastrophic event insurance
    B. Professional liability insurance
    C. Accident insurance
    D. Life insurance
    E. Primary insurance

114. Which of the following models of supervision for a head athletic trainer could be described as a "mentoring" approach?
    A. Developmental supervision
    B. Inspection supervision
    C. On-field supervision
    D. Clinical supervision
    E. None of the above

115. You have been asked to initiate an athletic training program in the high school in which you work. One of the areas you are covering is sexually transmitted diseases. The following topics relating to AIDS should include all of the following except:
    A. Blood-borne pathogens
    B. HIV testing
    C. Universal precautions
    D. Bacterial infections
    E. OSHA guidelines

116. An athletic trainer discovers that he is infected with HIV. All of the following would be prudent steps for the athletic trainer to take except:
    A. Avoid seeking medical care
    B. Inform, if or when it becomes appropriate to do so, his patients, coworkers, and supervisors of his status
    C. Take the necessary steps to avoid the possibility of infecting others
    D. Make sure he has ongoing medical evaluations
    E. B and D

117. The statute of limitations involving a negligence suit has a limit of how many years?
    A. Up to 2 years
    B. 4 to 5 years
    C. 7 to 10 years
    D. 10 to 15 years
    E. 1 to 3 years

118. Which type of insurance should the athletic trainer carry in case of a criminal complaint involving negligence?
    A. General secondary insurance
    B. Catastrophic insurance
    C. Accident insurance
    D. Professional liability insurance
    E. Primary insurance

119. An athlete and his coach from your wrestling program have been trying to convince you that the athlete, who has been diagnosed with impetigo, can return early to wrestle. Your response should be based upon which NATA *Code of Ethics* principle?
    A. I: "Members Shall Practice With Compassion, Respecting the Rights, Welfare and Dignity of Others"
    B. II: "Members Shall Comply With the Laws and Regulations Governing the Practice of Athletic Training, National Athletic Trainers' Association (NATA) Memberships Standards and the NATA Code of Ethics"
    C. III: "Members Shall Maintain and Promote High Standards in Their Provision of Services"
    D. IV: "Members Shall Not Engage in Conduct That Could be Construed as a Conflict of Interest, Reflects Negatively on the Athletic Training Profession or Jeopardizes a Patient's Health and Well-Being"
    E. None of the above

120. Which of the following are types of state regulation statuses for athletic trainers?
    I. Certification
    II. Licensing
    III. Active
    IV. Registration
    V. Inactive
    A. I, II, V
    B. II, III, IV
    C. I, II, IV
    D. II, IV, V
    E. I, II, III

121. All of the following are steps an athletic trainer can take to avoid litigation except:
    A. Develop a comprehensive emergency plan
    B. Establish a detailed, written job description
    C. Establish a yearly plan for modality maintenance
    D. Keep accurate records of all prescription medications dispensed
    E. A and B

122. An athletic trainer is working in a clinical setting. Which of the following populations is the athletic trainer best suited to treat?
    A. Neurologically impaired
    B. Mentally impaired
    C. Burn patients
    D. Geriatric patients
    E. Physically active

123. All of the following are violations of the BOC standards of practice except:
    A. Practicing as an athletic trainer without a license in a state that has an athletic trainer regulation
    B. Representing oneself as a BOC-certified athletic trainer using another individual's certification number
    C. Divulging the contents of a section of the certification exam to another certified athletic trainer or to a prospective student
    D. Functioning as a clinical athletic trainer in a sports medicine clinic within the confines of the individual state's practice act
    E. Prescribing medication

124. What is the state of being legally responsible for the harm one causes another person?
    A. Criminal intention
    B. Foreseeable harm
    C. Tort
    D. Negligence
    E. Liability

125. An athlete steps out of a whirlpool onto a slippery, wet floor and slips and falls, fracturing his wrist. The athletic trainer may be considered _____ in this case.
    A. Negligent
    B. Immune
    C. A plaintiff
    D. A witness
    E. Not guilty

126. The athletic trainer can avoid the risk of litigation by doing all of the following except:
    A. Keep medical records confidential
    B. Establish positive personal relationships with athletes
    C. Create a safe playing environment with documentation of such
    D. Keep an updated résumé on file with the athletic director
    E. B and C

127. A certified athletic trainer is observed to be intoxicated while at work at a major university. This is in violation of which principle of the NATA *Code of Ethics*?
    A. I: "Members Shall Practice With Compassion, Respecting the Rights, Welfare and Dignity of Others"
    B. II: "Members Shall Comply With the Laws and Regulations Governing the Practice of Athletic Training, National Athletic Trainers' Association (NATA) Memberships Standards and the NATA Code of Ethics"
    C. III: "Members Shall Maintain and Promote High Standards in Their Provision of Services"
    D. IV: "Members Shall Not Engage in Conduct That Could be Construed as a Conflict of Interest, Reflects Negatively on the Athletic Training Profession or Jeopardizes a Patient's Health and Well-Being"
    E. None of the above

128. A certified athletic trainer refuses to treat an athlete based on the athlete's ethnicity. This is in violation of which principle of the NATA *Code of Ethics*?
    A. I: "Members Shall Practice With Compassion, Respecting the Rights, Welfare and Dignity of Others"
    B. II: "Members Shall Comply With the Laws and Regulations Governing the Practice of Athletic Training, National Athletic Trainers' Association (NATA) Memberships Standards and the NATA Code of Ethics"
    C. III: "Members Shall Maintain and Promote High Standards in Their Provision of Services"
    D. IV: "Members Shall Not Engage in Conduct That Could be Construed as a Conflict of Interest, Reflects Negatively on the Athletic Training Profession or Jeopardizes a Patient's Health and Well-Being"
    E. None of the above

129. *Sports medicine* is a term that includes all of the following specializations related to the study of sport except:
    A. Exercise physiology
    B. Biomechanics
    C. Sports psychology
    D. Sports nutrition
    E. Recreational therapy

130. In what year were certified athletic trainers recognized by the AMA as "allied health care professionals"?
    A. 1988
    B. 1997
    C. 1994
    D. 2000
    E. 1990

131. Athletic training scope of practice parameters set by legislation fall into all of the following areas except:
    A. Restrictions regarding site of practice
    B. Modality use restrictions
    C. Restrictions regarding classroom teaching
    D. The definition of athletic training or athletic trainer
    E. Supervision of athletic trainers

132. Which of the following health care providers would be known as a primary care provider?
    A. A physical therapist
    B. An orthopedic technician
    C. A nurse
    D. An athletic trainer
    E. A physician

133. Which one of the following would be an example on a component of evidence-based practice?
    A. Defining a clinically relevant question
    B. Determine appropriate cost of supplies
    C. Decreasing the opportunity for third-party reimbursement
    D. Improve patient compliance
    E. None of the above

134. When taking a history from an athlete during the initial evaluation after an injury, at which of the following "levels of listening" should the athletic trainer be functioning?
    A. Passive
    B. Active
    C. Courteous
    D. Appreciative
    E. Analytical

135. _____ and _____ are 2 major components of "professionalism."
    A. Commitment, open-mindedness
    B. Status, narcissism
    C. Procrastination, decisiveness
    D. Job titles, upward mobility
    E. Dedication, upward mobility

136. Continuing education units may be obtained through all of the following methods except:
    A. Attending a BOC-approved seminar
    B. Completing a NATA journal quiz
    C. Completing postgraduate course work
    D. Writing a medical column in a local newspaper or popular magazine
    E. Home study courses

137. The only individuals who should have access to databases containing an athlete's medical records should be the _____ and _____.
    A. Athletic trainer, team physician
    B. Athletic trainer, school nurse
    C. Team physician, athletic director
    D. Parents, school nurse
    E. Athletic trainer, coach

138. _____ and _____ are 2 signs of occupational "burnout."
    A. Exhaustion, anger
    B. Excitement, creativeness
    C. Confusion, anxiety
    D. Paranoia, skepticism
    E. Anger, forgetfulness

139. Which of the following professionals possesses expertise in the analysis of human motion?
    A. A physiatrist
    B. An exercise physiologist
    C. A strength and conditioning specialist
    D. A biomechanist
    E. An athletic trainer

140. One of your patients is having significant pain as a result of a hallux valgus deformity. Which of the following individuals should the athletic trainer consult with in the care of this patient?
    A. A hand surgeon
    B. A physical therapist
    C. A podiatrist
    D. A dentist
    E. A neurologist

141. Although an athletic trainer has successfully passed the BOC exam, he or she must be educated on the rules and regulations of the state(s) in which he or she intends to practice. The individual must be knowledgeable of the state's:
    A. Certification guidelines
    B. Code of ethics
    C. Medical practice act
    D. Board of directors directives
    E. OSHA guidelines

142. Which of the following should a certified athletic trainer be concerned with when treating athletes?
    A. Foreseeable harm
    B. Tort
    C. Malfeasance
    D. The good samaritan act
    E. Malpractice

143. One of your high school baseball players is having elbow surgery at the end of the season. He is a major league prospect, and a scout has asked you to detail the surgery and outline the anticipated rehabilitation. When answering the scout's questions, the athletic trainer should do which of the following?
    A. Refer the scout to the athletic director
    B. Refer the scout to the team physician
    C. Refer the scout to the athlete
    D. None of the above
    E. All of the above

144. As a head athletic trainer at a Division I university, you are charged with designing a drug testing procedure. It is up to you how to design and implement the procedure and select the individuals being tested. The best way to select subjects is to use which of the following methods?
    A. Random timing
    B. Announced testing
    C. Preseason testing
    D. Random selection
    E. Scheduled weekly testing

145. All athletes should be required to participate in a pre-participation physical examination prior to any athletic-related activity. During this exam, an athlete should also be required to fill out pertinent paperwork. What is one of the most important forms the athlete must complete?
    A. Previous athletic experience form
    B. Assumption of risk form
    C. Statutes of limitations form
    D. Personal information form
    E. Health insurance form

146. What is a medical condition called that is not covered by health insurance?
    A. A rider
    B. A deductible
    C. A premium
    D. An exclusion
    E. A liability

147. The NATA *Code of Ethics* is defined as which of the following?
    A. Moral legal privileges inherent in being a member of a community
    B. Violation of commitment to privacy and protection of information or communications
    C. A set of rules by which an athletic trainer should conduct him- or herself
    D. The basis or explanation for an action taken by an athletic trainer
    E. None of the above

148. Which of the following is a way for an athletic trainer to protect him- or herself from negligence?
    A. Good documentation
    B. Testimony in court
    C. Sovereign immunity
    D. Having good malpractice insurance
    E. All of the above

149. Which of the following is a form of state credential, established by statute and intended to protect the public, that regulates the practice by specifying who may practice and what duties they may perform?
    A. Licensure
    B. Exemption
    C. Certification
    D. Registration
    E. None of the above

150. Which of the following is not one of the 4 principles of the NATA *Code of Ethics*?
    A. I: "Members Shall Practice With Compassion, Respecting the Rights, Welfare and Dignity of Others"
    B. II: "Members Shall Comply With the Laws and Regulations Governing the Practice of Athletic Training, National Athletic Trainers' Association (NATA) Memberships Standards and the NATA Code of Ethics"
    C. III: "Members Shall Maintain and Promote High Standards in Their Provision of Services"
    D. IV: "Members May Engage in Conduct That Constitutes a Conflict of Interest if the BOC Board of Supervisors Grants Prior Approval"
    E. A and C

151. Which of the following is a legal defense that attempts to claim that an injured plaintiff understood the risk of an activity and freely chose to undertake the activity regardless of the hazards associated with it?
    A. Sovereign immunity
    B. Comparative negligence
    C. Assumption of risk
    D. Statutes of limitations
    E. None of the above

152. Which of the following is not necessary when obtaining insurance information for a patient's medical records?
    A. The insured's name
    B. The insured's mother's maiden name
    C. The insurance company's phone number
    D. Policy numbers
    E. The insurance company's address

153. Which of the following is not an approach to ethical decision making?
    A. Egoism
    B. Utilitarianism
    C. Formalism
    D. Socialism
    E. A and C

154. Sports medicine encompasses all of the following fields of study related to sport except:
    A. Biomechanics
    B. Massage therapy
    C. Sports nutrition
    D. Sport psychology
    E. Coaching

155. All of the following are considered support personnel that work along with the athletic trainer to ensure the health and safety of the athlete except:
    A. Nurse
    B. Sport psychologist
    C. Social worker
    D. All of the above
    E. B and C

156. All of the following are guidelines and position statements released by the NATA except:
    A. Exertional heat illness
    B. Fluid replacement for patients
    C. Eye safety in sports
    D. Lightning safety for athletics and recreation
    E. Asthma in athletics

157. All of the following are considered members of the primary sports medicine team except:
    A. Coach
    B. Athletic trainer
    C. Physical therapist
    D. Team physician
    E. A and D

158. When was the NATA officially formed?
    A. 1948
    B. 1953
    C. 1955
    D. 1962
    E. 1950

159. Who is responsible for compiling medical histories and conducting physical examinations for each athlete on a team?
    A. The athletic trainer
    B. The team physician
    C. The athletic director
    D. All of the above
    E. None of the above

160. Which of the following is a possible employment setting for an athletic trainer?
    A. Industrial setting
    B. High school setting
    C. Hospital setting
    D. College or university
    E. All of the above

161. Which of the following is not a classification of regulation utilized when allowing an athletic trainer the right to practice within a specific state?
    A. Certification
    B. Licensing
    C. Delegation
    D. No Regulation
    E. Registration

162. Who is the accrediting body for entry-level athletic training programs?
    A. CAATE
    B. JRC-AT
    C. NATA
    D. BOC
    E. CAAHEP

163. Which of the following is not a domain of athletic training?
    A. Clinical Evaluation and Diagnosis
    B. Diagnosis of Athletic Injuries
    C. Immediate and Emergency Care
    D. Injury/Illness Prevention and Wellness Protection
    E. Organizational and Professional Health and Well-Being

164. Athletic trainers are which type of decision maker?
    A. Primary
    B. Secondary
    C. Tertiary
    D. Supplemental
    E. Definers

165. What is negligence?
    A. A situation in which an athletic trainer fails to act as a reasonably prudent athletic trainer would act under the same circumstances
    B. A legal wrong, other than breach of contract, for which a remedy will be provided, usually in the form of monetary damage
    C. An unexcused failure to perform the duties specified in a contract
    D. Liability generating conduct associated with the adverse outcome of a patient treatment
    E. None of the above

166. Part of professional development is networking within your profession. This is accomplished by which of the following?
    A. Going to professional meetings
    B. Having a professional appearance at all times
    C. Arriving late to a conference
    D. Not keeping in contact with colleagues in your profession
    E. All of the above

167. Using a best practices approach suggests that medical documentation of all physician referrals, initial evaluation, assessment, treatments, and dates of follow-up care for all patients is a good idea for all of the following reasons except:
    A. Professional standards of practice
    B. Legal protection if sued
    C. Improved communication between the team or family physician
    D. Protection against a possible malpractice suit
    E. B and C

168. All of the following are true about state certification and/or licensure with respect to athletic trainers except:
    A. Certification is a less restrictive form of professional regulation than licensure
    B. Licensure does not prohibit anyone from performing the tasks of an athletic trainer under state law
    C. The BOC is recognized as the certifying board
    D. Licensure is the most restrictive form of state credentialing
    E. A and C

169. The rules, standards, and principles that dictate proper conduct among members of a society or profession are known as which of the following?
    A. Rights of conduct
    B. Code of conduct
    C. Morality
    D. Professional demeanor
    E. Ethics

170. An athletic trainer shares a patient's electronic medical record (EMR) via email with a local podiatrist for his medical opinion without the patient's consent. This podiatrist has never met the patient. This violates which of the 4 principles of the NATA *Code of Ethics*?
    A. I: "Members Shall Practice With Compassion, Respecting the Rights, Welfare and Dignity of Others"
    B. II: "Members Shall Comply With the Laws and Regulations Governing the Practice of Athletic Training, National Athletic Trainers' Association (NATA) Memberships Standards and the NATA Code of Ethics"
    C. III: "Members Shall Maintain and Promote High Standards in Their Provision of Services"
    D. IV: "Members Shall Not Engage in Conduct That Could be Construed as a Conflict of Interest, Reflects Negatively on the Athletic Training Profession or Jeopardizes a Patient's Health and Well-Being"
    E. A and B

171. All of the following are components of outcome assessment methods from the Agreement-Trust Matrix except:
    A. Patient chart documentation
    B. Internal chart audits
    C. Randomized clinical trials
    D. Patient review
    E. A and D

172. All of the following are advantages of inspection-production supervision except:
    A. Helps ensure goal achievements
    B. Sets well-defined limits on job behavior
    C. Documents input and output of a sports medicine clinic
    D. Enhances common understanding of athletic roles
    E. A and D

173. What does it mean when one fails to act when there is a legal duty to do so?
    A. Negligence
    B. Malpractice
    C. Commission
    D. Misdemeanor
    E. Omission

174. Which word defines a person who is highly cooperative in a support plan?
    A. Bedfellow
    B. Opponent
    C. Plaintiff
    D. Adversary
    E. Ally

175. Athletic directors, owners, staff, and _____ are all part of a major inside interest group.
    A. Parents
    B. Clients
    C. Coaches
    D. Professional groups
    E. None of the above

176. A sports medicine program should include which of the following in order to be successful?
    A. Provide the best possible health care
    B. Good communication among members of the sports medicine team
    C. Good communication between the athletic trainer and parents
    D. All of the above
    E. None of the above

177. One of your soccer players is requesting to play in the conference championship in 2 days. This athlete is 2 days post concussion. Who should make the final decision of an athlete's eligibility for participation in organized athletic activity in this situation?
    A. Coach
    B. Athlete
    C. Parent
    D. School nurse
    E. Physician

178. The athletic administrator's role includes which of the following?
    A. Establishes the chain of command for the sports medicine team
    B. Makes certain that each member has appropriate credentials
    C. Is responsible for having appropriate personnel for the appropriate positions
    D. All of the above
    E. None of the above

RELATED ATHLETIC TRAINING SUBJECT MATTER

Human Anatomy

1. What is inflammation of the common flexor origin of the forearm musculature called?
    A. Lateral epicondylitis
    B. Cycler's wrist
    C. Tennis elbow
    D. Pronation overuse syndrome
    E. Medial epicondylitis

2. Where is the olecranon process located?
    A. Ulna
    B. Tibia
    C. Vertebrae
    D. Sternum
    E. Clavicle

3. Which muscle does not assist in plantarflexion of the ankle?
    A. Peroneus tertius
    B. Posterior tibialis
    C. Plantaris
    D. Soleus
    E. Gastrocnemius

4. Which muscle does the axillary nerve innervate?
    A. Deltoid
    B. Latissimus dorsi
    C. Pectoralis minor
    D. Trapezius
    E. Scalenes

5. The collateral ligaments of the knee are taut in which of the following?
    A. Flexion
    B. Extension
    C. Extension and flexion
    D. Genu varus
    E. Genu valgum

6. Which cranial nerve is injured if the athlete complains of a decrease in the sense of smell after a high velocity head injury?
    A. II
    B. IV
    C. III
    D. V
    E. I

7. The rotator cuff consists of all the following muscles except:
    A. Supraspinatus
    B. Infraspinatus
    C. Teres major
    D. Subscapularis
    E. Teres minor

8. The rectus femoris muscle performs what 2 actions?
    A. Hip flexion and knee extension
    B. Hip extension and knee flexion
    C. Hip flexion and hip internal rotation
    D. Knee extension and hip internal rotation
    E. None of the above

9. The pes anserinus is made up of the tendons of what 3 muscles?
   A. Biceps femoris, gracilis, semitendinosus
   B. Iliotibial band, sartorius, semimembranosus
   C. Sartorius, gracilis, semimembranosus
   D. Sartorius, gracilis, semitendinosus
   E. Tensor fasciae latae, gracilis, semitendinosus

10. The subscapularis muscle originates on the _____ and inserts into the _____.
    A. Subscapular fossa, lesser tubercle of the humerus
    B. Supraspinous fossa, greater tubercle of the humerus
    C. Distal two-thirds of the humerus, coronoid process of the ulna
    D. Scapula, middle third of the humerus
    E. None of the above

11. The gluteus maximus is responsible for what following motion(s)?
    A. Flexion and internal rotation of the thigh
    B. Extension of the hip
    C. External rotation of the hip
    D. Extension and external rotation of the hip
    E. Abduction of the hip

12. What is the nerve root that affects elbow extension?
    A. C4
    B. C8
    C. C5
    D. C6
    E. C7

13. Holding a vibrating tuning fork next to the athlete's ear to determine air conduction of sound is a test for the _____ cranial nerve.
    A. VIII
    B. VI
    C. V
    D. X
    E. III

14. To test the hypoglossal nerve, the athletic trainer should request the patient to perform what action?
    A. Shrug his or her shoulders
    B. Stick his or her tongue out
    C. Open his or her mouth wide
    D. Smile
    E. None of the above

15. "Handlebar palsy," which occurs in cyclists, presents with motor weakness of what nerve(s)?
    A. Ulnar
    B. Median
    C. Musculocutaneous
    D. Ulnar and median
    E. Radial

16. Where is the scaphoid bone of the wrist palpated?
    A. Proximal to the radial head
    B. Lateral to the cuboid bone
    C. Just distal to the styloid process of the radius
    D. Just distal to the styloid process of the ulna
    E. Just proximal to the styloid process of the ulna

17. All of the following muscles are innervated by the ulnar nerve except:
    A. Flexor carpi ulnaris
    B. Adductor pollicis
    C. All the hypothenar muscles
    D. Extensor carpi ulnaris
    E. None of the above

18. What type of joint is the hip joint?
    A. Fibrous
    B. Amphiarthrotic
    C. Synarthrotic
    D. Diarthrotic
    E. Semiarthrotic

19. Flexion and extension of the knee joint occurs in the _____ plane around a _____ axis.
    A. Sagittal, transverse
    B. Sagittal, coronal
    C. Frontal, anterior-posterior
    D. Transverse, longitudinal
    E. Sagittal, longitudinal

20. Which of the following describes an impacted fracture?
    A. A fracture that telescopes one part of the bone on the other
    B. The bone splits along its length
    C. The fracture is at a right angle to the shaft
    D. A fracture consisting of 3 or more fragments at the fracture site
    E. None of the above

21. Which of the following joints is classified as a uniaxial diarthrodial joint?
    A. The interphalangeal joints of the fingers
    B. Hip joint
    C. Carpometacarpal joint of the thumb
    D. Scapulothoracic joint
    E. None of the above

22. Which of the following muscles does not flex the hip?
    A. Tensor fasciae latae
    B. Pectineus
    C. Iliopsoas
    D. Rectus femoris
    E. Biceps femoris

23. Which of the following movements is greatest in the thoracic region?
    A. Lateral flexion of the spine
    B. Flexion and extension of the spine
    C. Rotation and extension of the spine
    D. Flexion of the spine
    E. None of the above

24. Which structures are located in the lateral compartment of the lower leg?
    A. Extensor digitorum longus, peroneus longus, and peroneus brevis muscles
    B. Peroneus longus and brevis muscles, the superficial branch of the peroneal nerve, and the peroneal artery
    C. Posterior tibialis muscle, posterior tibial artery, and the deep peroneal nerve
    D. Extensor digitorum longus, peroneal brevis, and peroneal tertius muscles
    E. Anterior tibialis, peroneal brevis, and Achilles tendon

25. Where would a Baker's cyst be located?
    A. In the popliteal fossa
    B. In the groin area
    C. On the breast
    D. On the lip
    E. The wrist

26. Which of the joints below compose the shoulder girdle?
    I. Sternoclavicular
    II. Acromioclavicular
    III. Glenohumeral
    IV. Scapulothoracic
    V. Costoclavicular
    VI. Scapulohumeral
    A. I, II, VI
    B. I, II, III, IV
    C. III, IV, V, VI
    D. III, V, VI
    E. I, II, V

27. The coracoclavicular ligaments consist of the _____ and _____ ligaments.
    A. Trapezoid, conoid
    B. Coracoacromial, conoid
    C. Acromioclavicular, trapezoid
    D. Costoclavicular, conoid
    E. Trapezoid, glenoid

28. Which of the following joints is a "mortise" joint?
    A. First metatarsophalangeal
    B. Elbow
    C. Sacroiliac
    D. Knee
    E. Ankle

29. What 2 structures pass through the tunnel of Guyon?
    A. The ulnar nerve and ulnar artery
    B. The radial and ulnar nerves
    C. The radial nerve and radial artery
    D. The ulnar nerve and radial artery
    E. None of the above

30. Which muscle is usually affected with tennis elbow?
    A. Extensor carpi radialis brevis
    B. Flexor carpi radialis
    C. Extensor carpi ulnaris
    D. Extensor pollicis brevis
    E. Coracobrachialis

31. All of the following muscles are intrinsic muscles of the hand except:
    A. The lumbricals
    B. The muscles of the thenar eminence
    C. The interossei
    D. The multifidi muscles
    E. All of the above are intrinsic muscles of the hand

32. What are the primary actions of the psoas major?
    A. Abduction of the hip
    B. Extension and internal rotation of the hip
    C. Hip flexion and internal rotation
    D. Trunk flexion
    E. Lateral flexion of the trunk

33. Where is the origin of the vastus lateralis located?
    A. Gerdy's tubercle
    B. The anterior inferior iliac spine
    C. The greater trochanter of the femur
    D. The lateral aspect of the femur
    E. Lister's tubercle

34. Which of the following muscle tendons form the borders of the anatomical snuff-box?
    I. Extensor hallucis longus
    II. Extensor pollicis brevis
    III. Flexor pollicis longus
    IV. Abductor pollicis longus
    V. Extensor pollicis longus
    A. I, III, V
    B. I, II, IV
    C. III, IV, V
    D. II, IV, V
    E. I, II, III

35. What is the structure that carries deoxygenated blood from the head and upper body to the heart?
    A. Descending aorta
    B. Superior vena cava
    C. Ascending aorta
    D. Jugular vein
    E. None of the above

36. At which of the following structures does gas exchange occur in the lungs?
    A. Terminal bronchiole
    B. The parietal pleura
    C. The pulmonary arteries
    D. The pulmonary veins
    E. The alveoli

37. All of the following structures pass through the popliteal fossa except:
    A. Tibial nerve
    B. Popliteal artery
    C. Popliteal vein
    D. Common peroneal nerve
    E. Peroneal artery

38. Where is the odontoid process located?
    A. Base of the sacrum
    B. Proximal end of the ulna
    C. Off the second cervical vertebra
    D. Base of the skull
    E. Distal to the olecranon process

39. Which of the following bones is not a carpal bone of the wrist?
    A. Lunate
    B. Cuneiform
    C. Hamate
    D. Pisiform
    E. Scaphoid

40. The plantar fascia or plantar aponeurosis is located where in the body?
    A. Base of the neck
    B. Lumbar region
    C. Lateral side of the thigh
    D. Sole of the foot
    E. Cervical spine

41. The sternocleidomastoid muscle originates on the _____ and inserts into the _____.
    A. Clavicle, mastoid process
    B. Clavicle and sternum, mastoid process
    C. Manubrium, occipital protuberance
    D. Manubrium, clavicle
    E. Third cervical vertebra, clavicle

42. Which of the following muscles is a strong extensor of the trunk?
    A. Gluteus maximus
    B. Erector spinae
    C. Quadratus lumborum
    D. Iliacus
    E. None of the above

43. Which structures pass through the femoral triangle?
    A. Femoral artery, femoral vein, femoral nerve
    B. Femoral artery, femoral nerve, iliac vein
    C. Deep circumflex vein, femoral nerve
    D. Great saphenous vein, femoral vein, iliac vein
    E. Superficial circumflex vein, femoral artery, femoral nerve

44. Which artery is closely involved with the brachial plexus and becomes the brachial artery at the lower border of the tendon of the teres major muscle?
    A. Subclavian
    B. Radial
    C. Axillary
    D. Subscapular
    E. None of the above

45. Which of the following muscles does not dorsiflex the ankle?
    A. Extensor digitorum longus
    B. Peroneus tertius
    C. Tibialis anterior
    D. Peroneus brevis
    E. A and C

46. Which of the following is not a bone of the middle ear?
    A. Malleus
    B. Cochlea
    C. Stapes
    D. Incus
    E. All of the above

47. Where is the C3,4 dermatome located?
    A. The top of the head
    B. Over the posterior upper arm area
    C. Over the lateral upper arm area
    D. The superior aspect of the shoulders and posterior neck area
    E. Anterior chest area

48. In what abdominal quadrant is the spleen located?
    A. Central
    B. Lower right
    C. Lower left
    D. Upper right
    E. Upper left

49. Your athlete comes to the athletic training facility after injuring his neck and left arm. You suspect involvement of the C5,6 nerve root. Which of the following actions would not be involved with an injury to a muscle with this innervation?
    A. Little finger abduction
    B. Elbow flexion
    C. Shoulder abduction
    D. Forearm supination
    E. Shoulder flexion

50. A soccer player has been kicked in the upper right quadrant of his abdomen. Which of the following internal organ(s) could have sustained a significant injury?
    A. Kidney
    B. Ureters
    C. Spleen
    D. Appendix and sigmoid colon
    E. Liver and gallbladder

Human Physiology

1. The bottom number of a blood pressure reading is the _____ pressure.
    A. Intrinsic
    B. Systolic
    C. Ejection fraction
    D. Venous
    E. Diastolic

2. The optimum time an ice pack should be applied to a body part is 10 minutes. This is to avoid the _____ response.
    A. Vasomotor
    B. Blocking
    C. Moro
    D. Belle
    E. Hunting

3. Redness and swelling during the inflammation process are caused by all of the following except:
    A. Histamine
    B. Prostaglandins
    C. Serotonin
    D. Acetylcholine
    E. Bradykinin

4. What is the level of desirable total cholesterol?
    A. Less than or equal to 200 mg/100 mL
    B. Greater than 250 mg/100 mL
    C. 55 mg/100 mL
    D. Less than 100 mg/100 mL
    E. None of the above

5. Which of the following is known as the separation of electrically charged particles causing a transmembrane electrical potential difference?
    A. Resting membrane potential
    B. Membrane permeability threshold
    C. Electrogenic pump
    D. Depolarization threshold
    E. Ion interference

6. When sodium ions move into a cell and the transmembrane potential is reduced (approaches zero), and when potassium ions rush out of the cell and the transmembrane potential is gradually re-established, an action potential is created. The 2 phases described above are known as what?
    A. Depolarization and repolarization
    B. Repolarization and depolarization
    C. Stimulation and propagation
    D. Propagation and repolarization
    E. Permability and repolarization

7. What is the primary component of striated skeletal muscle?
   A. Sarcomere
   B. Muscle fiber
   C. Myofibril
   D. Fascicle
   E. None of the above

8. What does a motor unit consist of?
   A. A cell body, axon, and dendrites
   B. The axon and single muscle fiber it innervates
   C. A motor neuron and the group of muscle fibers it innervates
   D. The motor neuron, muscle fiber, and muscle group
   E. The dendrite and the group of muscle fibers it innervates

9. What type of muscle fiber is more prevalent in a sprinter's lower extremity?
   A. Pink
   B. Type I
   C. Slow twitch
   D. Smooth
   E. Fast twitch

10. What mineral must be present in adequate amounts in the muscle fiber for a contraction to occur?
    A. Na^+
    B. Ca^{++}
    C. Cl-
    D. PO_4
    E. All of the above

11. In addition to the release of energy, the breakdown of ATP during a muscle contraction produces which of the following byproducts?
    A. $H_2O + CO_2$
    B. $Cr + PO_4$
    C. $ADP + PO_4$
    D. ADP + ATPase
    E. Bilirubin

12. During aerobic metabolism, enzymes reduce large molecules of carbohydrates, fat, and protein into smaller particles so they can be oxidized in a chain of chemical reactions. What is this series of chemical reactions collectively called?
    A. The Krebs cycle
    B. Oxidative carboxylic acid cycle
    C. Thermocaloric cycle
    D. Phosphocreatine reaction
    E. Electron transport cycle

13. Deep pain may originate from 3 specific areas when a nerve is injured. These areas are known as sclerotomes, myotomes, and dermatomes. Sclerotomic pain is transported by what type of nerve fiber?
    A. Unmyelinated C fibers
    B. Unmyelinated D fibers
    C. Myelinated A-Delta fibers
    D. Myelinated C fibers
    E. Myelinated B-Delta fibers

14. Muscular fiber arrangements may be known as _____ or _____.
    A. Fusiform, pennate
    B. Oblique, striated
    C. Striated, smooth
    D. Multinuclear, uninuclear
    E. Transverse, longitudinal

15. What is amenorrhea?
    A. Diminished flow during menses
    B. Absence of flow during menses
    C. Painful menses
    D. Late onset of menses
    E. None of the above

16. What should be avoided by an athlete who has frequent episodes of constipation?
    A. Laxatives or enemas
    B. High fiber diet
    C. Bland diet
    D. Calcium supplements
    E. B and D

17. Hemophilia occurs when which of the following blood factors is missing?
    A. Granulocytes
    B. Hemoglobin
    C. Factor IV
    D. Rh factor
    E. Factor VIII

18. In addition to the partial pressure of oxygen in the alveolar gas of the lungs, what other factors influence the rate of diffusion of oxygen into the bloodstream?
    A. The respiratory rate and pleural surface area
    B. The amount of CO_2 present in the alveoli and the pulmonary veins
    C. The respiratory rate and CO_2 partial pressure
    D. The thickness of the alveolar capillary membrane and the amount of surface area available for diffusion
    E. All of the above

19. A patient's pulmonary function is tested via spirometry. Several measurements are taken during this test. What is the maximum amount of air that can be expired after a maximum inspiration?
    A. Maximum expiratory flow rate
    B. Forced expiratory volume
    C. Residual volume
    D. Tidal volume
    E. Vital capacity

20. During what phase of the menstrual cycle does a graafian follicle mature?
    A. Second phase
    B. Ovulatory
    C. Luteal
    D. Menstrual
    E. Follicular

21. What are the 2 phases of menstruation?
    A. Anovulation, luteal
    B. Prolactin, menarche
    C. Follicular, luteal
    D. Menarche, follicular
    E. First phase, second phase

22. Which of the following structures is not innervated?
    A. Periosteum of bone
    B. Peritoneum of the abdomen
    C. Epithelium of the skin
    D. Enamel of a tooth
    E. All of the above are innervated

23. A football player sustained a large laceration to his lower leg 4 weeks ago. Which type of repair has taken place by this time?
    A. Callus formation
    B. Primary healing
    C. Margination
    D. Secondary healing
    E. Erythrocyte migration

24. Noxious stimuli that are created by musculoskeletal injury result in the release of endorphins and enkephalins during the mediation of pain. These opioids are produced by the stimulation of the _____ of the midbrain and _____ in the pons and medulla.
    A. Periaqueductal gray area, substantia gelatinosa
    B. Periaqueductal gray area, raphe nucleus
    C. Central cortex, substantia gelatinosa
    D. Raphe nucleus, red nucleus
    E. Periaqueductal white area, substantia gelatinosa

25. A female field hockey player reports to the athletic trainer complaining that her knee still hurts from a grade II medial collateral ligament sprain she suffered almost 3 months ago. How long may it take for a ligament to completely heal after a significant injury?
    A. Between 4 and 6 months
    B. Up to 1 year
    C. Up to 4 months
    D. Between 1.5 and 2 years
    E. Between 4 and 6 weeks

26. You are aware of a diabetic patient who has just self-administered his morning dose of insulin and has basketball practice within the following hour. Which of the following would be a prudent action to suggest to this patient before he begins exercising?
    A. Hyperhydrate prior to practice
    B. Eat a candy bar before practice
    C. Eat a slice of bread with peanut butter or cheese prior to practice
    D. Drink a soft drink before exercising
    E. None of the above

27. All of the following are physiological responses to cryotherapy except:
    A. Increased metabolism
    B. Decreased muscle spasm
    C. Analgesia
    D. Increased joint stiffness
    E. B and D

28. An athlete falls on an outstretched hand and injures his wrist. After evaluating the injury, the athletic trainer suspects a scaphoid fracture. Because this area has a poor blood supply, which of the following conditions may occur if the injury is mistreated?
    A. de Quervain's syndrome
    B. Aseptic necrosis
    C. Carpal tunnel syndrome
    D. Swan neck deformity
    E. Bennett's deformity

29. A soccer player gets kicked in the low back and is brought to the athletic training facility. During his examination, he goes to the bathroom and reports that there is blood in his urine. Which of the following terms describes this sign of an internal injury?
    A. Hyperpnea
    B. Hematoma
    C. Hypernatremia
    D. Hemarthrosis
    E. Hematuria

30. Smooth muscle tissue is found in all of the following structures except:
    A. Lungs
    B. Arterial walls
    C. Colon
    D. Intestines
    E. Scalenes

31. While performing an isometric contraction, a patient should be instructed to breathe normally to prevent the valsalva's effect. Which of the following occurs when the patient produces the valsalva's effect?
    A. The patient experiences dyspnea
    B. The patient will hyperventilate
    C. The patient becomes hypotensive
    D. There is a significant, rapid rise in blood pressure
    E. The patient will pass out

32. During ballistic stretching, the Golgi tendon organs are unable to produce a relaxing effect of the muscle because of the constant stimulation of which of the following structures?
    A. Muscle spindles
    B. Posterior horn of the spinal cord
    C. The antagonist muscle
    D. Cerebral cortex
    E. None of the above

33. The adrenal glands secrete which of the following substances?
    I. Cortisol
    II. Epinephrine
    III. Serotonin
    IV. Aldosterone
    V. Estrogen
    VI. Human growth hormone
    A. I, II, III, VI
    B. I, II, IV, V
    C. II, III, V, VI
    D. III, IV, V, VI
    E. I, II, III, IV

34. A male patient gets kicked in the groin area and sustains an injury to the testicles. The major function of the testes is to produce _____ and _____.
    A. Semen, urine
    B. Spermatozoa, testosterone
    C. Testosterone, estrogen
    D. Semen, spermatozoa
    E. Testosterone, progesterone

Exercise Physiology

1. What can be defined as the training effect on the cardiac system?
   A. Cardiac output (CO) = increased stroke volume (SV) + decreased heart rate (HR)
   B. CO = SV / HR
   C. CO = decreased SV – increased HR
   D. SV = CO x HR
   E. None of the above

2. When reading an exercise prescription, which of the following statements represents the frequency of exercise?
   A. 3 sessions a week
   B. 45 minutes of continuous exercises
   C. Running or cycling
   D. 80% of VO_2 max
   E. None of the above

3. What 3 different lipoproteins make up total cholesterol?
   A. Triglycerides, high-density lipoproteins (HDL), and low-density lipoproteins (LDL)
   B. LDL, HDL, and very-low-density lipoproteins (VLDL)
   C. LDL, VLDL, and triglycerides
   D. Alpha lipoprotein, LDL, and triglycerides
   E. Triglycerides, omega-3 fatty acids, HDL

4. During vigorous activity, accessory muscles come into play to aid respiration. During inspiration, these muscles include the _____ and _____.
   A. Upper trapezius, levator scapulae
   B. Sternocleidomastoid, scalenes
   C. Intercostals, abdominals
   D. Intercostals, levator scapulae
   E. Abdominals, sternocleidomastoid

5. In very cold environments, the athlete's body will attempt to produce heat through many different mechanisms. One of these methods is by hypothalamic stimulation of what?
   A. Posterior hypothalamus
   B. Sweat glands
   C. Pituitary glands
   D. Adrenal glands
   E. Thyroid gland

6. A basketball player comes limping off the court complaining of a hamstring spasm. Which of the following procedures would be the most effective in reducing the spasm?
    A. Massage the hamstring
    B. Moist heat pack followed by ultrasound
    C. Static stretch of the involved muscle
    D. Static stretch of the antagonistic muscle
    E. Ice massage followed by ballistic stretch

7. A patient who is hyperflexible (mobile beyond the joint's normal range) is subject to what types of injuries?
    A. Tendinitis and bursitis
    B. Fractures and ligament tears
    C. Sprains and strains
    D. Fractures and dislocations
    E. Tendinitis and adhesive capsulitis

8. Interval training would be appropriate for all the following sports except:
    A. Football
    B. Soccer
    C. Volleyball
    D. Basketball
    E. Archery

9. During what season would it be beneficial for an athlete to participate in a sport (other than his or her primary sport) to maintain an adequate level of fitness?
    A. Off-season
    B. Postseason
    C. In-season
    D. Preseason
    E. Transition phase of in-season

10. Which of the following principles must be adhered to when designing a training program for an athlete in order to obtain optimal training effects?
        I.   Overload
        II. Specificity
        III. Progression
        IV. Consistency
        V.   Environmental factors
        VI. Psychological well-being
    A. I, III, IV, V
    B. II, IV, V, VI
    C. I, II, III, IV
    D. II, III, V, VI
    E. I, II, IV, VI

11. All of the following effects are true regarding changes that take place as a result of resistive exercise except:
    A. Increased ligament strength
    B. Improved elasticity of skeletal muscle
    C. Increased mineral content of bone
    D. Improved maximal oxygen uptake
    E. Increased tendon strength

12. Under which of the following conditions is the tension created in a muscle the greatest during exercise?
    A. When the interaction between the cross-bridges of the actin and myosin myofilaments are at a maximum
    B. When the muscle position is at its shortest
    C. When a muscle is at its most lengthened point
    D. When the muscle insertion is at a 90-degree angle to the shaft of a bone
    E. None of the above

13. _____ and _____ determine the amount of blood that is pumped through the heart in a given period of time.
    A. Cardiac output, heart rate
    B. Respiratory rate, ventricular filling rate
    C. Stroke volume, cardiac output
    D. Heart rate, stroke volume
    E. Respiratory rate, cardiac output

14. If a 20-year-old patient is exercising at 80% of his or her maximal heart rate, his or her target heart rate could be calculated to equal what?
    A. 150 BPM
    B. 140 BPM
    C. 170 BPM
    D. 200 BPM
    E. 160 BPM

15. In order to improve a patient's flexibility, PNF techniques may be incorporated into a training program. Which of the following techniques involves an isotonic contraction during the "push" phase?
    A. Hold-relax
    B. Contract-relax
    C. Slow-reversal-hold-relax
    D. Fast-reversal-hold-relax
    E. Slow-hold-relax

16. When bench-pressing a barbell, the triceps and pectoralis major musculature contract in what manner during the "lift" phase?
    A. Isokinetically
    B. Isometrically
    C. Eccentrically
    D. Concentrically
    E. None of the above

17. Which type of training program is most beneficial if the coach or athletic trainer is trying to improve muscular strength and flexibility?
    A. Plyometric training
    B. Anaerobic training
    C. Circuit training
    D. Power lifting
    E. All of the above

18. If an athlete is not well hydrated, is in poor physical condition in the beginning of a sport season, and is exercising in a very hot, humid environment, he or she may be susceptible to heat injuries. What is the area of the body that is responsible for thermoregulation?
    A. Barioceptors
    B. Thymus
    C. Hypothalamus
    D. Pituitary gland
    E. Adrenal gland

19. Year-round sports conditioning is developed through the concept of periodization. Periodization is an approach that allows the athlete to train in stages so peak performance may be attained at the appropriate time and injuries are avoided. Which of the following describe the different phases in periodization?
    A. Fall season, winter season, spring season, off-season
    B. Postseason, off-season, preseason, in-season
    C. First, second, third, and fourth quarters
    D. Preparation phase, active phase, maintenance phase
    E. Active phase, prepatory phase, competition phase

20. The purpose of a proper cool-down period after exercising is to _____ and _____.
    A. Decrease the heart rate, decrease cardiac output
    B. Increase ventilation, prevent dizziness
    C. Help the blood return to the heart to be reoxygenated, decrease muscular lactic acid build-up
    D. Improve flexibility, decrease body temperature
    E. Decrease heart rate, restore thermoregulation

21. Which type of exercise utilizes a rapid stretch of the muscle eccentrically followed by a rapid concentric contraction and is used to develop explosive movements?
    A. Ballistic
    B. Isokinetic
    C. Isotonic
    D. Internal
    E. Plyometric

22. Developing significant muscle bulk is dependent on the levels present in the body of which of the following hormones?
    A. Epinephrine
    B. Cortisol
    C. Norepinephrine
    D. Estrogen
    E. Testosterone

23. To help prevent an athlete from developing hypothermia while playing in very cold weather, what should the athletic trainer advise the athlete to do?
    A. Wear a hooded sweatshirt
    B. Only stay out in the cold for brief periods of time
    C. Wear layers of clothing
    D. Wear lined pants
    E. B and D

24. One of your lacrosse players has blonde hair, light green eyes, and a very fair complexion. You suggest she wear a sunscreen with which of the following levels of SPF?
    A. 4
    B. 6
    C. 10
    D. 30
    E. 8

25. An asthmatic patient who lives and trains in an urban area is susceptible to the effects of air pollution. To avoid an asthma attack while training, the athletic trainer should recommend that the patient train at which of the following times of day?
    A. Predawn hours
    B. Mid-day
    C. Late afternoon
    D. On weekends and the evening
    E. None of the above

26. You have a Black patient with known sickle-cell disease who is training in high altitudes for a long-distance road race. This patient might be at risk for which condition?
    A. Ruptured spleen
    B. Enlarged gallbladder
    C. Cystic fibrosis
    D. Tinea corporis
    E. Hypertension

27. Unlimited access to fluids is critical during hot weather because the patient will sweat more. Sweat is hypotonic, which means the patient is likely to experience what imbalance?
    A. Water loss in excess of salt loss
    B. Salt loss in excess of water loss
    C. Water loss is equal to salt loss
    D. Sugar loss in excess of water loss
    E. Sugar loss equal to water loss

28. Delayed-onset muscle soreness (DOMS) can occur with high-intensity exercise. Which of the following types of exercise is most likely to cause DOMS?
    A. Endurance
    B. Isometric
    C. Plyometric
    D. PNF
    E. Isotonic

29. If a joint capsule is stretched beyond its physiological limitations causing a reflexive muscle contraction, which of the following laws is being demonstrated?
    A. Ohm's
    B. Harrod's
    C. Wolff's
    D. Newton's
    E. Hilton's

30. When performing a urinalysis with a dipstick (such as Clinistix or a similar product) for abnormal glucose and protein levels, which of the following are considered abnormal findings in the adolescent?
    A. +2
    B. +3
    C. +4
    D. All of the above
    E. None of the above

31. Why are men generally much stronger than women?
    A. Women have a lower strength:body weight ratio
    B. Men have a lower strength:body weight ratio
    C. Men have a greater strength:muscle mass ratio
    D. Women have a greater strength:fat percentage ratio
    E. Women have a lower strength:body mass ratio

32. Which of the following physiological adaptations does not occur in skeletal muscle during endurance training?
    A. Increased aerobic enzyme activity
    B. Increased myoglobin levels
    C. Increased mitochondrial density
    D. Decreased mitochondrial density
    E. A and B

33. During a 400-meter sprint, which of the following energy systems is predominant?
    A. Lactic acid system
    B. ATP-CP system
    C. Anaerobic glycolysis system
    D. Aerobic metabolic system
    E. Anaerobic metabolic system

34. What effect does aerobic exercise have on a patient's diastolic blood pressure?
    A. Diastolic blood pressure will increase at the same pace as systolic
    B. Diastolic blood pressure will significantly decrease at higher workloads
    C. It will remain closely the same level as at rest
    D. Diastolic blood pressure will significantly increase with increasing workloads
    E. None of the above

35. Footstrike anemia can be controlled by having the athlete wear well-cushioned shoes, limiting running to very soft surfaces, and teaching the athlete to land lightly on his or her feet while exercising. What is this condition called?
    A. Hemolysis
    B. Hyperkalemia
    C. Rubefacients
    D. Hemarthrosis
    E. Hemoptysis

Biomechanics

1. What is a contraction that occurs as the muscle shortens?
    A. Isotonic
    B. Eccentric
    C. Isometric
    D. Concentric
    E. Static

2. The foot becomes a "rigid lever" for push-off when it is in what position?
    A. Supination
    B. Pronation
    C. Dorsiflexion
    D. Adduction
    E. Plantar flexion

3. How many degrees of freedom does the knee have?
    A. 0
    B. 1
    C. 3
    D. 4
    E. 2

4.   How many degrees of movement does the scapula contribute to shoulder abduction?
     A.   30
     B.   80
     C.   100
     D.   180
     E.   60

5.   What role does the quadriceps musculature assume during active knee extension against gravity?
     A.   Antagonist
     B.   Agonist
     C.   Synergist
     D.   Stabilizer
     E.   None of the above

6.   In the human body, the point of attachment of the muscle causing the motion is almost always closer to the joint axis than the resisting motion. What type of lever system most commonly exists in the body?
     A.   Fourth
     B.   Second
     C.   Fifth
     D.   First
     E.   Third

7.   In what position will the movement arm of a force be the greatest?
     A.   When the movement arm is at a 45-degree angle to the applied force
     B.   When the force of gravity is 90 degrees to the applied force
     C.   When the lever being moved is parallel to the applied force
     D.   When the angle of application of the force is at 90 degrees to the lever being moved
     E.   None of the above

8.   Of the following statements, which is true about anatomic pulleys?
     A.   Anatomic pulleys change the direction of the muscle force but not the magnitude of the force
     B.   Anatomic pulleys always deflect the line of pull of a muscle away from the joint axis
     C.   Anatomic pulleys change the direction and magnitude of the force
     D.   Anatomic pulleys improve leverage and, therefore, increase the magnitude of the force
     E.   None of the above

9.   Muscular tension may be increased by increasing the _____ or _____.
     A.   Frequency of motor units firing, the number of motor units that are stimulated
     B.   External force, inert muscle force
     C.   Contractile tension, viscoelastic tension
     D.   Number of repetitions while weight lifting, the poundage of weight
     E.   Angle of applied force, frequency of motor units firing

10. What 3 motions compose pronation of the foot?
     A.   Inversion, abduction, dorsiflexion
     B.   Inversion, adduction, plantar flexion
     C.   Eversion, abduction, dorsiflexion
     D.   Eversion, adduction, plantar flexion
     E.   Eversion, abduction, plantar flexion

11. What class lever does the gastrocnemius use during plantar flexion?
     A.   First
     B.   Second
     C.   Third
     D.   Fourth
     E.   Fifth

12. Each lever has a _____, which is the perpendicular distance from the line of force to the axis, and a _____, which is the perpendicular distance from the resistance to the axis.
     A.   Force arm, rotary arm
     B.   Short arm, long arm
     C.   Force arm, resistance arm
     D.   Rotary arm, translatory arm
     E.   Force arm, translatory arm

13. Running utilizes _____ motion of the entire body and _____ motion of the arms and legs.
     A.   Decelerant, accelerant
     B.   Vertical, horizontal
     C.   Rotary, translatory
     D.   Linear, angular
     E.   Vertical rotary

14. Momentum is created by the combination of _____ and _____.
     A.   Speed, weight
     B.   Mass, velocity
     C.   Acceleration, weight
     D.   Torque, friction
     E.   Acceleration, inertia

15. A sprinter who is in the "ready" position at the start of a race has a lot of potential energy. What is his potential energy converted into as he takes off when the gun is heard?
    A. Lactic acid
    B. Thermal energy
    C. Work energy
    D. Kinetic energy
    E. Aerobic energy

16. Which of the following describes the plane and axis for cervical rotation?
    A. Horizontal, vertical
    B. Horizontal, sagittal
    C. Sagittal, anterior-posterior
    D. Frontal, vertical
    E. Frontal, horizontal

17. When manually resisting the tibia during knee extension, all of the following statements regarding the torque produced are true except:
    A. The torque of an external force (ie, the hand against the anterior tibia) can be increased by increasing the magnitude of the applied force
    B. The torque of an external force can be increased by applying the force perpendicular to the tibial crest
    C. The torque of an external force can be increased by moving the force distally near the ankle
    D. The torque of an external force can be increased by applying the force parallel to the tibial shaft
    E. A and B

18. An avulsion fracture of a bone is caused by which type of tissue stress?
    A. Compression
    B. Bending
    C. Shearing
    D. All of the above
    E. None of the above

19. A lever is considered in rotational equilibrium when any muscle acting on that lever is neither shortening nor lengthening. This results in what kind of contraction?
    A. Isometric
    B. Isotonic
    C. Passive
    D. Concentric
    E. Eccentric

20. What type of joint is the carpometacarpal joint of the thumb?
    A. Pivot
    B. Ball and socket
    C. Hinge
    D. Plane
    E. Saddle

21. What is the maximum number of degrees of freedom a joint can possess?
    A. 2
    B. 5
    C. 4
    D. 6
    E. 3

22. Which of the following joints is an example of a hinge joint?
    A. Acromioclavicular
    B. Atlantoaxial
    C. Talocrural
    D. Shoulder
    E. Elbow

23. The frontal plane divides the body into _____ and _____ parts.
    A. Top, anterior
    B. Right, left
    C. Top, bottom
    D. Anterior, posterior
    E. Superior, lateral

24. What is an example of an activity taking place with the upper extremity in a closed-chain position?
    A. Swinging a bat
    B. Performing a push-up
    C. Throwing a ball
    D. Running with closed fists
    E. All of the above

25. What occurs at the knee joint during the screw-home mechanism?
    A. The tibia externally rotates on the femur during knee extension
    B. The femur externally rotates on the tibia during knee flexion
    C. The femur internally rotates on the tibia during knee extension
    D. The tibia internally rotates on the femur during knee extension
    E. The tibia externally rotates on the femur during knee flexion

26. What occurs at the articulating surfaces of a joint that is subjected to a compressive load?
    A. The joint surfaces are brought closer together
    B. The joint surfaces are forcefully separated
    C. There is a "twisting" movement at the joint surfaces
    D. There is a "bending" motion that occurs at the joint surfaces
    E. There is a "gliding" motion that occurs at the joint surfaces

27. Loading of a joint that is unstable due to a ligament rupture produces which of the following stresses on the joint cartilage?
    A. No change at all
    B. Rolling/pivoting stress
    C. Tension forces
    D. Abnormally low stress
    E. Abnormally high stress

28. Shoulder abduction occurs in the _____ plane and moves around a _____ axis.
    A. Frontal, sagittal
    B. Horizontal, vertical
    C. Frontal, anterior-posterior
    D. Sagittal, medial-lateral
    E. Frontal, superior-inferior

29. Hip internal/external rotation occurs in the _____ plane around a _____ axis.
    A. Sagittal, medial-lateral
    B. Horizontal, anterior-posterior
    C. Frontal, anterior-posterior
    D. Horizontal, vertical
    E. Sagittal, anterior-posterior

30. While covering a football game, a player gets tackled and sustains a spiral fracture of the tibial shaft. Which of the following force(s) comes into play when a bone is fractured in this manner?
    A. Compression, tension
    B. Torsion
    C. Compression, shearing
    D. Impaction
    E. Shearing, distraction

31. Repeated rubbing over the epidermis may cause which of the following conditions?
    A. Avulsion
    B. Blisters
    C. Contusions
    D. Bursitis
    E. Impetigo

Psychology

1. A patient comes to the athletic trainer just prior to his first soccer game complaining of nausea and informs the athletic trainer that he is really nervous. Which of the following is an appropriate method to relax a nervous patient?
    A. Yoga
    B. Progressive muscle relaxation
    C. Have the coach calm the patient
    D. Resting in a warm sauna for 10 minutes
    E. Pilates

2. The coach confers with the athletic trainer concerning a difficult athlete on his team. During his description of the athlete's behavior, he complains of the athlete's lack of assertiveness, procrastination, constant criticism of others, and evasiveness. What type of behavior does this profile?
    A. Obsessive-compulsive
    B. Passive-aggressive
    C. Anxiety disorder
    D. Depression
    E. Post-traumatic stress disorder

3. Which of the behaviors below are seen with abuse of anabolic steroids?
    I. Mania
    II. Depression
    III. Anxiety
    IV. Psychosis
    V. Hyperactivity
    VI. Insomnia
    A. III, V, VI
    B. I, II
    C. V, VI
    D. I, II, III, VI
    E. II, III, IV, V

4. Which of the following is not a stage of the general adaptation syndrome (response phases of stress)?
    A. Exhaustion
    B. Anger
    C. Resistance
    D. Alarm
    E. All of the above

5. A patient who is "burned out" may display which of the following symptoms?
    A. Negative self-concept
    B. Chronic fatigue
    C. Negative attitude toward his or her teammates
    D. Headaches
    E. All of the above

6. At the time of injury, the patient experiences a great deal of stress. The patient responds to this stressor by passing through 3 psychophysiological phases. During which of the following phases is the adrenal gland most active?
    A. Exhaustive
    B. Resistance
    C. Anger
    D. Alarm
    E. Frustration

7. You notice one of your basketball players is showing signs of overtraining. Which of the following would not be an appropriate response to an overtrained athlete by the athletic trainer?
    A. Listening to the athlete's fears
    B. A tapered decrease in training over a period of 1 week
    C. An abrupt cessation of training
    D. Counseling the athlete in relaxation techniques
    E. All of the above

8. Which of the following must the patient feel if he or she is to have a good rapport with the athletic trainer?
    A. Neglect
    B. Empathy
    C. Pity
    D. Love
    E. Trust

9. How might an athletic trainer assist the patient in helping him- or herself heal after an injury?
    A. Provide the patient access to painkillers
    B. Help the patient "visualize" the healing process through imagery
    C. Give the patient articles to read about his or her injury
    D. Make sure therapeutic modalities are applied in the correct sequence
    E. Move the patient through rehabilitation as rapidly as possible

10. After a wrestler is injured, you notice he has developed a very negative attitude and is generally depressed. Two methods of redirecting this patient's negative and angry ideas are _____ and _____.
    A. Thought stopping, refuting irrational thoughts
    B. Meditation, progressive relaxation
    C. Therapeutic imagery, attention diversion
    D. Thought stopping, mediation
    E. None of the above

11. While rehabilitating a patient, you find he is excessively willing to do "whatever it takes" to recover fully and as quickly as possible. In doing so, you often have to remind the patient not to push himself too hard and do too much. Which of the following is not a possible cause of overcompliance?
    A. Obsessive-compulsive behavior
    B. Slight feelings of denial
    C. Masking an underlying fear
    D. Manic-depressive behavior
    E. B and C

12. During a football player's rehabilitation of a fractured lower leg, he will experience moments of intense pain. What may the athletic trainer suggest to the patient as a means of controlling his own pain?
    A. Rehearse various plays in his mind
    B. Scream at the top of his lungs
    C. Tell the athletic trainer to stop when he feels a little discomfort
    D. Only come to therapy when no other patient or coach is in the facility
    E. Tell him it is going to hurt and not to complain

13. You notice that a gymnast you have been treating becomes sarcastic, loses her appetite, and appears unusually fatigued all the time after a severe wrist injury. These are all symptoms of what?
    A. Denial
    B. Anxiety
    C. Bulimia
    D. Anorexia
    E. Depression

14. A patient must be _____ and take _____ if he or she is to completely rehabilitate an injury.
    A. Emotionless, time off
    B. Passive, all prescribed medications
    C. Cooperative, responsibility
    D. Dependent, time off
    E. Aggressive, responsibility

15. Purging is a major symptom of what?
    A. Bulimia
    B. Anorexia nervosa
    C. Obsessive-compulsive disorder
    D. Manic depression
    E. None of the above

16. Just before a big game, one of your patients is demonstrating symptoms of moderate anxiety. Which of the following responses would be appropriate when caring for the patient?
    A. Tell the patient to "get a grip on himself"
    B. Tell the patient you feel sorry for him
    C. Tell the patient to talk to the coach
    D. Tell the patient it is okay to be nervous but to focus on his goal
    E. Tell the patient you will ask the team physician to prescribe an antidepressant

17. While treating a patient for chronic patellar tendinitis, his coach tells you it is tough to get the patient motivated to practice and his performance has significantly declined since the beginning of the season. What problem might the athletic trainer suspect?
    A. Undertraining
    B. Staleness
    C. A personality disorder
    D. The patient is accident prone
    E. Bipolar disorder

18. A patient who will be experiencing a long rehabilitation process and may have his or her position filled by another player may be at risk for which problem?
    A. Schizophrenia
    B. Mania
    C. Severe depression
    D. Bipolar disorder
    E. Personality disorder

19. What would be an appropriate action for the athletic trainer to take to relax a patient who is very anxious about his or her injury?
    A. Teach the patient about his or her injury
    B. Teach the patient about controlled breathing
    C. Have the patient speak with the school nurse
    D. Downplay the injury
    E. All of the above

20. An athlete is injured during an ice hockey game and, after being examined by the team physician, is diagnosed with a complete anterior cruciate ligament tear. You have been told by the doctor that this athlete cannot compete the rest of the season. When you see the athlete the next day he states, "The doctor doesn't know what he is talking about. I'll be fine." This athlete is demonstrating what behavior?
    A. Hysteria
    B. Depression
    C. Anger
    D. Bargaining
    E. Denial

21. Which of the following actions taken by the athletic trainer can help make the patient more compliant with rehabilitation of an injury?
    A. Have the coach threaten to kick him or her off the team if he or she does not cooperate
    B. Have the patient bring a friend to the rehabilitation session
    C. Plan the rehabilitation sessions around the patient's daily routine
    D. Make the rehabilitation sessions "fun"
    E. All of the above

22. Which of the following factors has a significant impact on the amount of stress a patient will experience during his or her recovery from an injury?
    A. Whether or not soothing music is played in the athletic training facility
    B. Whether or not the coach is present during treatment
    C. Whether or not the same athletic trainer renders care
    D. The degree to which the patient perceives he or she has control over his or her care
    E. The amount of pressure the patient's family places on him or her to play

23. An athlete who wipes off his golf clubs after every shot and constantly makes sure each club is returned to exactly the same spot in his bag every time it is used is demonstrating which of the following behaviors?
    A. Obsessive-compulsive
    B. Anxiety disorder
    C. Staleness
    D. Overachievement
    E. Obsessive-defiant disorder

24. Which of the following techniques allows the patient to assess his or her own efforts at controlling a specific physiological response, such as muscular tension?
    A. Moist heat pack
    B. Biofeedback
    C. Massage
    D. PNF
    E. Imagery

25. The anorexic female is usually a _____ and an _____.
    A. Hypochondriac, underachiever
    B. Perfectionist, overachiever
    C. Type B individual, underachiever
    D. Neurotic individual, antisocial personality
    E. Type A individual, amusing personality

26. A patient becomes hysterical after learning she has suffered a severe shoulder injury and cannot compete in her sport anymore. She is crying, screaming, and generally appears out of control. The appropriate response from the athletic trainer would be which of the following?
    A. Find her coach and have him deal with her
    B. Call her parents and have one of them calm her down
    C. Give the patient "space"
    D. Allow the patient to express her fears but remain calm and demonstrate understanding. Assist the patient in seeing the problem in proportion to the situation
    E. Tell the patient she is acting like a 3 year old

27. You have a patient who comes to your office and is very depressed. He is not doing well academically, his parents are in the process of a divorce, and the coach just cut him from the baseball team after tryouts. He tells you he wants to kill himself. What is your appropriate response?
    A. Tell the patient he should see a psychiatrist
    B. Listen to the patient, take him seriously, and consult the team doctor immediately
    C. Tell the patient he is not normal
    D. Ignore the patient and hope he will not do anything
    E. Tell the patient he is just looking for attention

28. An associated complex of pathologies affecting active women that includes disordered eating, amenorrhea, and osteoporosis is known as which of the following?
    A. Premenstrual syndrome
    B. Female athlete triad
    C. Female athlete trifecta
    D. Athletic perimenstrual syndrome
    E. None of the above

29. Eliminating negative thoughts that are connected to the effects of anxiety by substituting a positive thought in its place is known as which of the following?
    A. Dissociation
    B. Autogenic training
    C. Redirection
    D. Thought stopping
    E. Thought substitution

30. Substance abuse, as defined by the DSM-IV-TR (*Diagnostic and Statistical Manual of Mental Disorders*), is manifested by which of the following criteria (occurring within a 12-month work period)?
    A. Recurrent substance abuse resulting in a failure to fulfill a major role obligation at school, work, or home.
    B. Recurrent substance abuse in situations where it is physically hazardous (ie, driving a car while impaired)
    C. Recurrent substance abuse–related legal problems (ie, arrests for substance-related disorderly conduct)
    D. Continued substance abuse despite having persistent or recurrent social or interpersonal problems caused by the effects of the substance (ie, arguments or fighting)
    E. All of the above

31. Somatically based strategies to manage stress include all of the following except:
    A. Rhythmic breathing
    B. Concentration breathing
    C. Desensitization
    D. Progressive relaxation
    E. "5 to 1" count

32. A victim of sexual abuse may demonstrate all of the following interpersonal problems except:
    A. Negative self-concept
    B. Low self-esteem
    C. Mania
    D. Anxiety and guilt about sexuality
    E. A distorted body image

33. Signs and symptoms of addiction for a physically active individual may include all of the following except:
    A. Attendance problems
    B. Deterioration of athletic performance
    C. Escalating issues with school, job, and team
    D. Belligerent behavior
    E. Desire to stay close to the team and coach when away from the performance venue

34. A patient who uses mood-altering substances on a frequent basis in the belief that the substance helps him or her perform better in any key area of life such as school, sports, relationships, or otherwise may be developing which of the following?
    A. Psychological dependence
    B. Physical dependence
    C. Somatic dependence
    D. Psychological binge
    E. None of the above

35. In order to be diagnosed with anorexia nervosa, a patient must be underweight by _____ or below what is considered normal weight for him or her.
    A. 70%
    B. 50%
    C. 25%
    D. 85%
    E. 65%

36. Bulimia nervosa typically results in feelings of _____ after a binge.
    A. Guilt
    B. Elation
    C. Anger
    D. Depression
    E. Peace

37. An athletic trainer should make a psychological referral under all of the following circumstances except:
    A. When the athletic trainer does not have time or resources to meet the needs of the patient
    B. When the patient becomes a danger to him- or herself and others, including the athletic trainer
    C. When the athletic trainer does not have the support system or supervision to address the psychological needs of the patient
    D. When the patient with psychological issues is affecting him- or herself in a way that it is counterproductive to proper life functioning.
    E. When the patient displays a bad mood that cannot be tempered by the athletic trainer or close friends

38. A stress management technique that involves systemic, purposeful tension followed by relaxation of predetermined muscle groups is known as which of the following?
    A. Autogenic training
    B. Contract-relax-release-contract
    C. Progressive relaxation
    D. Rhythmic relaxation
    E. None of the above

39. Achieving a deep state of relaxation by disciplining the mind against encroaching thoughts is known as:
    A. Dissociation
    B. Autogenic training
    C. Desensitization
    D. Meditation
    E. Reframing

40. After what period of time should an individual demonstrating symptoms of depression be referred to a mental health professional?
    A. 24 hours
    B. 2 days
    C. 1 week
    D. 2 weeks
    E. 100 hours

41. Anxiety is often manifested by all of the following symptoms except:
    A. Tachycardia
    B. Nausea
    C. Intense worry
    D. Paranoia
    E. Sleepiness

42. When educating an injured patient about the rehabilitative process, all of the following steps taken by the athletic trainer are appropriate except:
    A. Clearly explain to the patient what is covered or not covered by insurance
    B. Educate the patient about the injury, using charts or visual aids
    C. Explain how the healing process occurs with estimated time frames
    D. Explain the consequences of not following the recommended protocol
    E. Explain the overall rehabilitation plan

43. Which of the following is an example of an overreaction to a recent injury?
    A. Trembling
    B. Nausea
    C. Anxiety
    D. Tachycardia
    E. Inappropriate joke telling

44. When providing "emotional first aid" to a newly injured patient, if the athletic trainer notices the patient failing to answer questions, looks confused, and is lacking emotion, how should the athletic trainer appropriately respond?
    A. Give the patient "space" and let him or her come to you
    B. With empathy and encourage the patient to express feelings
    C. Be direct and firm with questioning
    D. Ask the patient if he or she is "on any medication"
    E. None of the above

45. Factors to incorporate into goal setting for a patient include all of the following except:
    A. Set specific and measurable goals
    B. Use positive language
    C. Make goals challenging but realistic
    D. Set a reasonable time frame
    E. Connect the outcome to the effort

46. When is seasonal affective disorder (SAD) most likely to occur?
    A. Winter
    B. Spring and summer
    C. Fall
    D. Summer into the Fall
    E. None of the above

47. An individual who has sustained a psychologically traumatic event may experience a numbing of general responsiveness, insomnia, or increased aggressiveness. This is known as which of the following?
    A. Paranoia
    B. Obsessive-compulsive disorder
    C. Tourette syndrome
    D. Post-traumatic stress disorder
    E. Bipolar disorder

Nutrition

1. In which of the following foods is a high concentration of vitamin A found?
    A. Liver, yogurt, milk
    B. Red meat, oranges, tea
    C. Nuts, cereals, fish
    D. Liver, carrots, greens
    E. None of the above

2. What is also known as vitamin C?
    A. Retinol
    B. Thiamine
    C. Ascorbic acid
    D. Niacin
    E. Folic acid

3. Besides sources such as fortified milk and fatty fish oils (such as in tuna fish), what is another major mode of obtaining vitamin D?
    A. Topical creams
    B. Sunlight
    C. Artichokes
    D. Fried beef liver
    E. None of the above

4. What is the conversion of glucose to lactic acid called?
    A. Photosynthesis
    B. Glycolysis
    C. Lactolysis
    D. The Krebs cycle
    E. Glycogenosis

5. When is the best time for an athlete to eat carbohydrate-rich foods?
    A. Within 2 hours after training
    B. 1 hour prior to training
    C. In small amounts while training
    D. A half-hour prior to training and throughout the training session
    E. 4 to 6 hours after training

6. At low workloads, muscle cells use _____ for fuel, while _____ is used for periods of intense exercise of short duration.
    A. Fat, protein
    B. Carbohydrate, fat
    C. Fat, phosphocreatine
    D. Protein, carbohydrate
    E. Glycogen, protein

7. In which of the following foods would be a high concentration of the mineral phosphorus be found?
    A. Potatoes
    B. Dark green vegetables
    C. Oranges
    D. Table salt
    E. Milk and cheese

8. Which of the following are the "building blocks" of protein?
    A. Sugars
    B. Amino acids
    C. Triglycerides
    D. Sterols
    E. All of the above

9. The loss of _____ and _____ account for the greatest percentage of electrolytes lost through sweat.
    A. Potassium, chloride
    B. Magnesium, potassium
    C. Sodium, potassium
    D. Potassium, zinc
    E. Sodium, chloride

10. All of the following statements regarding fluid replacement during performance are appropriate except:
    A. The athlete should drink cold fluids to decrease body core temperature
    B. It is best for the athlete to consume small amounts of fluids frequently rather than large amounts of fluid infrequently
    C. Water is the ideal fluid replacement
    D. Do not force fluids on the athlete; he or she will seek out fluid replacement when thirsty
    E. A and B

11. Which of the categories below are not considered one of the 6 classes of nutrients?
    I. Carbohydrates
    II. Proteins
    III. Antioxidants
    IV. Water
    V. Fats
    VI. Vitamins
    A. I, IV
    B. II, V
    C. V, VI
    D. III
    E. I, II

12. Which of the following nutrients is absolutely necessary for every body chemical reaction to take place normally?
    A. Vitamins
    B. Amino acids
    C. Water
    D. Fats
    E. All of the above

13. Nutrition labels that are found on food packages allow the purchaser to compare nutritional values of food and are expressed in "percent daily values" (based on a 2000-calorie diet) that follow a new nutrient label, which used to be known as the US recommended daily allowance. What new standards does the new label now follow?
    A. Recommended percent nutrients
    B. US recommended daily allowance
    C. Reference daily intakes
    D. US advised allowances
    E. None of the above

14. All of the following are methods of measuring body composition except:
    A. Measuring muscle and fat girths
    B. Hydrostatic weighing
    C. Electrical impedance
    D. Measuring skin-fold thickness
    E. C and D

15. Weight loss occurs when which of the following conditions exists?
    A. Less than 1000 calories are expended per day
    B. There is a negative caloric balance
    C. There is a positive caloric balance
    D. There is perfect caloric balance
    E. None of the above

16. Fat is a nutrient that is utilized as an energy source in the form of triglycerides. Triglycerides are stored in what type of cell?
    A. Striated
    B. Lipoma
    C. Beta
    D. White blood cells
    E. Adipose

17. A football player desires to increase his body weight and wants to know how he should go about it in a safe manner. To increase his muscle mass without causing negative results, both his _____ and _____ should increase appropriately.
    A. Fat intake, carbohydrate intake
    B. Muscular exercise, dietary intake
    C. Dietary intake, caloric expenditure
    D. Caloric expenditure, water intake
    E. None of the above

18. One of your female cheerleaders has been diagnosed by your team physician with a combination of anorexia, osteoporosis, and amenorrhea. You recognize this combination as signs of what?
    A. Marfan syndrome
    B. The unhappy triad
    C. Female triad syndrome
    D. Paget's disease
    E. Bone cancer

19. One of your gymnasts had a bone density test that came back positive for mild osteoporosis. Which of the following minerals should be supplemented to prevent osteoporosis in a high-risk athlete?
    A. Folate
    B. Niacin
    C. Folic acid
    D. Fluoride
    E. Calcium

20. One of your male cross-county runners is a committed lactovegetarian. Which of the following minerals may be deficient with this type of diet?
    A. Calcium, fluoride
    B. Iron, zinc
    C. Folic acid
    D. Copper, iron
    E. None of the above

21. One of your athletes goes out of his way to avoid eating carbohydrates, such as bread and potatoes, because of his fear of becoming fat. Which of the following substances will the body begin to utilize for energy if there is a significant lack of carbohydrates in the diet?
    A. Protein
    B. Fat
    C. Glucose
    D. Antioxidants
    E. None of the above

22. A patient routinely complains of bloating, flatulence, and diarrhea after ingesting milk or ice cream. What might be the cause of this patient's symptoms?
    A. Proteinuria
    B. Rickets
    C. Scurvy
    D. Lactase deficiency
    E. None of the above

23. Significant losses of electrolytes, such as sodium, chloride, potassium, or magnesium, during heavy exercise may lead to symptoms such as _____ or _____.
    A. Drop in pressure, diuresis
    B. Muscle strains, ligament strains
    C. Dyspnea, indigestion
    D. Muscular cramps, heat illness
    E. None of the above

24. Which 2 structures regulate water excretion?
    A. Kidneys, brain
    B. Kidneys, bladder
    C. Stomach, small intestines
    D. Kidneys, ureters
    E. Adrenal glands, thyroid

25. One of your baseball players reports that he is having difficulty playing in the outfield under lights and has similar difficulty seeing at night while driving. While evaluating him you find out he hates vegetables and drinks milk infrequently. He "enjoys hamburgers and French fries." What substance might this athlete be lacking in his diet?
    A. Carbohydrates
    B. Protein
    C. Vitamin A
    D. Phosphorus
    E. None of the above

Pharmacology

1. Lomotil is what type of medication?
   A. Antibiotic
   B. Antidiarrheal
   C. Antifungal agent
   D. Antiemetic
   E. Antipyretic

2. Which of the following medications is often used for depression?
   A. Relafen
   B. Lithium
   C. Midol
   D. Ritalin
   E. Prozac

3. All of the following substances have stimulant properties except:
   A. Nicotine
   B. Theophylline
   C. Pseudoephedrine
   D. Caffeine
   E. Pepcid

4. Ibuprofen is available in which of the below dosages?
   I. 400 mg
   II. 200 mg
   III. 600 mg
   IV. 50 mg
   V. 100 mg
   VI. 800 mg
   A. II, IV, V
   B. II, III, V
   C. III, V, VI
   D. I, II, III, VI
   E. III, IV, V

5. What is the brand name for the NSAID diclofenac?
   A. Indocin
   B. Voltaren
   C. Orudis
   D. Feldene
   E. Relafen

6. What is the recommended dosage for the NSAID Naprosyn?
   A. 250 to 500 mg twice a day
   B. 500 to 750 mg twice a day
   C. 50 to 100 mg twice a day
   D. 200 mg once a day
   E. None of the above

7. Frequently abused drugs include stimulants such as amphetamines (speed), cocaine (coke or crack), and depressants (alcohol or downers). An athlete who has overdosed on a stimulant would manifest all of the following signs except:
   A. Agitation
   B. Decreased reaction time
   C. Rapid pulse and respirations
   D. Convulsions
   E. Arrhythmias

8. Beta-blockers inhibit the action of catecholamines and decrease cardiac output. In which of the following sports would the effects of beta-blockers potentially enhance performance?
   A. Swimming
   B. Long-distance running
   C. Archery
   D. Baseball
   E. All of the above

9. In moderation, caffeine stimulates the _____ and _____ centers of the brain, causing increased alertness.
   A. Cerebral cortex, medulla
   B. Reticular formation, medulla
   C. Hypothalamus, midbrain
   D. Cerebellum, midbrain
   E. Brain stem, midbrain

10. Which of the following is not an adverse effect associated with the abuse of human growth hormone?
    A. Laryngeal thickening
    B. Hypercalciuria
    C. Hypertrophic neuropathy
    D. Mandibular growth
    E. Diarrhea

11. When 2 drugs are combined and there is a response that is 2 times the response as when each drug is used alone, this is known as what type of effect?
    A. Antagonistic
    B. Mutually exclusive
    C. Agonistic
    D. Synergistic
    E. None of the above

12. Drugs may be classified according to all of the following except:
    A. Chemical classification
    B. Mechanism of action
    C. Therapeutic effect
    D. Legal classification
    E. Route of administration

13. Which of the following may be linked to Reye's syndrome in children and teenagers when treating a viral infection?
    A. Aspirin
    B. Acetaminophen
    C. Pencillin
    D. Amoxicillin
    E. Lotrimin

14. What is the primary mechanism of action of penicillin?
    A. Inhibits DNA synthesis
    B. Inhibits cell wall synthesis
    C. Inhibits protein synthesis
    D. It is a metabolic inhibitor
    E. It enhances protein catabolism

15. Opioid analgesics do all of the following except:
    A. Causes drowsiness
    B. Reduces anxiety and distress
    C. Causes constipation
    D. Increases heart rate
    E. Suppresses coughing

16. Symptoms of caffeine withdrawal include all of the following except:
    A. Fatigue
    B. Headache
    C. Irritability
    D. Yawning
    E. Drowsiness

17. Which of the following drugs are anticonvulsants?
    A. Xanax, Valium
    B. Benadryl, Phenegran
    C. Klonopin, Tegretol
    D. Thorazine, Clozaril
    E. Dilaudid, Demerol

18. The abbreviation GERD stands for which of the following?
    A.   Gastroesophageal reflux disease
    B.   Gall bladder esophageal reflux disease
    C.   Gastroesophageal renal disease
    D.   Gastrointestinal entero-renal disease
    E.   None of the above

19. The abbreviation IBS stands for which of the following?
    A.   Irregular bowel syndrome
    B.   Inflammatory bowel disease
    C.   Internal bowel syndrome
    D.   Irritable bowel syndrome
    E.   None of the above

20. Diuretics increase the excretion of:
    A.   Sodium (Na+) and Potassium (K+) ions
    B.   Sodium (Na+) and Chloride (Cl-) ions
    C.   Potassium (K+) and Chloride (Cl-) ions
    D.   Magnesium (Mg) and Potassium (K+) ions
    E.   None of the above

21. All of the following are medication routes of administration except:
    A.   Oral
    B.   Rectal
    C.   Parenteral
    D.   Aerosol
    E.   Buccal

22. Hemorrhoids may be treated by all of the following except:
    A.   Corticosteriods
    B.   Local anesthetics
    C.   Astringents
    D.   Vasoconstrictors
    E.   Antihistamines

23. According to the hypertension guidelines set in 2014 by the Joint National Committee (JNC8) panel, the blood pressure threshold for initiating drug therapy for an individual younger than 60 years old is:
    A.   Systolic Bp ≥ 140 mm Hg, diastolic ≥ 90 mm Hg
    B.   Systolic Bp ≥ 130 mm Hg, diastolic ≥ 90 mm Hg
    C.   Systolic Bp = 120 mm Hg, diastolic = 80 mm Hg
    D.   Systolic Bp = 150 mm Hg, diastolic ≤ 80 mm Hg
    E.   Systolic Bp ≥ 130 mm Hg, diastolic ≥ 70 mm Hg

24. Which of the following drugs is an appropriate treatment for a panic disorder?
    A.   Ritalin
    B.   Depakote
    C.   Warfarin
    D.   Xanax
    E.   Theophylline

25. Which of the following drugs is used to treat Type 2 diabetes?
    A.   Dilantin
    B.   Prozac
    C.   Zocor
    D.   Glucophage
    E.   Coumadin

26. Which of the following drugs is used to treat the herpes simplex virus?
    A.   Penicillin G (Bicillin LA)
    B.   Doxycycline (Vibramycin)
    C.   Azithromycin (Zithromax)
    D.   Acyclovir (Zovirax)
    E.   Permethrin (Elimite)

27. To avoid gastric upset, NSAIDS should be taken with which of the following?
    A.   Food or milk
    B.   A glass of wine
    C.   Gatorade
    D.   An energy drink
    E.   Cranberry juice

28. Adverse reactions related to skeletal muscle relaxants include all the following except:
    A.   Drowsiness
    B.   Dizziness
    C.   Hyperventilation
    D.   Decreased liver and kidney function
    E.   Physical dependence

29. Which of the following drugs is commonly used to treat hyperlipidemia?
    A.   Flonase
    B.   Crestor
    C.   Wellbutrin
    D.   Tagamet
    E.   None of the above

30. Adverse effect of insulin use include all of the following except:
    A.   Hypoglycemia
    B.   Weight gain
    C.   Immune-based responses
    D.   Lipohypertrophy
    E.   Hyperglycemia

Physics

1. The area of the applicator that emits ultrasound and is expressed in square centimeters is known as what?
   A. The transducer head surface area
   B. Effective emitting area
   C. Effective radiating area
   D. Direct-contact area
   E. The sound head

2. What is the frequency range of therapeutic ultrasound?
   A. 1.0 to 3.0 MHz
   B. 0.1 to 1.0 MHz
   C. 10,000 to 20,000 Hz
   D. 10,000 to 30,000 Hz
   E. None of the above

3. An object immersed in water experiences an upward force that is equal to the weight of the water displaced by the object. What law of physics is this?
   A. Archimedes' principle
   B. Wolff's law
   C. Pascal's law
   D. Bernoulli's law
   E. Newton's third law

4. A TENS unit is based on the _____ of pain control.
   A. Counter irritant theory
   B. Gate control theory
   C. Beta-endorphin theory
   D. Opiate theory
   E. Distraction theory

5. A pulsed current may be _____ or _____.
   A. Monophasic, biphasic
   B. Alternating, direct
   C. Direct, monophasic
   D. Alternating, biphasic
   E. None of the above

6. What is the most commonly used frequency in short-wave diathermy?
   A. 10 MHz
   B. 27.33 MHz
   C. 4068 Hz
   D. 2450 MHz
   E. None of the above

7. Which modality produces electromagnetic radiation with a frequency above 300 MHz and a wavelength shorter than 1 m?
   A. Infrared diathermy
   B. Short-wave diathermy
   C. Microwave diathermy
   D. Induction field diathermy
   E. None of the above

8. All of the following may be settings on a TENS unit except:
   A. Modulating
   B. Burst
   C. Continuous
   D. Ramp
   E. Surge

9. What kind of current is needed for iontophoresis?
   A. Interferential
   B. Alternating
   C. Alternating or direct
   D. Ionized
   E. Direct

10. Which of the following is the correct definition of work?
    A. W = distance x velocity
    B. W = force x power
    C. W = force x distance
    D. W = pressure x distance
    E. None of the above

11. To perform iontophoresis, the medication used must be _____.
    A. Diluted
    B. Neutralized
    C. In powder form
    D. Mixed with a gel
    E. Ionized

12. According to Joule's law, heat produced by high-frequency electrical currents is directly proportional to all of the following except:
    A. Power output
    B. Square of the current strength
    C. Resistance of the conductor
    D. Time during which the current flows
    E. C and D

13. In the application of electrotherapy, the strength of an electrical current in a circuit is directly proportional to the applied electromotive force and inversely proportional to the resistance of the current. What law does this describe?
    A. Cosine's
    B. Cowling's
    C. Joule's
    D. Wolff's
    E. Ohm's

14. By what means does heat transfer to the skin with the use of a hot pack?
    A. Conduction
    B. Convection
    C. Radiation
    D. Evaporation
    E. All of the above

15. What type of waveform is produced when the current flow direction reverses on regular intervals?
    A. Galvanic current
    B. Pulsed current
    C. Alternating current
    D. Faradic current
    E. None of the above

16. The temperature of a thermometer reading is given in degrees Celsius. What formula must be used to convert the temperature from Celsius to Fahrenheit?
    A. (Temperature in Fahrenheit – 32) x 5/9
    B. (Temperature in Celsius – 32) x 5/9
    C. (Temperature in Celsius x 9/5) + 32
    D. (Temperature in Celsius + 32) x 5/9
    E. None of the above

17. What is the impedance of an electrical circuit?
    A. The pathway in which a current will flow
    B. The magnitude of the current flow
    C. The resistance within the circuit
    D. The direction of current flow
    E. The frequency of current flow

18. An athlete is evaluated by the athletic trainer and it is determined that he has acute supraspinatus tendinitis. Which of the following modalities is not appropriate to decrease pain and inflammation of the tendon?
    A. Phonophoresis
    B. Iontophoresis
    C. Ice packs
    D. Ice massage
    E. Moist heat packs

19. The strength of a current flow is known as what?
    A. Rheobase
    B. Resistance
    C. Amperage
    D. Voltage
    E. None of the above

20. According to Poiseuille's law, the _____ and _____ of a blood vessel are very critical in terms of resistance to blood flow.
    A. Length, radius
    B. Muscle type, contractility
    C. Length, thickness
    D. Direction, temperature
    E. Direction, radius

21. Which of the following intensities is considered medium intensity when treating an area with ultrasound?
    A. 0.8 to 1.5 watts per square cm
    B. 1.5 to 2.0 watts per square cm
    C. 1.0 to 3.0 total watts
    D. 5.0 to 8.0 total watts
    E. < 0.8 watts per square cm

22. How far from the skin surface should the ultrasound transducer head be kept when utilizing the underwater technique?
    A. Between 1 and 3 inches
    B. 3 inches
    C. 5 inches
    D. 0.5 to 1 inch from the skin surface
    E. 3 to 5 inches

23. What is the polarity of an anode in an electrical stimulator?
    A. Disperse
    B. Negative
    C. Positive
    D. Neutral
    E. The anode has no polarity

Evidence-Based Practice

1. The PICOT format can be used to construct a clinical question. The acronym "PICOT" stands for which of the following?
   A. Plan, Implementation, Clinical hypothesis, Outcome(s), Type of interest
   B. Patient population, Intervention of interest, Comparison intervention or issue of interest, Outcome(s) of interests, Time of interest
   C. Purpose, Implementation, Clientele, Outcome(s), Time of study
   D. Patient population, Intervention of interest on issue, Outcome(s) of interest, Type of study
   E. None of the above

2. All of the following are considered "Descriptive Study Designs" except:
   A. Case reports
   B. Case series
   C. Time series
   D. Cross- sectional studies
   E. Retrospective reports

3. All of the following are databases commonly used by health care professionals except:
   A. Google Scholar
   B. Cochrane Database
   C. Cumulative Index to Nursing and Allied Health Literature (CINAHL)
   D. Medline
   E. Jeffline

4. Controlled vocabulary searching utilizes which of the following?
   A. Medical Subject Headings (MeSH)
   B. Keywords
   C. A Boolean operator
   D. A Mapping feature
   E. None of the above

5. Data are classified as all of the following except:
   A. Nominal
   B. Ordinal
   C. Dependent
   D. Interval
   E. Ratio

6. A variable that is measured by an investigator is known as:
   A. An independent variable
   B. A dependent variable
   C. A hypothesis
   D. A null variable
   E. None of the above

7. A statement made by an investigator indicating his or her expectations about the differences or relationships among variables being investigated is known as:
   A. A predictable hypothesis
   B. A null hypothesis
   C. A research hypothesis
   D. A differential hypothesis
   E. A descriptive hypothesis

8. Data that are continuous and primarily cluster around a central value, such as the mean, is known as what?
   A. Skewness
   B. Quantitative data
   C. Bell curve
   D. Normal distribution
   E. Homogeneity of variance

9. Researchers use a threshold value, known as ___, to determine if the results of a study are significant.
   A. Q value
   B. A beta level
   C. Confidence interval
   D. Standard deviation
   E. Significance level

10. A Type I error is made during a research project when:
    A. A researcher makes an incorrect decision to REJECT the Null Hypothesis when it is actually true.
    B. A researcher makes an incorrect decision to ACCEPT the Null Hypothesis.
    C. A researcher makes an incorrect decision to REJECT the Research Hypothesis when it is actually true.
    D. A researcher makes an incorrect decision to ACCEPT the Research Hypothesis.

11. What type of participant sampling allows for every person in the population of interest to have an equal chance of being chosen?
    A. Cluster sampling
    B. Systematic random sampling
    C. Random sampling
    D. Proportional stratified sampling
    E. Convenience sampling

12. A blinding process is put into place by a researcher to eliminate which of the following from a study?
    A. An interval validity threat
    B. An external validity threat
    C. Attrition
    D. Bias
    E. Violated assumptions of a statistical test

13. Which of the following defines "Critical Appraisal"?
    A. The critical evaluation of a research article that rates the quality of evidence based on the research design of the study
    B. The process of carefully and systematically examining research to judge its trustworthiness as well as its value and relevance in a particular context
    C. The process by which a clinician offers an opinion whether literature supports a particular research study
    D. A peer-review process that assures a study is valid
    E. A peer-review process that assures a study is reliable

14. The variable that will be measured by the Boolean operator during a study is called:
    A. A dependent variable
    B. An independent variable
    C. A quantitative variable
    D. An outcome variable
    E. None of the above

15. An internal validity threat can include which of the following, jeopardizing a researcher's ability to draw an accurate conclusion?
    A. Treatments, procedures, or participant experience
    B. Participant history and maturation
    C. Participant maturation and attrition
    D. Experimental procedures and error rate
    E. None of the above

16. Confidence intervals commonly range from _____ to _____.
    A. 10% to 50%
    B. 85% to 99%
    C. 75% to 100%
    D. 0.05% to 0.25%
    E. 80% to 100%

17. The consistency of a specific measurement is known as:
    A. Strata
    B. Validity
    C. Predictive validity
    D. An interval
    E. Reliability

18. The validity of a clinical diagnostic test is measured through mathematical equations that compare it to which of the following?
    A. An error rate
    B. Exclusion criteria
    C. A reference or "gold standard" finding
    D. A functional outcome
    E. The null hypothesis

19. Which are the 2 most commonly utilized scales for examining evidence?
    A. The adjectival and binary response scales
    B. An original and nominal scale
    C. The Cronbach's alpha and weighted Kappa statistic
    D. The JADAD and appraisal scales
    E. The Oxford Centre for Evidence-Based Medicine (CEBM) Scale and the Strength of Recommendation Taxonomy (SORT)

20. When there is a negative clinical diagnostic finding but a positive reference standard finding, the result is known as a:
    A. False negative finding
    B. False positive finding
    C. True negative finding
    D. True positive finding
    E. None of the above

21. When there is a positive clinical diagnostic finding and a positive reference standard finding, the result is known as a:
    A. False negative finding
    B. False positive finding
    C. True negative finding
    D. True positive finding
    E. None of the above

22. Percent accuracy of a clinical diagnostic test can be derived by which of the following formulas?
    A. True positive finding + true negative finding ÷ total number of patients × 100
    B. True positive finding + false negative finding ÷ total number of patients × 100
    C. False positive finding + true negative finding ÷ total number of patients × 100
    D. False positive finding + false negative finding ÷ total number of patients × 100
    E. None of the above

23. Prevalence is defined as:
    A. The observation of a participant or group of participants over multiple time instances
    B. The number of cases of a condition existing in a given population at any one time
    C. The odds or probability that a patient has a condition based on clinical presentation before a diagnostic test is conducted
    D. Pretest odds times likelihood ratio
    E. None of the above

24. A feature in which a database will automatically attempt to match a keyword entered in the search box to a MeSH (Medical Subject Heading) term that already exists is known as:
    A. Filtering
    B. Mapping
    C. Truncating
    D. Matching
    E. Pairing

25. When the subject or characteristic fits into only one category, it is known as being:
    A. Incidental
    B. Nominal
    C. Singular
    D. Mutually exclusive
    E. Mutually inclusive

26. Which of the following is a disablement model that utilizes a biopsychosocial perspective of disability?
    A. The Nexus Disablement Model
    B. The Ottawa Disablement Model
    C. NAGI Disablement Model
    D. Patient-Centered Outcome Model
    E. Integrated Disablement Model

27. A letter rating system assigned to a body of evidence by examination of a group of articles relating to the same topic is known as:
    A. A grade of recommendations
    B. Numeric assignment
    C. Strength of recommendation taxonomy
    D. A level of evidence
    E. None of the above

28. Which of the following is NOT a commonly used response scale for a patient-rated outcome (PRO) instrument?
    A. Binary response scale
    B. Visual analog scale
    C. Adjectival scale
    D. Likert response scale
    E. Criterion-based response scale

29. Which of the following is NOT a patient-rated outcome (PRO) instrument?
    A. Short Form 12
    B. Disablement in the Physically Active Scale
    C. Pediatric Quality of Life Inventory
    D. Physiotherapy Evidence Database (PEDro)
    E. Patient-Reported Outcomes Measurement Information System

30. An incidence rate (also known as *injury rate*) can be defined by which of the following equations?
    A. Number of New Injuries ÷ Total Exposure Time
    B. Number of Total Injuries ÷ Total Number of Participants
    C. Total Number of Participants × Total Exposure Time
    D. Number of Total Injuries × Number of Participants in the Control Group
    E. Number of Participants in the Treatment Group ÷ Total Exposure Time

31. The midpoint in which 50% of the values fall on either side of the value is known as the:
    A. Mode
    B. Mean
    C. Standard deviation
    D. Confidence interval
    E. Median

32. An "Alpha Value," which is a significance level assigned by the researcher to represent a threshold at which the results will be declared significant or not, is typically which of the following?
    A. 1.0
    B. 0.05
    C. 10.0
    D. 0.25
    E. 0.75

33. What are the 3 main types of clinical prediction rules used in health care?
    A. Preventative, prognostic, and therapeutic
    B. Prognostic, diagnostic, and therapeutic
    C. Interventional, prognostic, and diagnostic
    D. Suggestive, diagnostic, and therapeutic
    E. Preventive, evaluative, and interventional

34. A 1- to 2-page summary that focuses on appraising a single research study to help determine if the reported results are valid, reliable, and clinically applicable is called what?
    A. Summary of best evidence
    B. Summary of key evidence (SKE)
    C. Clinical bottom line (CBL)
    D. Critically appraised paper (CAP)
    E. None of the above

35. The Disabilities of the Arm, Shoulder and Hand (DASH) questionnaire, the Modified Oswestry, and Lower Extremity Functional Scale (LEFS) are all considered which of the following?
    A. Disease-oriented outcome instruments
    B. Specific patient-reported outcome instruments
    C. Condition-oriented outcome instruments
    D. Functional ability instruments
    E. None of the above

36. An aggregate of legal medical records from multiple entitles (ie, an AT, MD, Sports Psychologist, etc) is known as which of the following?
    A. Electronic health record (EHR)
    B. Patient flow chart
    C. Electronic medical record (EMR)
    D. Athletic health record
    E. None of the above

37. All of the following are basic components of an electronic medical record (EMR) except:
    A. Clinical documentation
    B. Data storage
    C. Clinical messaging between providers and patients
    D. Results reporting for clinical tests
    E. Patient satisfaction surveys

38. A level I validation of a Clinical Prediction Rule (CPR) study is described by which of the following?
    A. It can be used in a variety of settings with confidence that it improves outcomes
    B. The CPR can be used with confidence in one setting only
    C. The CPR should be used with caution and only in settings similar to those used in the study
    D. The CPR should not be used until further validation occurs
    E. None of the above

39. An 11-item scale that was developed by physiotherapists to rate the methodological quality of randomized controlled trials is known as a _____ scale?
    A. Quorum scale
    B. Consort scale
    C. PRISMA scale
    D. PEDro scale
    E. STARD scale

40. A Critically Appraised Topic (CAT) is an appraisal tool that is used to synthesize numerous research articles that review the same general topic of interest. Most CATs include all of the following sections except:
    A. Clinical scenario
    B. Focused clinical question
    C. Strength of recommendation
    D. Summary of best evidence
    E. Opinion of application

41. What is the first step in the use of evidence-based practice?
    A. Searching the medical literature
    B. Appraising published studies
    C. Developing an answerable clinical question
    D. Integrating the evidence into clinical practice
    E. Evaluating the EBP process and patient outcomes

42. The "5 S" model of health care research evidence provides a strategy to search within an organized model of evidence-based information that is more relevant to point of fare application. Which of the following is NOT a level of the "5 S" model?
    A. Systems
    B. Standards
    C. Summaries
    D. Synopses
    E. Syntheses

43. A systematic review in which the data from the included studies are pooled for additional analyses and a summary estimate of effect is known as a:
    A. Clinical practice guideline
    B. Meta-analysis
    C. Critical appraisal checklist
    D. Cross-sectional study
    E. Evidence hierarchy

44. All of the following are critical appraisal checklists except:
    A. CONSORT
    B. STOBE
    C. STARD
    D. PRISMA
    E. ELK

45. EBP in athletic training does all of the following except:
    A. Ensures higher reimbursement for athletic training treatments
    B. Ensures a scientific foundation for athletic training practice
    C. Improves critical thinking
    D. May elevate the athletic training profession in the medical community
    E. Can lead to the development of best practice guidelines

46. Detailed searches of a body of literature may be assigned a Strength of Recommendation (SOR) represented by a grade depending on the quality, quantity, and consistency of the included studies. All of the following are accepted SOR Grades except:
    A. A
    B. B
    C. C
    D. D
    E. E

47. A collection of data on a single patient is known as a:
    A. Case report
    B. Case series
    C. Cohort study
    D. Clinical report
    E. Singular study

48. Clinical questions can be categorized into which of the following types of questions?
    A. Alpha and beta
    B. Background and foreground
    C. Simple and complex
    D. Singular and multi-factorial
    E. Ying and yang

49. Foreground questions are developed by using the _____ Format:
    A. SROBE
    B. STRAND
    C. CAT
    D. PICOT
    E. CAP

50. A variable that is manipulated by a researcher is known as a(n)?
    A. Alternative variable
    B. Variable of interest
    C. Comparative variable
    D. Dependent variable
    E. Independent variable

TRUE/FALSE QUESTIONS

The athletic training education competencies are designed to serve as an outline for the required knowledge that students enrolled in approved athletic training programs should master. The entry-level athletic trainer should have the ability to provide athletic training services to a variety of patients across the spectrum of the lifespan. The content areas are reflected throughout the text with this section focused on evaluating your knowledge of the content areas. Although you will not have true/false questions on the exam, these will serve as a basis of evaluation of pure facts.

EVIDENCE-BASED PRACTICE

1. Evidence-based practice is important to athletic training solely to improve the third-party reimbursement rates that athletic trainers receive. ☐ T ☐ F

2. Personal experiences or those of colleagues are basis enough to utilize a specific treatment method without utilizing scientific validity. ☐ T ☐ F

3. Evidence-based practice is best defined as the use of the consensus of scientific evidence to indicate the best clinical practices for managing specific conditions. ☐ T ☐ F

4. Weak evidence should not be given greater weight on the basis of numerous weak studies. One randomized controlled trial is better than numerous quasi-experimental studies. ☐ T ☐ F

5. A clinical trial is any research project that prospectively assigns human subjects to intervention or comparison groups to study the cause-effect relationship between a medical intervention and a health-related outcome. ☐ T ☐ F

6. A controlled experimental lab study that is conducted in an artificial environment is said to be an in vivo study. ☐ T ☐ F

7. Using a cookbook approach for clinical practice that ignores clinician experience or the circumstances of a specific patient is acceptable as long you utilize the same treatment on all patients of similar injuries. ☐ T ☐ F

8. A cross-over (within-group) experimental research design allows for each subject to receive every condition in succession but provides a random treatment administration while at least 2 conditions are being evaluated simultaneously. ☐ T ☐ F

9. A group of people with a common experience over a defined period of time is a cohort. ☐ T ☐ F

10. The practice of using treatment methodologies that are a result of a research study is acceptable since a research study was completed and an article was published. ☐ T ☐ F

PREVENTION AND HEALTH PROMOTION

1. Fibroids of the uterus always develop into cancer. ☐ T ☐ F

2. Type 1 diabetes can be prevented from developing with a proper diet and exercise. ☐ T ☐ F

3. A daily regimen of calcium, vitamin D (as per recommended daily allowance), exercise, and a balanced diet is critical in preventing osteoporosis in women who are at risk for the disease. ☐ T ☐ F

4. Trichomonas can be prevented by thoroughly cooking any raw pork products. ☐ T ☐ F

5. Men who have an undescended or partially descended testicle are at a higher risk of developing testicular cancer than men with fully descended testicles. ☐ T ☐ F

6. To prevent dehydration and the possibility of heat stroke during activity on hot, humid days, for every pound of water that is lost, 24 ounces of fluid should be replaced. ☐ T ☐ F

7. Otitis externa can be prevented by using ear plugs while swimming and a drying agent in the ear canal immediately after swimming. ☐ T ☐ F

8. Conjunctivitis can be prevented through good hand washing and proper eyelid hygiene. ☐ T ☐ F

9. The cure rate for skin cancer exceeds 95% with early detection and treatment. ☐ T ☐ F

10. Although the best way for an athletic trainer to avoid litigation is to exactly follow the manufacturer's instruction for the use and maintenance of a piece of equipment, if an athletic trainer modifies a piece of equipment to make it fit better for the athlete and he or she is still injured during an event, the manufacturer will then be solely liable for the injury. ☐ T ☐ F

CLINICAL EXAMINATION AND DIAGNOSIS

1. Huntington's chorea is a genetic disorder. ☐ T ☐ F

2. Cerebral palsy is diagnosed by skeletal muscle biopsy. ☐ T ☐ F

3. Decorticate posturing is caused by the lack of dopamine in the brain. ☐ T ☐ F

4. Hallmark signs of endometriosis are severe abdominal cramping and heavy menstrual bleeding. ☐ T ☐ F

5. A patient with Wernicke's aphasia can understand the spoken word, but cannot verbally communicate properly. ☐ T ☐ F

6. Emphysema is a result of the deterioration of the bronchioles and bronchi. ☐ T ☐ F

7. Anterior compartment syndrome may be addressed without consequence up to 72 hours after the initial insult. ☐ T ☐ F

8. The basal metabolic rate is increased in individuals with hyperthyroidism. ☐ T ☐ F

9. Graves' disease, systemic lupus erythematosus, and rheumatoid arthritis are all autoimmune diseases. ☐ T ☐ F

10. Cranial nerve V has been injured if the athlete cannot masticate. ☐ T ☐ F

THERAPEUTIC INTERVENTIONS

1. A C6 quadriplegic is unable to independently operate a manual wheelchair. ☐ T ☐ F

2. It is contraindicated to strengthen the abdominals of a patient who has been diagnosed with spondylolisthesis. ☐ T ☐ F

3. Grade III joint mobilization is an appropriate technique when treating a patient with adhesive capsulitis. ☐ T ☐ F

4. Strength training in the D2 flexion PNF pattern should be done with caution in a patient who has been diagnosed with anterior shoulder instability. ☐ T ☐ F

5. When performing an interval throwing program, the progression of throwing distances of 45 feet, then 60 feet, then 90, 120, 150, and 180 feet are appropriate provided there is no increased pain or soreness the next day. ☐ T ☐ F

6. Proprioception is the ability to detect movement of a joint; kinesthesia is the ability to determine the position of a joint in space. ☐ T ☐ F

7. The proper sequence for a functional progression program following an ankle sprain includes walking, jogging, running, lunges, sprints, lateral shuffles, and cariocas. ☐ T ☐ F

8. Conservative treatment for a mild case of thoracic outlet syndrome includes strengthening of the trapezius, rhomboids, serratus anterior, and erector spinae and stretching of the pectoralis minor and scalene muscles. ☐ T ☐ F

9. A patient with multiple sclerosis should exercise in the morning rather than in the afternoon. ☐ T ☐ F

10. Patients who are on heparin, such as a patient who has had a recent total knee replacement, need to avoid vegetables high in vitamin K. ☐ T ☐ F

11. Maximal effect occurs when an energy source raised (such as ultrasound) strikes the body at a 90-degree angle. ☐ T ☐ F

12. A major disadvantage of using an instant (chemical) coldpack is the chemical inside the pack has an alkaline pH, which can cause burns if it comes in contact with the skin. ☐ T ☐ F

13. Mr. Wheaton is an overweight referee with hypertension and seasonal allergies. During a recent conversation, he tells you he takes over-the-counter sinus medications for his allergies. You should be concerned that the parasympathetic actions may increase his blood pressure. ☐ T ☐ F

14. A patient was administered morphine for pain control. Assessment reveals a decreased level of consciousness and shallow respirations at a rate of 8 per minute. The physician decided to prescribe an opiate antagonist. Narcan (naloxone hydrochloride) would be an example of this type of drug. ☐ T ☐ F

15. Albuterol (beta 2 adrenergic agonist) would be a common drug for a 16-year-old female who is suffering from depression. ☐ T ☐ F

PSYCHOSOCIAL STRATEGIES AND REFERRAL

1. The correct order of the Kübler-Ross classic model of reactions to death and dying is depression, anger, bargaining, denial, and acceptance. ☐ T ☐ F

2. A patient suffering from burnout may be experiencing feelings and thoughts of emotional instability, depression, a reduced sense of accomplishment, and lack of interest in activity or sport. ☐ T ☐ F

3. Seasonal affective disorder (SAD) is identified by an individual being overly jovial at inappropriate times. SAD usually occurs in men and can be treated by rest and relaxation. ☐ T ☐ F

4. When training a patient to utilize mental techniques to aid in the process of healing following an injury, an athletic trainer might encourage the patient to recline or be seated in a chair and progressively contract and relax his or her muscles. The contracting of each muscle group should last from 5 to 10 seconds and then relax for 20 to 30 seconds. This technique is known as progressive meditation. ☐ T ☐ F

5. All of the following are described as psychological barriers to rehabilitation: anxiety, denial, sleep disturbance, and depression or grief. ☐ T ☐ F

6. There are 3 progressive, reactive phases of rehabilitation: reaction to injury, reaction to rehabilitation, and reaction to return. When the rehabilitation length is of short duration (less than 4 weeks) the patient's reaction to injury is one of shock and relief. ☐ T ☐ F

7. When a patient is injured and there is an abrupt withdrawal from training, this can lead to a condition known as sudden exercise abstinence syndrome. ☐ T ☐ F

8. You have a lacrosse player who has been injured and displays anxiety and worry regarding her rehabilitation, often stating she "cannot do this" and "this is a waste of time." This type of thinking can be reframed into positive thoughts by the use of a technique known as thought stopping. □ T □ F

9. According to the DSM V, an individual who is observed to have episodes of abnormally elevated, expansive, or irritable moods lasting a week or more would be characterized as having bipolar disorder. □ T □ F

10. When counseling a patient regarding his or her nutritional health, it is important that the athletic trainer take into consideration the patient's social influences and his or her attitudes in philosophy toward life. □ T □ F

Acute Care of Injury and Illness

1. A spontaneous anterior epistaxis is a medical emergency. □ T □ F

2. A patient should be referred to a physician after a concussion when there is a loss of consciousness on the field; amnesia lasting longer than 15 minutes; deterioration of neurologic function; unequal, dilated, or unreactive pupils; irregularity in respirations; or vomiting. □ T □ F

3. A patient complains of nocturnal itching, and he presents with dark lines between his fingers, toes, the volar aspect of his wrists, and the genitalia. Permethrin 5% cream would be an appropriate treatment for this scenario. □ T □ F

4. When a patient has a seizure, it is important to restrain his or her movements so he or she does not hurt him- or herself and gently awaken the patient after the convulsions have stopped. □ T □ F

5. A patient with paronychia should soak the affected finger or toe in Epsom salts or boric acid a few times a day and apply a topical antibiotic to the affected area between soakings. □ T □ F

6. When using lumbar traction, a good guideline to use when selecting an initial force high enough to cause vertebral separation is to use a force that is equal to one-half the athlete's body weight. □ T □ F

7. When covering an athletic event that is taking place in a pool, it is important that the athletic trainer have access to a rescue tube and an aquatic spine board. □ T □ F

8. The rapid form vacuum immobilizer is the best splint to use if an athlete has sustained a fracture with a deformity. □ T □ F

9. When there is a luxation of a tooth, the athletic trainer should make every effort to reimplant the tooth into its normal place or get the tooth to a dentist as soon as possible for reimplantation. □ T □ F

10. Treatment of a hordeolum consists of the application of hot, moist compresses and the application of an ointment of 1% yellow oxide or mercury to the affected area. □ T □ F

Health Care Administration

1. An athletic trainer should be aware that all insurance plans have an out-of-network benefit. These benefits cover services by providers not contracted with their insurance company. □ T □ F

2. An MCO is a maintenance care organization. This type of insurance plan is used only for long-term illnesses and injuries (ie, "maintenance care"). □ T □ F

3. A zero-based budget allows the athletic trainer to spend money freely within his or her budget without having to justify spending. □ T □ F

4. A certified athletic trainer can be sued for negligence if he or she decides to suture an athlete with a laceration during a game. □ T □ F

5. All preferred provider organization health insurance companies require the policyholder to select a primary care physician. □ T □ F

6. Ground fault interrupters are no longer necessary to use with modalities and whirlpools as long as there are high-voltage electrical plugs available. □ T □ F

7. Current Procedural Terminology was established by the American Medical Association to allow for uniformity in billing. □ T □ F

8. An athletic trainer who is in a management position should exhibit the elements of leadership, including decision making, planning, coordination of employees, and organization. □ T □ F

9. NOCSAE is the organization that certifies football helmets to make sure they are able to withstand repeated blows of high mass and low velocity. □ T □ F

10. All of the following are human resources issues: job description, hiring practices, vacation policies, benefits, and release of medical records. □ T □ F

11. As long as an athletic trainer is BOC certified, he or she can practice for up to 1 year in any state without a license. □ T □ F

12. All certified athletic trainers are expected to uphold Principle 1 of the NATA *Code of Ethics*, which states, "Members shall practice with compassion, respecting the rights, welfare and dignity of others." □ T □ F

13. Any individuals, including athletic trainers, doctors, coaches, and administrators, who are supportive of both a program and a particular plan relative to the specific program are considered to be adversaries. ☐ T ☐ F

14. Omission is a failure to act when an athletic trainer has a legal duty to do so. ☐ T ☐ F

15. The athletic trainer can automatically release medical information of a collegiate athlete to professional organizations, the media, and anyone else who requests the information upon the athlete's completion of a school-conducted physical examination. ☐ T ☐ F

16. In a health maintenance organization, policyholders are allowed to see any physician or utilize any medical service as long as the services are provided in the state in which the policyholder lives. ☐ T ☐ F

17. Point-of-service plans are very similar to preferred provider organizations except that a primary care physician is assigned to the policyholder to coordinate care. ☐ T ☐ F

18. Athletic insurance that pays for medical expenses only after all other insurance policies have reached their limit is referred to as secondary coverage insurance. ☐ T ☐ F

19. Feirman State University has a large percentage of student-athletes who do not have primary insurance coverage. In this situation, it would benefit the institution to have a large group primary policy to keep medical costs down. ☐ T ☐ F

20. As the athletic trainer closely reviews the insurance policy that has been selected for his or her respective institution, he or she must pay special attention to the exemptions and exclusions within the policy. With most accident policies, only acute, short term injuries are considered "exclusions." ☐ T ☐ F

Professional Development and Responsibility

1. The code of ethics governing the practice of athletic training is the same code for both the NATA and the BOC. ☐ T ☐ F

2. The BOC Standards of Professional Practice are designed to ensure specific patient outcomes. ☐ T ☐ F

3. A certified athletic trainer can hold any level of cardiopulmonary resuscitation, from any provider, as long as automated external defibrillator competency is validated. ☐ T ☐ F

4. The BOC Practice Analysis is intended to provide the sole guidelines for practicing athletic training and supersedes all state laws governing the profession. ☐ T ☐ F

5. The state practice acts for athletic trainers are the same in all 50 states as long as the individual holds the BOC credential for athletic training. ☐ T ☐ F

6. As a certified athletic trainer, you must willingly accept the professional organization position statements that relate directly to the practice of athletic training. ☐ T ☐ F

7. More than 25 of the 50 states offer registration as part of their regulatory acts for athletic training. ☐ T ☐ F

8. In a situation where there is a conflict between the NATA *Code of Ethics* and the law, the law prevails. ☐ T ☐ F

9. Athletic injury surveillance systems collect and analyze data that relate to the relationship of various factors that influence the frequency and distribution of sports injuries. ☐ T ☐ F

10. The athletic trainer can significantly reduce the risk of litigation by developing and following an emergency plan, documenting efforts to create a safe playing environment, have a detailed job description in writing, and maintaining confidentiality of medical records. ☐ T ☐ F

Applied Decision Making

This section is designed to allow you to utilize your judgment in making patient care decisions in a simulated situation. Although this format is not utilized in the BOC examination, your ability to know what to do when presented with a patient with specific complaints or when in a critical situation is invaluable.

A passing mark for each section of the following problems must be 80%. The passing mark is calculated by the number of correct responses encompassing 80% of the total number of questions per section. The authors recommend that if you do not pass a section at an 80% level, you review the material that is relevant to that particular section.

Assign the appropriate value from the list identified below.

++ = Most appropriate answer
+ = Appropriate, but not first priority
0 = No relevance to the problem
- = Not a priority/harmful
-- = Detrimental

EXAMPLE

Opening Scene

One of your wrestlers comes to the athletic training facility complaining of severe itching and a burning sensation on the top of his scalp. He has noticed a lot of skin flaking with some hair loss.

Section A

How will you begin your evaluation of this patient's condition? (Please select and prioritize your choices.)

_____ 1. Ask the patient if he has had this problem before.

_____ 2. Put gloves on and examine the patient's scalp.

_____ 3. Ask the patient if he has had a recent cold.

_____ 4. Administer an oral antibiotic medication from your athletic training kit.

_____ 5. Use the patient's teammate's towel to clean the area.

Answer Key

The current situation: You know that your patient has a dermatological problem.

Your immediate responsibility: To perform your initial evaluation to determine the type and extent of the problem.

_+_ 1. It is appropriate to ask the patient if he has had this problem before because he may be able to provide you with important information regarding this condition.

_++_ 2. It is necessary and proper to don gloves and examine the patient's scalp to determine the type and extent of this lesion.

_0_ 3. Asking the patient if he has had a recent cold has no relevance to this problem.

_--_ 4. It is not within the athletic trainer's scope of practice to administer a prescription drug without the direction of a supervising medical doctor.

Van Ost L, Lew Feirman K, Manfré K. *Athletic Training Exam Review: A Student Guide to Success, Sixth Edition* (pp 131-151).
© 2017 SLACK Incorporated.

___ 5. This is an inappropriate action because this condition could be contagious and using another individual's towel is not sanitary.

Problem I

Opening Scene

A gymnast injures his right lower leg after a dismount off the rings. He appears to be in a lot of pain and has not stood up. He is lying on his left side. You did not witness this event.

Section A

How will you begin your initial evaluation of the patient's condition? (Please select and prioritize your choices.)

_____ 1. Ask the patient what happened.
_____ 2. Ask the patient if he heard a snap.
_____ 3. Check the right knee range of motion.
_____ 4. Observe the leg for edema or bleeding.
_____ 5. Palpate the leg for deformity.
_____ 6. Check the patient's vital signs.
_____ 7. Palpate the patient's popliteal pulse.
_____ 8. Place a moist heat pack directly on the injury.
_____ 9. Elevate the right leg.
___ 10. Have a coach call for an ambulance.
___ 11. Check the rest of his body for any other injuries.
___ 12. Cut away the gymnast's pant leg (uniform).
___ 13. Immediately immobilize the lower right leg.

Section B

You have ruled out a compound fracture but suspect a fracture of both the tibia and fibula. With this information, how would you proceed at this time? (Please select and prioritize your choices.)

___ 14. If there is an obvious deformity of the bony shaft, try to reduce it to get good alignment.
___ 15. Remove the patient from the mat to apply an immobilizer.
___ 16. Direct others to clear the area of people and equipment.
___ 17. Pack the right leg in ice.
___ 18. Check pulses in the ankle and foot.
___ 19. Check for Volkmann's contracture.
___ 20. Allow the competition to continue.
___ 21. Position the patient in a supine position.
___ 22. Palpate the right hip joint.
___ 23. Elevate the entire leg.
___ 24. Check for crepitus.
___ 25. Immobilize the right lower leg.
___ 26. Massage the injured area.

Section C

The EMS team has arrived, and the patient is about to be transported to the emergency room. What are your final steps before he leaves with the EMS team? (Please select and prioritize your choices.)

___ 27. Check the lower extremity for numbness.
___ 28. Have the patient walk to the ambulance with crutches.
___ 29. Issue NSAIDs for swelling.
___ 30. Have the coach follow the patient to the hospital.
___ 31. Allow the patient to eat and drink whatever he wants.
___ 32. Notify the coach that the patient will no longer be permitted to participate for the rest of the season.
___ 33. Call ahead to the emergency room to make arrangements for his arrival.
___ 34. Check the patient for symptoms of shock.
___ 35. Assure the patient he will be taken care of before he departs.
___ 36. Fit the patient for crutches.
___ 37. Call the patient's parents.
___ 38. Fill out an injury report.

Problem II

Opening Scene

A field hockey player who is playing defense gets hit in the eye with a ball during a direct shot at the goal. She is lying on her side with her hands on her face.

Section A

How will you begin to evaluate the severity of the injury? (Please select and prioritize your choices.)

_____ 1. Remove the facemask.
_____ 2. Check the patient's fine motor skills.
_____ 3. Test the patient's balance.
_____ 4. Use an ammonia capsule to revive the patient.
_____ 5. Have the patient walk off the field.
_____ 6. Remove the mouthguard.
_____ 7. Ask who made the shot.
_____ 8. Ask the patient where the pain is located.
_____ 9. Palpate the patient's shoulders.
___ 10. Perform a primary survey.

___ 11. Gently palpate the area around the orbit and nose for crepitus.

___ 12. Don latex gloves.

___ 13. Observe for Battle's sign.

___ 14. Ask the patient if she has a scholarship.

___ 15. Check the area for bleeding and lacerations.

___ 16. Ask the patient if her vision is blurred.

Section B

The patient has a deep laceration above the left eyebrow. Based on this information, what are your next steps? (Please select and prioritize your choices.)

___ 17. Check the pupil for reflex movements with a penlight.

___ 18. Apply moist heat to the eye.

___ 19. Rinse the wound with saline solution.

___ 20. Apply antiseptic ointment to the laceration.

___ 21. Cover both eyes with gauze pads.

___ 22. Have the patient tell you what happened.

___ 23. Apply ice to the injury.

___ 24. Use butterfly strips to close the laceration.

___ 25. Ignore the patient if she asks if there will be a scar.

___ 26. Use sutures to close the wound.

___ 27. Call for an ambulance.

___ 28. Have the patient wait outside for the ambulance.

___ 29. Apply compression directly to the eye once you have "closed" the laceration.

___ 30. Perform a secondary survey.

Section C

You now have the laceration "closed" and are awaiting the ambulance. What are your final steps going to include? (Please select and prioritize your choices.)

___ 31. Keep the patient calm.

___ 32. Announce the patient's status over the public address system.

___ 33. Check the patient's insurance plan.

___ 34. Call the school nurse to accompany the patient to the hospital.

___ 35. Constantly change the bandage.

___ 36. Allow the patient to speak to her coach.

___ 37. Allow the press access to the patient.

___ 38. Wash your hands.

___ 39. Document the incident on an accident report form.

___ 40. Give the patient a vitamin E pill.

___ 41. Report your findings and treatment plan to the patient's coach.

PROBLEM III

Opening Scene

While covering a state track meet, you observe a high jumper land incorrectly on the crash mat. When you get to the high jump pit, you see him lying on his right side and he is not moving.

Section A

Given the above information, what would your initial steps be in evaluating the condition of this patient? (Please select and prioritize your choices.)

___ 1. Call for an ambulance.

___ 2. Ask the patient where he has pain.

___ 3. Do a primary survey.

___ 4. Make a mental note as to how the patient is positioned.

___ 5. With assistance from an athletic training student, turn the patient onto his back.

___ 6. Ask the patient to wiggle his fingers and toes.

___ 7. Ask the patient what occurred.

___ 8. Place an ice pack on the patient's neck.

___ 9. Palpate the patient's knees for deformity.

___ 10. Check the patient for any areas of bleeding on his face.

___ 11. Send for the patient's parents.

___ 12. Check the patient's level of consciousness.

Section B

After speaking to the patient and completing your initial evaluation, you suspect a potentially serious neck injury. What would your next steps be in caring for this patient? (Please select and prioritize your choices.)

___ 13. With assistance, carry the patient to the sidelines.

___ 14. To determine the severity of the injury, see if the patient can rotate his head.

___ 15. Ask the patient if he has any numbness or tingling down either upper extremity.

___ 16. Tell the patient to not move his head.

___ 17. Check the patient's pupillary response with a penlight.

___ 18. Do a check of cranial nerves IV through XII.

___ 19. With the assistance of at least 2 to 4 other people and while maintaining the head in neutral, log-roll the patient into a supine position.

___ 20. Ask the officials to stop the meet.

___ 21. Secure the patient on a spine board.

___ 22. Ask someone to call an ambulance.

___ 23. Place the patient in a cervical collar.

___ 24. Monitor the patient's vital signs.

Section C

The patient is brought by ambulance to the hospital. What would be your next actions? (Please select and prioritize your choices.)

___ 25. Contact your team physician.

___ 26. Fill out an accident report form.

___ 27. Return to the meet and follow up with the patient at a later time.

___ 28. Check your records to see if the patient is allergic to any medications.

___ 29. Check with the coach to see if the patient is on a scholarship.

___ 30. Contact the patient's parents to inform them of the accident.

___ 31. Follow the ambulance to the hospital and leave your senior athletic training student to cover the meet.

___ 32. Suggest to the athletic director that the school should eliminate the high jump event next time because it is too dangerous.

PROBLEM IV

Opening Scene

One of your female cross-country runners comes into the athletic training facility complaining of chronic left anterior knee pain, which comes and goes with activity.

Section A

Your initial evaluation of this problem would include which of the following actions? (Please select and prioritize your choices.)

___ 1. Put an ice pack on the patient's knee.

___ 2. Observe the patient's posture.

___ 3. Palpate the anteromedial joint line for tenderness and swelling.

___ 4. Perform a bilateral Ober's test.

___ 5. Ask the patient if she feels a popping sensation while walking or running.

___ 6. Ask the patient if she has ever injured her foot before.

___ 7. Perform a Patrick's test.

___ 8. Ask the patient if the knee hurts going up and down stairs.

___ 9. Tell the patient to stop running when it hurts.

___ 10. See how the patient responds to temporary orthotics.

___ 11. Observe the left knee for swelling.

___ 12. Palpate the patellar area for tenderness.

___ 13. Perform a KT-1000 test.

Section B

After your initial evaluation, you conclude this patient has a chronically subluxing patella. What steps would you take at this time to treat this patient? (Please select and prioritize your choices.)

___ 14. Recommend the patient wear a soft brace to stabilize the patella during running.

___ 15. Teach the patient exercises to strengthen her hamstrings.

___ 16. Teach the patient exercises to strengthen her left vastus medialis obliquus.

___ 17. Tell the patient to perform deep squatting exercises 2 to 3 times per day.

___ 18. Evaluate the effect of patellar taping with activity.

___ 19. Teach the patient iliotibial band stretching exercises.

___ 20. Tell the patient to consistently stretch her hamstrings.

___ 21. Give the patient Voltaren.

___ 22. Tell the patient to avoid soft, flat surfaces while running.

Section C

To speed up this patient's rehabilitation, you decide she should come to see you on a daily basis for treatment in the athletic training facility. Which activities/treatments would you perform for this condition? (Please select and prioritize your choices.)

___ 23. Apply a TENS unit to the left knee for pain.

___ 24. Perform PNF exercises, which emphasize hip flexion, abduction, and internal rotation.

___ 25. Apply ultrasound treatments to promote healing.

___ 26. Instruct the patient in plyometric activities.

___ 27. Have the patient perform both open- and closed-chain quadriceps exercises.

___ 28. Evaluate the patient's running gait on a treadmill.

___ 29. Have the patient perform exercises that strengthen the hip adductors.

___ 30. Routinely apply ice packs to the affected knee after activity.

PROBLEM V

Opening Scene

The pitcher from your baseball team comes to the athletic training facility with complaints of a deep ache in his right shoulder, which occurs after pitching and lingers for a number of hours after he stops the activity. He also states his right arm feels unusually fatigued after throwing a short period of time. He reports his shoulder feels the best when he has his right hand in his pants pocket. You have seen him voluntarily sublux his shoulders in the past as he was telling his friends he is double-jointed.

Section A

What questions would be appropriate to ask during the history portion of your initial exam? (Please select and prioritize your choices.)

_____ 1. How long has he had this problem?

_____ 2. When was the last time his right shoulder was injured?

_____ 3. What specific actions/positions make the pain worse?

_____ 4. If he is eating enough protein?

_____ 5. If his shoulder feels like it slips with activity?

_____ 6. If he is double-jointed?

_____ 7. If he is taking his vitamins?

_____ 8. What the intensity of the pain is on a scale of 0 to 10 (0 representing no pain, 10 representing excruciating pain)?

_____ 9. If his father had the same problem when he played baseball?

_____ 10. If he is taking any medications for the pain?

Section B

With the information obtained from the history, which of the following special tests would be appropriate when examining his shoulder? (Please select and prioritize your choices.)

_____ 11. Phalen's test.

_____ 12. Clunk test.

_____ 13. Pivot shift test.

_____ 14. Patrick's test.

_____ 15. Thompson's test.

_____ 16. Apprehension test (anterior and posterior).

_____ 17. Hawkins-Kennedy test.

_____ 18. Neer's sign.

_____ 19. Posterior drawer test (of the shoulder).

_____ 20. Ober's test.

_____ 21. Trendelenburg's test.

_____ 22. Sulcus sign.

Section C

After completing your evaluation, you suspect the patient has multidirectional instability of the right shoulder. Knowing what you do about this condition, which of the following exercises would be appropriate to specifically strengthen the scapular stabilizers and rotator cuff musculature? (Please select and prioritize your choices.)

_____ 23. Shoulder shrugs.

_____ 24. Biceps curls.

_____ 25. Shoulder abduction exercises with free weights.

_____ 26. Cervical isometric exercises.

_____ 27. Internal/external rotation of the shoulder using a Theraband.

_____ 28. Manual PNF exercises (D2 extension pattern).

_____ 29. Triceps curls.

_____ 30. Rowing exercises.

_____ 31. Serratus anterior strengthening exercises.

_____ 32. Partial sit-ups.

_____ 33. Prone trunk extensions.

_____ 34. Calf raises.

PROBLEM VI

Opening Scene

You are covering a tennis match when one player runs to the net for a volley, stops and sets for the shot, and suddenly falls to the court while grabbing his left lower leg. He is in severe pain.

Section A

With the information you have available, how will you begin your initial evaluation of this injury? (Please select and prioritize your choices.)

_____ 1. Establish if the patient is breathing.

_____ 2. Ask the patient to walk off the court.

_____ 3. Ask the patient what happened.

_____ 4. Determine the patient's level of consciousness according to the Glasgow Coma Scale.

_____ 5. Check the patient's leg for bleeding.

_____ 6. Ask the patient where the pain is located.

_____ 7. Observe the left lower extremity for any deformity.

_____ 8. Ask the patient if he felt a snap or pop.

____ 9. Have an athletic training student apply an ice bag to the leg.

____ 10. Ask the patient if he has ever injured his right leg before.

____ 11. Ask the patient if he can hop on the left leg.

Section B

You assist the patient off the court and have him sit on a bench. What actions would you perform at this time? (Please select and prioritize your choices.)

____ 12. Palpate the calf for pain, swelling, or deformity.

____ 13. Perform a Lachman's test bilaterally.

____ 14. Perform a Thomas test bilaterally.

____ 15. Check active range of motion of both ankles.

____ 16. Measure the Q-angle of the right leg.

____ 17. Check to see if the patient has bunions.

____ 18. Perform a Thompson's test bilaterally.

____ 19. Perform a Hawkin's test bilaterally.

____ 20. Perform an anterior drawer test bilaterally on both ankles.

____ 21. Palpate the left femoral pulse.

____ 22. Test the patellar tendon reflex bilaterally.

____ 23. Manually muscle test the ankle plantar flexors bilaterally.

Section C

Based on your initial assessment, you determine the patient has a torn gastrocnemius muscle. The patient is transported to the athletic training facility in a golf cart. What would your initial treatment consist of during week 1? (Please select and prioritize your choices.)

____ 24. Warm whirlpool treatments.

____ 25. Applying ice packs to the lower leg.

____ 26. Applying a compression wrap.

____ 27. High-volt galvanic stimulation.

____ 28. Posterior lower leg splint.

____ 29. Range of motion exercises on the BAPS board.

____ 30. Calf raises.

____ 31. Fitting the patient with crutches.

____ 32. Applying an antibiotic ointment to the defect.

____ 33. Begin hamstring curls with weight.

____ 34. Start ultrasound treatments.

____ 35. Begin gentle active range of motion exercises for the right ankle.

Section D

Four weeks have passed since the initial injury. The patient has minimal/no discomfort with active plantar flexion, but the movement is still weak against resistance (4/5). All other ankle and knee motions are within normal ranges. Which of the following exercises would be appropriate? (Please select and prioritize your choices.)

____ 36. Stationary bike.

____ 37. Uphill jogging.

____ 38. Push-ups.

____ 39. Progressive-resistance ankle exercises.

____ 40. Plyometric exercises.

____ 41. Upper body ergometer.

____ 42. Proprioception exercises.

____ 43. Calf raises.

____ 44. Partial squats.

____ 45. Progressive-resistance hamstring exercises.

____ 46. Progressive-resistance quadriceps exercises.

____ 47. General lower extremity flexibility exercises.

____ 48. Biceps curls.

____ 49. Shoulder press.

____ 50. Agility exercises.

Section E

Six weeks have passed since the initial injury. The patient has done very well during his rehabilitation. What specific criteria would you use to determine that this patient is fully recovered and ready to participate in tennis? (Please select and prioritize your choices.)

____ 51. The patient can walk 50 feet without a limp.

____ 52. The patient has no complaints of lower extremity pain at rest or during activity.

____ 53. There is no visible swelling or ecchymosis.

____ 54. There is no pain with palpation of the injured area.

____ 55. The patient has no pain while performing a hamstring curl.

____ 56. The patient has full ankle and knee range of motion.

____ 57. The coach demands the patient's return to competition.

____ 58. The patient can hop on the injured leg without pain.

____ 59. The patient can jog on the treadmill for 20 minutes without pain.

____ 60. The patient is getting bored with his rehabilitation program.

____ 61. The strength of the patient's left ankle and leg is equal to the right side.

____ 62. The team physician clears the patient to return to full activity.

____ 63. The patient can bench press 50 pounds or more.

PROBLEM VII

Opening Scene

You are covering a men's varsity basketball game when one of your players is observed injuring his right knee while rebounding a ball. He is able to limp off the court unassisted. He reports his knee bent sideways when he landed. He states he felt a sharp pain but cannot recall feeling a pop or snap.

Section A

What actions would you take during your initial assessment of this injury? (Please select and prioritize your choices.)

_____ 1. Ask the patient to point to where he feels pain.

_____ 2. Observe the right knee for swelling or deformity.

_____ 3. Apply an ice pack to the knee.

_____ 4. Apply a knee immobilizer to the injured extremity.

_____ 5. Issue a cane to the patient.

_____ 6. Palpate the right knee anterolateral/anteromedial joint line.

_____ 7. Palpate the right gluteus medius muscle.

_____ 8. Have the patient perform 10 calf raises.

_____ 9. Check the range of motion of both knee joints.

_____ 10. Ask the patient if he has ever injured his right knee before.

_____ 11. Manually muscle test the strength of the hip flexors bilaterally.

_____ 12. Manually muscle test the strength of the quadriceps bilaterally.

_____ 13. Manually muscle test the strength of the hamstrings bilaterally.

_____ 14. Check the patient's pupillary reaction.

Section B

What special tests would you perform during your evaluation of this injury? (Please select and prioritize your choices.)

_____ 15. Lachman's test bilaterally.

_____ 16. Vertebral artery test bilaterally.

_____ 17. Tinel's test bilaterally.

_____ 18. Valgus stress test bilaterally.

_____ 19. Varus stress test bilaterally.

_____ 20. Posterior drawer test bilaterally.

_____ 21. Empty can test bilaterally.

_____ 22. Finkelstein's test bilaterally.

_____ 23. Yergason's test bilaterally.

_____ 24. McMurray's test bilaterally.

_____ 25. Anterior drawer test bilaterally.

_____ 26. Pivot shift test bilaterally.

_____ 27. Patellar apprehension test bilaterally.

Section C

After being examined by the team physician, the patient is diagnosed with a second-degree medial collateral sprain. What actions would you take to control the pain and swelling and address the limitations in range of motion? (Please select and prioritize your choices.)

_____ 28. Apply moist heat packs to the right knee.

_____ 29. Massage the knee joint.

_____ 30. Have the patient use a rowing machine.

_____ 31. Fit the patient with crutches.

_____ 32. Manually muscle test the quadriceps.

_____ 33. Begin isotonic hamstring strength exercises.

_____ 34. Apply ice packs to the knee.

_____ 35. Have the patient perform active knee extension and flexion range of motion exercises as tolerated.

_____ 36. Have the patient elevate his left leg during the course of the day.

_____ 37. Give the patient Tylenol with codeine for pain.

_____ 38. Use high-volt galvanic stimulation.

Section D

The team physician recommends the patient begin rehabilitation in 1 week. Knowing the patient will be unable to return to basketball for approximately 4 to 5 weeks, how would you go about beginning a functional exercise program and maintaining his aerobic condition during weeks 1 to 2 postinjury? (Please select and prioritize your choices.)

_____ 39. Swimming (regular crawl).

_____ 40. Calf raises.

_____ 41. Running on the treadmill.

_____ 42. Stairmaster (low resistance).

_____ 43. Upper body ergometer.

_____ 44. Wall pulley exercises (upper extremity).

_____ 45. Stationary bicycling.

_____ 46. Fartlek training.

_____ 47. Plyometric exercises.

_____ 48. Rowing machine.

PROBLEM VIII

Opening Scene

A soccer player jumps up to head a ball. While he is in the air, he is kicked in the abdominal area by an opponent. He curls up in pain on the ground.

Section A

What steps would you take during your initial evaluation of this patient? (Please select and prioritize your choices.)

_____ 1. Perform a primary survey.

_____ 2. Give the patient oxygen.

_____ 3. Auscultate the patient's heart.

_____ 4. Palpate the abdominal area.

_____ 5. Ask the patient where the pain is located.

_____ 6. Have the patient stand and jog a little.

_____ 7. Have the patient count backward from 100.

_____ 8. Have an athletic training student bring out a stretcher.

_____ 9. Put on a glove before touching the patient.

_____ 10. Observe the abdominal area for edema or ecchymosis.

_____ 11. Ask if the pain radiates anywhere.

Section B

Following your initial evaluation, you have determined this patient has sustained a contusion to the lower right quadrant. What actions would you take at this time? (Please select and prioritize your choices.)

_____ 12. Apply an ice pack to the injured area.

_____ 13. Apply a compression wrap to the injured area.

_____ 14. Massage the patient's lumbar area.

_____ 15. Massage the patient's abdominal area.

_____ 16. Assist the patient to walk off the field if he is able to do so.

_____ 17. Apply a neoprene rib belt.

_____ 18. Position the patient in supine with his knees bent.

_____ 19. Monitor the patient for any changes in pain intensity.

_____ 20. Take the patient's pulse and blood pressure.

Section C

You follow up with the patient the next day in the athletic training facility. He states he is sore but has less pain today. How would you treat this patient at this time? (Please select and prioritize your choices.)

_____ 21. Continue to apply ice to the injured area.

_____ 22. Begin to apply moist heat packs.

_____ 23. Manually muscle test the abdominal muscles.

_____ 24. Re-evaluate the injury.

_____ 25. Have the patient drink a glass of Gatorade.

_____ 26. Pad the area for activity.

_____ 27. Have the patient begin exercises on an upper body ergometer.

PROBLEM IX

Opening Scene

Two soccer players collide head-on during a game. You are called onto the field by the referee after your player does not get up off his back. You did not witness the collision.

Section A

How will you begin your initial evaluation of the patient's condition? (Please select and prioritize your choices.)

_____ 1. Ask the patient where his pain is located.

_____ 2. Immediately roll the patient onto his side.

_____ 3. Check to see if the patient can move his fingers and toes.

_____ 4. As you approach the field, ask any witnesses what occurred.

_____ 5. Check the patient for any areas that may be bleeding.

_____ 6. Instruct an athletic training student to call for an ambulance.

_____ 7. Evaluate the patient's level of consciousness.

_____ 8. Perform a primary survey.

_____ 9. Ask the patient if he has ever had a prior head injury.

_____ 10. Note the position of the patient.

_____ 11. Ask if the patient can stand and walk.

_____ 12. Check the patient's pupillary reactions with a penlight.

_____ 13. Place an ice pack on the patient's left shoulder.

_____ 14. Remove the patient from the playing field.

_____ 15. Ask the patient if he can remember what happened and ask him to explain.

_____ 16. Assess the patient's pulse rate and blood pressure.

_____ 17. Ask the athletic training student to get a spine board.

_____ 18. Sit the patient up to make breathing easier.

Section B

The patient is able to get up and walk off the field to the sidelines without assistance. Based on the information you now have, what would you do next? (Please select and prioritize your choices.)

____ 19. Perform a secondary survey.

____ 20. Ask the patient if he knows where he is, the date, and the name of his coach.

____ 21. Escort the patient to the athletic training facility and let him sleep.

____ 22. Give the patient aspirin for a headache.

____ 23. Palpate the patient's cervical area.

____ 24. Palpate the patient's left upper trapezius muscle.

____ 25. Check the patient's bilateral grip strength.

____ 26. Tell the coach the patient is not to return to the game.

____ 27. Observe the patient's posturing as he walks off the field.

____ 28. Note the patient's skin color.

____ 29. Ask the patient's parents what type of medical insurance they have.

____ 30. Call the team physician to gain guidance.

____ 31. Call the patient's parents to make sure they arrange a doctor's visit the next day.

____ 32. Elevate the patient's feet.

____ 33. Give the patient a pair of crutches.

Section C

Your athletic training staff has escorted the patient to the athletic training facility. You meet the patient there and reassess his injury. (Please select and prioritize your choices.)

____ 34. Record the patient's vital signs every 10 minutes.

____ 35. Manually muscle test the upper trapezius muscle.

____ 36. Perform an Adson's test.

____ 37. Manually muscle test the deltoids.

____ 38. Manually muscle test the rotator cuff musculature.

____ 39. Have the patient sit with his head between his knees.

____ 40. Have the patient do a couple of deep squats.

____ 41. Ask the patient to count backward from 50.

____ 42. Check the deep tendon reflex of the triceps bilaterally.

____ 43. Give the patient oxygen via a mask.

____ 44. Have the team physician come to the athletic training facility to reassess the injury.

____ 45. Have the patient drive himself home.

____ 46. Check the patient's sensation of the left upper arm.

____ 47. Check the active range of motion of the patient's neck.

____ 48. Test for a Tinel's sign.

____ 49. Palpate the lateral epicondyle of the elbow for any tenderness.

____ 50. Manually muscle test the biceps.

____ 51. Manually muscle test the triceps.

Section D

The team physician has arrived and re-evaluated the athlete. He determines the athlete has a concussion and a left-sided "burner." What would you do at this time? (Please select and prioritize your choices.)

____ 52. Put an ice pack on the athlete's left shoulder.

____ 53. Assess if the athlete still has sensory changes in his left upper arm or hand.

____ 54. Let the coach know the athlete has a minor injury and will play tomorrow.

____ 55. Have the physician write a note to keep the athlete home the next 2 days for observation by his parents.

____ 56. Give the athlete shoulder strengthening exercises.

____ 57. See if the athlete can do a few push-ups.

____ 58. Monitor the athlete the next few days for any changes in his condition.

____ 59. Make sure the team physician clears the athlete first before he returns to playing soccer.

____ 60. Give the athlete a soft neck collar to wear.

Problem X

Opening Scene

A wrestler from an opposing high school was elbowed in the nose prior to his arrival to your school for a county tournament. Throughout the tournament, he has been experiencing recurrent nosebleeds. He approaches you during an active nosebleed.

Section A

How will you begin your initial evaluation and treatment of the patient's condition? (Please select and prioritize your choices.)

____ 1. Ask the patient how hard he was hit.

____ 2. Ask the patient if he has had a similar problem in the past.

____ 3. Ask the patient if his parents are aware of his current problem.

____ 4. Ask the patient if he has any allergies.

____ 5. Have the patient put his head between his knees.

____ 6. Ask the patient if he is dizzy.

____ 7. Take the patient's pulse and blood pressure.

___ 8. Ask the patient if his athletic trainer has given him a noseguard.

___ 9. Place a warm compress on his nose.

___ 10. Ask the patient if he has high blood pressure.

___ 11. Apply pressure to the patient's right cheek.

___ 12. Palpate the patient's nose and surrounding areas for pain and swelling.

___ 13. Observe the nose for swelling or deformity.

___ 14. Put an ice pack behind the patient's neck.

___ 15. Allow the patient to blow his nose to clear the nostril.

___ 16. Place a cotton nose plug under the patient's top lip.

Section B

The nosebleed is beginning to stop. With this information, what would be your next steps? (Please select and prioritize your choices.)

___ 17. Perform a primary survey.

___ 18. Keep the patient lying down with his legs elevated.

___ 19. Allow the patient to apply finger pressure to the bridge of his nose.

___ 20. Allow your athletic training student to find the patient's coach or a responsible adult so your assessment can be shared.

___ 21. Do not let the patient return to the competition for the rest of the day.

___ 22. Apply a nose splint.

___ 23. Have the patient sit with his head tilted back.

___ 24. Call the patient's home athletic trainer.

___ 25. Use a cotton nose plug to stop the bleeding.

___ 26. Give the patient aspirin for the swelling.

___ 27. Make sure there is no blood present on the patient, his clothing, the mat, and the floor.

Section C

The nosebleed has stopped. What would be your final actions, and what instructions would you provide the patient with at this time? (Please select and prioritize your choices.)

___ 28. Call your team doctor to report what happened.

___ 29. Call the patient's team doctor to report what happened.

___ 30. Have the patient's parents come to your athletic training facility.

___ 31. Limit the patient's fluid intake.

___ 32. Allow the patient to return to the competition.

___ 33. Send the patient for x-rays.

___ 34. Call the patient's athletic trainer to report what happened.

___ 35. Have the patient do 10 sit-ups.

___ 36. Use a biohazard bag for any contaminated materials.

___ 37. Maintain close contact with the patient during the remainder of the competition.

___ 38. Tell the patient to keep an ice pack on his nose while he is not competing.

PROBLEM XI

Opening Scene

You are covering a basketball game when one of your players steps on another player's foot. You see the patient twist his left ankle. He is jogging with an obvious limp. The coach calls a time-out.

Section A

What will your initial evaluation include? (Please select and prioritize your choices.)

___ 1. Check the patient's low back for an injury.

___ 2. Get a wheelchair.

___ 3. Check the patient's hamstring flexibility.

___ 4. Observe both ankles for swelling/deformity.

___ 5. Have the patient jog off the court.

___ 6. Gently bang on the heel of the injured ankle.

___ 7. Perform a Lachman's test.

___ 8. Perform an anterior draw test on both ankles.

___ 9. Palpate the ankle and foot for areas of tenderness.

___ 10. Check the range of motion of the left ankle.

Section B

You have completed your initial evaluation and suspect that he has a second-degree lateral ankle sprain of his left ankle. With assistance, the patient is brought into the athletic training facility. What is your initial treatment going to include? (Please select and prioritize your choices.)

___ 11. Keep the patient in nonweightbearing.

___ 12. Dispense aspirin to the patient.

___ 13. Begin RICE.

___ 14. Call the team doctor with your assessment.

___ 15. Begin ultrasound treatments.

___ 16. Place the left ankle in a hot whirlpool.

___ 17. Fit the patient with crutches.

___ 18. Set up an appointment for an x-ray.

___ 19. Begin an upper body exercise program.

___ 20. After the game, present your findings to the coach.

___ 21. Begin a Theraband strengthening program for the left ankle.

Section C

The team doctor is scheduled to be in the athletic training facility tomorrow morning. What instructions will you give the patient for home? (Please select and prioritize your choices.)

___ 22. If he still has mild/moderate pain tonight, have the patient go to the nearest emergency room.

___ 23. Call the patient's parents with information on what happened.

___ 24. Begin lower extremity closed-chain exercises as tolerated.

___ 25. Keep ice packs on the ankle frequently and elevate it when the patient is not ambulating.

___ 26. Keep a compression wrap on the ankle except when the patient is sleeping.

___ 27. Have the patient wear high-top sneakers.

___ 28. Have the patient try to hop on the affected leg the next day to see if it still hurts.

PROBLEM XII

Opening Scene

The women's gymnastics coach reports to your office to discuss the behavior of one of her patients. After reviewing what the coach has observed over the past month, you both suspect the patient may be showing signs of anorexia nervosa.

Section A

With the information you now have available, how would you advise the coach to proceed? (Please select and prioritize your choices.)

___ 1. Confront the patient with her problem and do not allow her to compete until the team physician evaluates her.

___ 2. Do not overemphasize the impact of lower body weight on the patient's performance.

___ 3. Tell the coach to keep a diary of when the patient eats.

___ 4. Have the coach encourage the patient to maintain good nutritional habits to optimize her performance.

___ 5. Keep the athletic training staff informed if the patient dramatically changes her behavior.

Section B

The patient has talked with the coach and comes to your office to express her fear of being cut from the team. With the information available, how would you proceed? (Please select and prioritize your choices.)

___ 6. Assist the patient in setting practical goals pertaining to safe means of dieting and determining a sensible target weight.

___ 7. Use "scare" tactics to discourage the use of laxatives and diuretics.

___ 8. Encourage the patient to express her fears and concerns regarding her weight and athletic abilities.

___ 9. Address the issue with your athletic director.

___ 10. Discuss the patient's options in case she is cut from the gymnastics team.

___ 11. Tell the patient she has nothing to worry about and you will talk to the coach for her.

___ 12. Tell the patient she should think about getting professional counseling to overcome her problem.

___ 13. Set up a meeting between the coach, patient, and yourself to discuss what has been observed and how it will be managed.

Section C

The patient concedes to you and the coach that she may have an eating disorder. With this information available, what are your next steps? (Please select and prioritize your choices.)

___ 14. Call the team physician.

___ 15. Set up an appointment with a psychologist.

___ 16. Put the patient on a strict diet emphasizing weight gain.

___ 17. Weigh the patient on a daily basis.

___ 18. Arrange for the patient to be hospitalized for a week to force feed her.

___ 19. Arrange counseling meetings for the patient with a sports nutritionist.

___ 20. Put the patient on a diet consisting of Ensure, bananas, and red meat at least twice a day.

PROBLEM XIII

Opening Scene

You are traveling with your school's men's basketball team when one of your patients comes to you complaining he has been having abdominal cramping and intermittent diarrhea for the past 2 days.

Section A

Based on the preceding information, how would you proceed with your initial assessment of this patient? (Please select and prioritize your choices.)

_____ 1. Ask the patient what his diet has consisted of (food and drink) during the past 2 to 3 days.

_____ 2. Ask the patient if he is nervous about playing.

_____ 3. Ask the patient if he has had this problem before.

_____ 4. Check the patient's blood pressure.

_____ 5. Take the patient's oral temperature.

_____ 6. Check the patient's body fat levels.

_____ 7. Palpate the patient's abdomen.

_____ 8. Have the patient run on a treadmill for 20 minutes.

Section B

Assuming from your evaluation that this patient has a gastrointestinal upset because of precompetition anxiety, what might your next steps be in assisting in this patient's recovery? (Please select and prioritize your choices.)

_____ 9. Speak with the coach and have the patient refrain from practice until the symptoms disappear.

_____ 10. Weigh the patient before and after practices and games.

_____ 11. Give the patient antimotility drugs, such as Imodium.

_____ 12. Make sure the patient eats a lot of green vegetables, like broccoli and cabbage.

_____ 13. Give the patient milk, soda, or tea to rehydrate.

_____ 14. Buy a water-testing kit and evaluate the hotel's drinking water.

_____ 15. Have the patient drink only bottled water.

PROBLEM XIV

Opening Scene

A soccer player injures his knee during practice. He is assisted into the athletic training facility by 2 teammates. Upon your initial observation, you notice he is limping and his right knee is visibly swollen.

Section A

Given the above information, how would you proceed with your initial evaluation of this patient? (Please select and prioritize your choices.)

_____ 1. Palpate the knee joint and surrounding areas for point tenderness.

_____ 2. Ask the patient if he can do a deep squat without pain.

_____ 3. Ask the patient what happened.

_____ 4. Check the dorsalis pedis pulse of the affected limb.

_____ 5. Ask the patient if he heard or felt a snap or pop.

_____ 6. Perform a Speed's test.

_____ 7. Perform a Lachman's test.

_____ 8. Check the knee for crepitus.

_____ 9. Ask the patient if he has had a prior injury to the affected knee.

_____ 10. Measure the range of motion of the affected knee.

_____ 11. Assess the strength of the patient's hip abductors.

_____ 12. Ask the patient to perform toe raises.

_____ 13. Perform a pivot shift test on the involved knee.

Section B

After evaluating the patient's knee, you suspect the patient has injured his anterior cruciate ligament. What steps would you take at this time? (Please select and prioritize your choices.)

_____ 14. Issue crutches to the patient and instruct him in toe-touch weightbearing.

_____ 15. Wrap the patient's knee in ice and elevate his leg.

_____ 16. Call the team physician.

_____ 17. Apply McConnell taping to the injured knee.

_____ 18. Instruct the patient to use a heating pad on his knee when he is at rest at home.

_____ 19. Order a functional brace for use during activity.

_____ 20. Apply ultrasound (pulsed) to the injured knee.

Section C

The team physician comes to the athletic training facility and, after examining the patient, agrees with your assessment and recommends the patient have an MRI to confirm the physical findings. Until the severity of the injury is known, he asks you to instruct the patient in the appropriate treatments for home. (Please select and prioritize your choices.)

_____ 21. Instruct the patient in knee and hip active range of motion exercises as tolerated.

_____ 22. Have the patient apply ice to the knee every few hours to minimize swelling.

_____ 23. Tell the patient to wean himself from the crutches to a cane over the next 24 hours.

_____ 24. Work on proprioception by having the patient practice balancing on the unaffected leg twice a day.

_____ 25. Instruct the patient to perform isometric quadriceps and hamstring exercises.

_____ 26. Give the patient a TENS unit for home use.

_____ 27. Have the patient practice going up and down stairs and jog as normally as possible.

Problem XV

Opening Scene

A football player comes to you requesting help in improving his general lower body strength and overall conditioning.

Section A

What suggestions would you make in assisting this patient in a preseason training program? (Please select and prioritize your choices.)

____ 1. Give the patient anabolic steroids.

____ 2. Instruct the patient in a general flexibility program.

____ 3. Have the patient run up and down the stadium stairs in pads.

____ 4. Monitor the patient's respiratory rate while at rest.

____ 5. Incorporate warm-up and cool-down periods.

____ 6. Make the exercises sport-specific.

____ 7. Have the patient participate in other sports, such as basketball or tennis.

____ 8. Have the patient perform progressive-resistance lower extremity exercises 3 days a week.

____ 9. Put the patient on a red meat and legume diet.

____ 10. Mix the training schedule to keep it interesting.

____ 11. Keep the training schedule intense and emphasize training for long periods of time (eg, 3 to 4 hours).

____ 12. Progress the conditioning program gradually as the patient improves his tolerance for work.

____ 13. Help the patient adjust to working in the heat.

Section B

As the football season begins, the patient continues to seek your advice to keep him fit and healthy. What types of things might you emphasize to keep him in condition during the season? (Please select and prioritize your choices.)

____ 14. Have the patient run 2 miles 3 times a week.

____ 15. Continue strength training exercises for the lower body.

____ 16. Make sure the patient takes 2 to 3 days off a week so he gets adequate rest.

____ 17. Monitor the patient's blood pressure on a daily basis.

____ 18. Have the patient perform plyometric activities for power.

____ 19. Establish a maintenance conditioning program to be performed on a regular basis.

____ 20. Put the patient on a clear liquid diet.

____ 21. Have the patient participate in a cross-training program.

____ 22. Give the patient a tennis ball so he can work on grip strengthening.

____ 23. Encourage the patient to take a class in judo.

Section C

What types of activities might you suggest the patient participate in as part of an off-season program? (Please select and prioritize your choices.)

____ 24. Continue a general flexibility program.

____ 25. Have the patient participate in a cross-training program.

____ 26. Have the patient jog 4 to 5 times a week.

____ 27. Have the patient eat a high-calorie diet to build up muscle strength.

____ 28. Have the patient meet with a sport psychologist to learn visual imagery.

____ 29. No physical activity. This is the period during which the patient should rest and recover.

____ 30. Give the patient time during his training schedule to participate in nonathletic events.

____ 31. Have the patient take up another sport to stay in shape.

Problem XVI

Opening Scene

An ice hockey player slams head first into the boards during practice. He is lying face down on the ice and is not moving. You have witnessed this event and no other players are involved.

Section A

How will you begin your initial evaluation of this patient's condition? (Please select and prioritize your choices.)

____ 1. Perform a secondary survey of the patient's entire body.

____ 2. With assistance, roll the patient onto his back while maintaining the head and neck in neutral.

____ 3. Remove the patient's helmet.

____ 4. Perform a primary survey.

____ 5. Establish the level of consciousness.

____ 6. Begin chest compressions.

____ 7. Have the coach get a vacuum splint.

____ 8. Ask the other players what happened during the last play.

____ 9. Sit the patient up so he can breathe.

Section B

You have determined the patient is unconscious and is not breathing, but he has a pulse. What are your next steps in treating this patient? (Please select and prioritize your choices.)

___ 10. Perform a secondary survey.

___ 11. Have the coach call for an ambulance.

___ 12. Vigorously shake the patient to try and get a response.

___ 13. Take the patient's blood pressure.

___ 14. Cut off the facemask.

___ 15. Log-roll the patient onto his side.

___ 16. Check the patient for a positive Romberg's sign.

___ 17. Perform abdominal thrusts to clear the airway.

___ 18. Begin artificial respiration.

___ 19. Establish if the patient is in cardiac arrest.

___ 20. Remove the patient's mouthguard.

___ 21. Use a jaw-thrust to open the patient's airway.

Section C

The EMS team has arrived. The patient begins breathing again and becomes responsive. He states he cannot feel anything. With this information, what will be your next actions? (Please select and prioritize your choices.)

___ 22. Perform a secondary survey.

___ 23. Continue to monitor breathing, pulse, and blood pressure.

___ 24. Tell the patient not to worry, that he should feel something soon, and it is a temporary problem.

___ 25. With assistance, secure the patient onto a spine board while maintaining the head and neck in neutral.

___ 26. Call your team doctor.

___ 27. Check pupillary response with a penlight.

___ 28. Argue with the EMS team about whether or not the patient's helmet should be removed.

___ 29. Tell the coach you will be at the emergency room and you will be in touch with him later.

___ 30. Fill out an incident report to document what happened.

Section D

After practice, you go to the hospital to check on the patient's condition. The emergency room physician informs you the patient will probably be a C5,6 quadriplegic. With this information available, what would you do next? (Please select and prioritize your choices.)

___ 31. Check on the patient to see how he is doing.

___ 32. Call the team physician to inform him what has happened.

___ 33. Contact the patient's parents.

___ 34. Tell the patient sometimes doctors make mistakes and not to give up hope.

___ 35. Check your liability insurance.

___ 36. Call the local newspaper to give them the story.

___ 37. Return to school and inform the coach.

___ 38. With the coaching staff, inform the team what has happened.

___ 39. Have the emergency room physician contact your athletic director.

Problem XVII

Opening Scene

A wrestler stops by the athletic training facility after practice complaining of chronic low back pain that increases a few hours to a day after a workout. He states he has had this pain before and has seen an orthopedic surgeon who had diagnosed him with a chronic low back strain. The patient denies having any radicular signs and states the pain is localized to the lumbar area.

Section A

With the information that is available to you, what would your initial evaluation include? (Please select and prioritize your choices.)

___ 1. Observe the patient's posture in standing.

___ 2. Ask the patient to describe his pain.

___ 3. Check the range of motion of both knees.

___ 4. Perform a Scour test of the right hip.

___ 5. Palpate the lumbar erector spinae.

___ 6. Observe the low back for signs of atrophy.

___ 7. Palpate the posterior superior iliac spine bilaterally.

___ 8. Check the patient for genu varum.

___ 9. Check the patient for a leg-length discrepancy.

___ 10. Have the patient do a partial squat.

___ 11. Evaluate the range of motion of the lumbar spine.

___ 12. Measure hip abduction with a goniometer.

___ 13. Check the flexibility of the hamstrings and hip flexors.

Section B

Your findings from the initial evaluation are consistent with a chronic lumbar strain. The patient does not appear to be in severe pain but does seem uncomfortable with active lumbar movement. Which of the following modalities would be appropriate to decrease this patient's pain? (Please select and prioritize your choices.)

___ 14. Friction massage.

___ 15. Ice packs.

___ 16. Warm whirlpool treatments (full body).

___ 17. Ultrasound.

___ 18. Iontophoresis.

___ 19. Ice massage.

___ 20. Chiropractic treatments.

___ 21. TENS therapy.

___ 22. Moist heat packs.

___ 23. Short-wave diathermy.

___ 24. Stationary bicycling.

___ 25. Functional electric stimulation.

___ 26. Cervical traction.

___ 27. Paraffin bath.

___ 28. Effleurage.

___ 29. Neoprene lumbar support.

Section C

Regarding the initial phases (I and II) of the rehabilitation program, which of the following exercises would be most appropriate? (Please select and prioritize your choices.)

___ 30. Active trunk extensions in prone.

___ 31. Gentle active-assisted low back stretching.

___ 32. Resisted knee extensions.

___ 33. Passive hamstring stretching.

___ 34. Active posterior pelvic tilts.

___ 35. Passive iliopsoas stretching.

___ 36. PNF exercises to the hip and lower extremity.

___ 37. Lower trunk rotations in supine.

Section D

Regarding the later phases (III and IV) of the rehabilitation program, which of the following exercises would be most appropriate? (Please select and prioritize your choices.)

___ 38. PNF exercises to the trunk.

___ 39. Resistive abdominal strengthening.

___ 40. Resistive cervical strengthening.

___ 41. Resistive prone hip extension.

___ 42. Achilles stretching exercises.

___ 43. Groin stretching exercises.

___ 44. Shoulder press.

___ 45. Jogging.

___ 46. Swimming.

___ 47. Resistive bridging exercises.

___ 48. Trunk extensions in prone.

PROBLEM XVIII

Opening Scene

One of your swimmers comes to your office complaining of severe ear pain that is accompanied by intense itching and a mild discharge.

Section A

Upon examining the patient's ear, you notice the ear canal is inflamed, and the patient has partial hearing loss. Based on these findings, you determine the patient has external otitis (swimmer's ear). What should you do to begin treatment of this condition? (Please select and prioritize your choices.)

___ 1. Dispense penicillin.

___ 2. Clear out the ear with a cotton swab soaked in epinephrine.

___ 3. Arrange for the patient to see the team physician.

___ 4. Cover the ear with a sterile gauze pad.

___ 5. Advise the patient to wear a hood in cold environments.

___ 6. Use a TENS unit for pain.

___ 7. Apply a moist heat pack to the affected ear.

___ 8. Allow the patient to continue swimming as tolerated.

Section B

The team physician comes to the athletic training facility, examines the patient, and makes a diagnosis of external otitis. He dispenses an oral antibiotic and ear drops (3% boric acid and alcohol) to be administered daily. In addition to these treatments, you instruct the patient in which of the following measures? (Please select and prioritize your choices.)

___ 9. Protect the patient's ear while swimming with a plug of lamb's wool soaked with lanolin.

___ 10. Have the patient wear a bathing cap when swimming.

___ 11. Have the patient cross-train to prevent frustration from not swimming.

___ 12. Instruct the patient to wear goggles while swimming.

___ 13. Instruct the patient not to stick any object into his ears.

PROBLEM XIX

Opening Scene

You are covering a high school field hockey game when one of your players gets hit hard in the mouth with a stick. She comes running off the field with her hand covering her mouth. There is a copious amount of blood on her face and hands.

Section A

What steps would you take during your initial evaluation of this patient? (Please select and prioritize your choices.)

_____ 1. Rinse the patient's mouth out with water.

_____ 2. Clean the patient's mouth out with a paper towel.

_____ 3. Don gloves.

_____ 4. Ask the patient why she is crying.

_____ 5. Ask the patient if she was wearing a mouthguard.

_____ 6. Review the school's liability insurance.

_____ 7. Observe the mouth, lips, and surrounding structures for lacerations or abrasions.

_____ 8. Palpate the mouth and surrounding structures for deformity.

_____ 9. Ask an athletic training student to get a cervical collar.

_____ 10. Have the patient open and close her mouth.

Section B

During your initial evaluation, you observe the patient is missing a front tooth. One of the patient's teammates comes to the sidelines with the tooth in her hand. What actions would you take at this time? (Please select and prioritize your choices.)

_____ 11. Ask the officials to stop the game.

_____ 12. Have an athletic training student take the patient to the school nurse.

_____ 13. Discuss your findings with the patient's parents.

_____ 14. Call your team physician for guidance.

_____ 15. Apply an ice pack to the mouth area.

_____ 16. Apply a cotton plug between the lip and injured gum.

_____ 17. Place the tooth in a container of sterile saline solution.

_____ 18. Rinse the tooth off with water.

_____ 19. Send the patient with the tooth to a dentist in less than 30 minutes.

_____ 20. Discard the tooth.

_____ 21. Place the patient in a side-lying position.

PROBLEM XX

Opening Scene

A wrestler comes to the athletic training facility during his off-season and asks you to help him lose 15 pounds. This patient had attempted to lose a significant amount of weight before and failed.

Section A

How would you advise the wrestler in his initial steps to lose the weight safely? (Please select and prioritize your choices.)

_____ 1. Have the patient consume a protein drink once a day in addition to his regular diet.

_____ 2. Measure the patient's percent body fat using calipers.

_____ 3. Have the patient read the _American Heart Association Cookbook_.

_____ 4. Send the patient to an acupuncturist.

_____ 5. Have the patient keep a log of what he eats on a daily basis.

_____ 6. Monitor the patient's weight loss progress once a week.

_____ 7. Put the patient on a fasting diet for 2 days.

_____ 8. Make sure the patient drinks 8 glasses of water daily.

_____ 9. Weigh the patient prior to beginning his program.

_____ 10. Have the patient sit in a sauna.

_____ 11. Monitor the patient's exercise program.

_____ 12. Assist the patient in developing a balanced diet.

_____ 13. Have the patient wear a rubber suit while running.

_____ 14. Put the patient on a lower extremity strengthening program.

Section B

The patient successfully loses the weight. How would you go about advising the patient in maintaining his current weight? (Please select and prioritize your choices.)

_____ 15. Continue to monitor the patient's food intake via a log.

_____ 16. Have the coach monitor the patient's food intake.

_____ 17. Have the patient drink 8 glasses of water a day.

_____ 18. Have the patient double his exercise session in duration.

_____ 19. Have the patient take laxatives.

_____ 20. Refer the patient to a sports nutritionist.

_____ 21. Encourage the patient to eat 4 to 6 small balanced meals a day.

_____ 22. Put the patient on an upper body strength program.

PROBLEM XXI

Opening Scene

A wide receiver gets a hard hit from the front while catching a football and lands hard on his right leg. He is lying on his back and is in severe pain. You immediately observe that his injured lower extremity is in a flexed, adducted, and internally rotated position.

Section A

How will you begin to evaluate the severity and nature of this injury? (Please select and prioritize your choices.)

_____ 1. Immediately straighten the leg and splint it in neutral.

_____ 2. Check the patient's vital signs.

_____ 3. Immediately cut away the patient's pant leg.

_____ 4. Perform a Lachman's test.

_____ 5. Remove the facemask.

_____ 6. Ask the patient where his pain is located.

_____ 7. Sit the patient upright.

_____ 8. Test bilateral lower extremity sensation.

_____ 9. Move the patient off the playing field.

_____ 10. Elevate both legs.

_____ 11. Have the coach call for an ambulance.

_____ 12. Check the rest of the patient's body for other injuries.

_____ 13. Ask the patient what happened.

_____ 14. Tell the patient not to move.

_____ 15. Palpate the rest of the right lower extremity for any deformities.

Section B

You have ruled out a knee injury and suspect the patient has sustained a traumatic right hip dislocation. With this information how would you proceed? (Please select and prioritize your choices.)

_____ 16. Call the patient's parents.

_____ 17. Check the patient for symptoms of shock.

_____ 18. Allow the competition to continue.

_____ 19. Keep the area clear of players.

_____ 20. Get the patient up on crutches.

_____ 21. Apply a vacuum splint to the entire lower extremity.

_____ 22. Put an ice pack on the right thigh and groin.

_____ 23. Give the patient aspirin for pain.

_____ 24. Check the hip for crepitus.

_____ 25. Ask the patient if he can actively extend his right leg.

_____ 26. Palpate the popliteal and dorsalis pedis pulses.

_____ 27. Keep the patient calm and encourage him not to move.

Section C

The ambulance has arrived with the EMS team, and the patient is going to be transported to the emergency room of the local hospital. What are your final steps before he leaves with the paramedics? (Please select and prioritize your choices.)

_____ 28. Call ahead to the emergency room to make arrangements for his arrival.

_____ 29. Allow the patient to drink some Gatorade.

_____ 30. Have a coach follow the patient to the hospital.

_____ 31. Reassure the patient that he will be taken care of before he departs.

_____ 32. Take the patient's helmet off.

_____ 33. Move the patient onto a spine board.

_____ 34. Fill out an injury report.

_____ 35. Call the patient's parents to let them know what has happened.

_____ 36. Contact the athletic director to give him a verbal report.

PROBLEM XXII

Opening Scene

As the second half of a high school basketball game begins, you are returning to the court when you find one of the referees kneeling down. He states that he is nauseous, and he is sweating profusely. He also tells you that he has "a heavy pressure in his chest."

Section A

How will you begin your initial evaluation of the referee's condition? (Please select and prioritize your choices.)

_____ 1. Ask the referee what happened.

_____ 2. Send someone for an ACE.

_____ 3. Tell the referee "not to worry about it" and that "he's just a little out of shape."

_____ 4. Have the referee remove his shirt.

_____ 5. Ask the other referee to stop the game.

_____ 6. Check the referee's vital signs.

_____ 7. Ask the referee if he is taking any medications.

_____ 8. Administer nitroglycerine.

_____ 9. Walk the referee to the men's locker room.

_____ 10. Ask the referee if he has ever experienced this before.

_____ 11. Ask the referee if he smokes.

_____ 12. Ask the referee if he has pain going down the left arm.

Section B

Based on the above information, you suspect the referee might be having a myocardial infarction. How will you proceed at this time? (Please select and prioritize your choices.)

___ 13. Send someone for the team doctor.

___ 14. Send someone for the automated external defibrillator.

___ 15. Lie the referee on his back.

___ 16. Inform the referee that he is having a heart attack.

___ 17. Call the referee's wife to inform her that her husband is having a heart attack and you are "sending for a squad."

___ 18. Put ice on the back of the referee's neck.

___ 19. Ask the referee to cough.

___ 20. Ask the referee is he is short of breath.

___ 21. Check the capillary refill of the fingers and toes.

___ 22. Try to put the referee at ease; speak to him with confidence, and let him know what you are doing to keep him calm.

___ 23. Activate the EMS.

Section C

The referee suddenly clutches his chest and collapses onto the court. What would your next actions be? (Please select and prioritize your choices.)

___ 24. Check the referee for responsiveness.

___ 25. Look for a doctor in the stands.

___ 26. Conduct a primary survey.

___ 27. Scream at the referee to "wake up!"

___ 28. Place the referee on a spine board with assistance from the coaches.

___ 29. Check for facial droop.

___ 30. Apply the automated external defibrillator.

___ 31. Perform abdominal thrusts.

___ 32. Begin CPR until the automated external defibrillator arrives.

___ 33. Roll the referee onto his right side.

Section D

The referee responds to the use of the automated external defibrillator. He is breathing on his own and has a palpable carotid pulse. The paramedics have just arrived at the field house and are preparing to take him to the hospital. What actions would you take after the referee leaves the school? (Please select and prioritize your choices.)

___ 34. Contact the local newspaper to inform them of the incident so they have the correct information.

___ 35. Fill out an incident report.

___ 36. Contact your athletic director.

___ 37. Follow the ambulance to the hospital.

___ 38. Return to the basketball game as play resumes.

PROBLEM XXIII

Opening Scene

You are covering a soccer game on a cold day when you notice one of your players is having difficulty breathing about 7 minutes into the game. He comes off the field coughing and complaining of "chest tightness."

Section A

How will you begin your initial evaluation of this player's condition? (Please select and prioritize your choices.)

___ 1. Ask if the patient is a diabetic.

___ 2. Ask the patient if this has ever happened to him before.

___ 3. Give the patient Imodium.

___ 4. Lie the patient in supine, and flex his knees to his chest.

___ 5. Ask the patient if he has an inhaler.

___ 6. Talk with the patient to keep him calm.

___ 7. Tell the coach you are going to send the patient to the team doctor.

Section B

You suspect that the patient has exercise-induced bronchospasm. What would your next steps be when caring for this patient? (Please select and prioritize your choices.)

___ 8. Have the patient breathe slowly through the nose.

___ 9. Check the patient's pulse rate.

___ 10. Have the patient breathe into a paper bag.

___ 11. Have the patient take 2 puffs of a short-acting inhaler.

___ 12. Have the patient slow to a less intense pace by performing a slow jog and/or stretch on the sidelines.

___ 13. Give the patient a warm drink like tea or hot chocolate.

___ 14. Have the patient sit down to rest.

___ 15. Tell the coach you are taking the patient out of the game.

___ 16. Monitor the patient's symptoms until they subside, and continue to monitor the patient for up to 12 hours after exercise.

Problem XXIV

Opening Scene

A football player comes to the athletic training facility complaining of severe low back pain that is radiating down his right leg. He is very guarded and is slightly forward flexed at the waist. He states that he was lifting in the weight room and his pain started after he lowered a dumbbell to the floor.

Section A

Your initial evaluation of this problem would include which of the following actions? (Please select and prioritize your choices.)

____ 1. Use iontophoresis on the patient's back.

____ 2. Put a moist heat pack on the patient's back.

____ 3. Palpate the lumbar erector spinae, sacroiliac areas, and both posterior superior iliac spine for tenderness.

____ 4. Observe the patient's trunk to see if there is a "lateral shift" present.

____ 5. Perform an Apley compression test.

____ 6. Perform a Slump test.

____ 7. Ask the patient how far the pain is felt down his leg.

____ 8. Ask the patient if he has a history of low back problems.

____ 9. Give the patient a back massage.

____ 10. Lie the patient in supine with his knees in full flexion.

Section B

The patient reports significant increasing pain down his leg to the level of his foot when he tries to bend forward. You suspect the patient has a lumbar herniated nucleus propulsus. What steps would you take at this time to treat this patient? (Please select and prioritize your choices.)

____ 11. Have the patient lie in prone.

____ 12. Teach the patient a series of Williams' flexion exercises.

____ 13. Tape the patient's lower back for support.

____ 14. Give the patient a muscle relaxant like Flexeril.

____ 15. Call the team physician, and suggest he order a MRI.

____ 16. Send the patient to a chiropractor.

____ 17. Teach the patient how to perform prone press-ups.

____ 18. Place an ice pack on the patient's back after exercise.

Section C

After a couple of days of treatment, the patient's radicular signs begin to centralize. What recommendations would you make to this patient to prevent another episode of lumbar pain? (Please select and prioritize your choices.)

____ 19. Keep his quadratus lumborum flexible.

____ 20. Avoid lifting heavy objects.

____ 21. Make sure he is using proper body mechanics while lifting.

____ 22. Maintain good hamstring flexibility.

____ 23. Take Advil on a regular basis before playing football.

____ 24. Make sure he bends at the waist when lifting.

____ 25. When sitting for prolonged periods of time, make sure he sits with his pelvis posteriorly rotated.

____ 26. Have the patient perform standing extensions when moving from a seated to a standing position.

Problem XXV

Opening Scene

You have been assigned to the medical tent located at the finish line of a half-marathon. As one of the runners crosses the line, you notice he appears somewhat ashen in color and is looking confused. As you escort him to the tent, you notice that his skin is cool and clammy to the touch.

Section A

How will you begin your initial evaluation of this patient's condition? (Please select and prioritize your choices.)

____ 1. Immediately administer an IV of glucose and water.

____ 2. Ask the patient what medications he is taking.

____ 3. While maintaining the patient's privacy with a light blanket/sheet, obtain a core temperature measurement.

____ 4. Take the patient's blood pressure and pulse rate.

____ 5. Perform a cranial nerve check.

____ 6. Check the patient for a positive Homan's sign.

____ 7. Check the patient's fingernails for good capillary refill.

____ 8. Ask the patient's name, the date, and where he is right now.

Section B

Based on your initial evaluation, you determine the patient is experiencing an episode of heat exhaustion. How would you proceed in treating this patient? (Please select and prioritize your choices.)

_____ 9. Have the patient rebreathe into a paper bag.

_____ 10. Move the patient into a cool area.

_____ 11 Place the patient in supine and elevate his feet.

_____ 12. Give the patient a massage to relax him.

_____ 13. Restrict the patient's fluid intake for at least 1 to 2 hours.

_____ 14. Continue to monitor the patient's vital signs.

_____ 15. Cover the patient with a cotton blanket

_____ 16. Cool the patient by sponging or toweling him with cold water, by use of a fan, or by placing ice packs around the neck and in the axilla and/or groin area.

_____ 17. Advise the patient not to run again until he is cleared by a doctor.

Problem XXVI

Opening Scene

You are covering a collegiate women's lacrosse game when you observe 2 players collide as they try to catch a ball in the air. One of the players is struck by her opponent's stick in the side of the chest. She falls to the ground and is in obvious pain. She is clutching her right side.

Section A

How will you begin to evaluate the severity of this injury? (Please select and prioritize your choices.)

_____ 1. Observe the patient for cyanosis.

_____ 2. Immediately move the patient off the field.

_____ 3. Ask the patient to move her fingers and toes.

_____ 4. Ask the patient to cough a couple of times to check respiratory competency.

_____ 5. Perform a primary survey.

_____ 6. Perform an Adson's maneuver.

_____ 7. Perform an upper quarter screen.

_____ 8. Look for coughing up of blood.

_____ 9. Palpate the thorax for point tenderness and crepitus.

Section B

You are able to assist the patient to the sidelines. She complains of significant pain during inspiration and continues to try to splint her chest with her arms. After a few minutes, you notice her lips look cyanotic. What steps would you take at this time to treat this patient? (Please select and prioritize your choices.)

_____ 10. Record the rate and depth of respirations.

_____ 11. Monitor vital signs.

_____ 12. Tightly and continuously wrap the chest with an elastic bandage.

_____ 13. Use a vapocoolant spray such as fluoromethane to reduce spasm.

_____ 14. Apply a sling and swathe, using the patient's arm as a splint and support with the forearm supported across the chest.

_____ 15. Observe the rib cage for any areas of deformity.

_____ 16. Check the patient's shoulder for active range of motion to make sure there is no injury to the scapula.

_____ 17. Perform an Allen's test.

_____ 18. Perform a Phalen's test.

_____ 19. Activate the EMS.

_____ 20. Apply a pad over the suspected fracture site.

_____ 21. Refer the patient to a physician as soon as possible.

Problem XXVII

Opening Scene

It is 1:00 pm and you are rehabilitating a volleyball player for a shoulder injury when you notice he is "slumping" in his chair as he is working on an upper body ergometer. When you ask him if he is all right, he responds slowly, and his speech appears to be slurred. You know this patient is a type 1 diabetic.

Section A

How will you begin to evaluate this patient's condition? (Please select and prioritize your choices.)

_____ 1. Ask if the patient if he is having difficulty breathing.

_____ 2. Observe for diaphoresis.

_____ 3. Take the patient's pulse rate.

_____ 4. Ask the patient when he last injected himself with insulin.

_____ 5. Observe for facial drooping.

_____ 6. Perform a cranial nerve assessment.

_____ 7. Perform a Romberg's test.

_____ 8. Bring the patient into your office and gently approach him about substance abuse.

_____ 9. Check for fruity smelling breath.

Section B

Based on your initial assessment, you determine the patient is experiencing insulin shock. What would your next steps be in treating this patient? (Please select and prioritize your choices.)

____ 10. Administer short-acting insulin.

____ 11. Have the patient eat a protein bar.

____ 12. Lie the patient in supine, and elevate his feet.

____ 13. Monitor vital signs.

____ 14. Give the patient a drink with high levels of sugar.

____ 15. Keep the patient warm with a blanket.

____ 16. Give the patient a drink that is high in electrolytes.

Section C

The patient recovers well after drinking some orange juice that is mixed with added sugar. What advice would you provide the patient with to prevent further episodes of hypoglycemia? (Please select and prioritize your choices.)

____ 17. Advise the patient to consume sufficient carbohydrates prior to exercising.

____ 18. Remind the patient to inject himself with high dosages of insulin on a regular basis before exercising to avoid "crashing" during periods of intense activity.

____ 19. Make sure he knows to inject himself in the muscles that will not be very active during a particular sporting event.

____ 20. Advise the patient to keep small amounts of candy with him in case he feels the symptoms of hypoglycemia occurring.

____ 21. Tell the patient to attend a diabetic support group.

ATTENTION STUDENTS!

Three practice applied decision-making exams of 2 problems each are available online at www.healio.com/books/atexam6E.

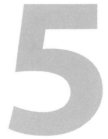

Skills Assessment

Although the BOC exam no longer requires you to perform actual skills or applications as part of the certification examination, we encourage you to be familiar with all skills relative to athletic training. This chapter will serve as an important practice tool for you to use in preparing for practical exams within your athletic training program.

You will need 2 partners and a stopwatch or wristwatch to practice for this section of the exam. One partner will play the role of the model, and the other partner will be the examiner. Have the partner who is playing the examiner read through a few of the questions to him- or herself first and collect any necessary items to complete the tasks on which you intend to work. For example, if you are required to tape a knee, you will need the appropriate selection of supplies. Try to avoid having your partners "help" you by giving you hints, either verbally or nonverbally, along the way. The idea is for you to become confident in your skills and speed of execution. Go over any mistakes you have made after you have completed this practice section.

Each task will be assigned a specific time limitation. You must correctly perform 90% of the steps to pass each task, except for Problems X and XIV, which must be correctly demonstrated in full.

PROBLEM I

A soccer player mildly strains his right hip flexor during a game. The athlete needs his leg wrapped in an elastic bandage to make him more comfortable prior to returning to play. You have 2 minutes to perform this task.

A. Is the athlete positioned in standing with the involved leg slightly flexed and internally rotated?

Yes ___   No ___

B. Was a double 6-inch elastic wrap selected?

Yes ___   No ___

C. Was the elastic wrap started at the upper part of the inner thigh and brought around to the posterior aspect of the thigh?

Yes ___   No ___

D. Was the wrap anchored onto the opposite iliac crest?

Yes ___   No ___

E. Does the wrap prevent excessive hip extension?

Yes ___   No ___

Passing score = 4 questions correctly answered

PROBLEM II

A patient comes to the athletic training facility after undergoing an arthroplasty of his left shoulder. Using a goniometer, measure the range of motion of shoulder flexion (normal active range of motion is 0 to 180 degrees). Please report your measurement to the examiner. (Note: The examiner should take the initial reading.) You have 2 minutes to perform this task.

A. Is the patient positioned in supine?

Yes ___   No ___

Van Ost L, Lew Feirman K, Manfré K. *Athletic Training Exam Review: A Student Guide to Success, Sixth Edition* (pp 153-161). © 2017 SLACK Incorporated.

B.   Is the axis of the goniometer aligned through the lateral aspect of the humeral head?

Yes ___   No ___

C.   Is the stationary arm of the goniometer aligned parallel to the trunk?

Yes ___   No ___

D.   Is the movable arm aligned parallel to the humeral shaft, siting the lateral epicondyle?

Yes ___   No ___

E.   Is the athletic trainer's recording within 5 degrees of the examiner's reading?

Yes ___   No ___

Passing score = 4 questions correctly answered

PROBLEM III

This next task is to test your palpation skills. With a skin marker or small pieces of athletic tape, place a mark on the following anatomical landmarks of the lower extremity. You have 2 minutes to perform this task.

A.   The anterior talofibular ligament.
      (Correct?) Yes ___   No ___
B.   Gerdy's tubercle.
      (Correct?) Yes ___   No ___
C.   The anterior superior iliac spine.
      (Correct?) Yes ___   No ___
D.   The popliteal fossa.
      (Correct?) Yes ___   No ___
E.   The quadriceps tendon.
      (Correct?) Yes ___   No ___
F.   The lateral collateral ligament of the knee.
      (Correct?) Yes ___   No ___
G.   The medial malleolus.
      (Correct?) Yes ___   No ___
H.   The deltoid ligament of the ankle.
      (Correct?) Yes ___   No ___
I.   The greater trochanter of the femur.
      (Correct?) Yes ___   No ___
J.   The medial border of the patella.
      (Correct?) Yes ___   No ___
K.   The lateral head of the gastrocnemius.
      (Correct?) Yes ___   No ___
L.   The first ray of the foot.
      (Correct?) Yes ___   No ___
M.   The navicular of the foot.
      (Correct?) Yes ___   No ___

N.   The base of the fifth metatarsal.
      (Correct?) Yes ___   No ___
O.   The tendon of the biceps femoris.
      (Correct?) Yes ___   No ___
P.   The fibular head.
      (Correct?) Yes ___   No ___

Passing score = 14 questions correctly answered

PROBLEM IV

A gymnast reports to the athletic training facility after sustaining a knee injury during practice. To test the integrity of the medial collateral ligament, you must perform a valgus stress test. Demonstrate this test just as you would on an injured patient. You have 3 minutes to perform this test.

A.   Is the patient positioned in supine?
      Yes ___   No ___
B.   Is the involved leg extended?
      Yes ___   No ___
C.   Has the athletic trainer stabilized the distal limb with one hand?
      Yes ___   No ___
D.   Has the athletic trainer placed his or her other hand over the lateral joint line?
      Yes ___   No ___
E.   Has the athletic trainer applied adequate force in the appropriate direction with the knee in full extension?
      Yes ___   No ___
F.   Has the athletic trainer applied adequate force in the appropriate direction at 30 degrees of flexion?
      Yes ___   No ___
G.   Has the athletic trainer performed the valgus stress test bilaterally?
      Yes ___   No ___

Passing score = 6 questions correctly answered

PROBLEM V

A basketball player has been participating in a rehabilitation program for a hamstring strain. Prior to allowing the player to return to playing, the athletic trainer should test the strength of the hamstrings to be sure they are of equal strength to the uninvolved side and are pain free to resistance. Demonstrate a manual muscle test for the hamstrings just as you would on a patient. You have 2 minutes to perform this task.

A. Is the patient positioned in prone?

Yes ___ No ___

B. Did the athletic trainer have the patient first move the limb actively from full knee extension to full knee flexion?

Yes ___ No ___

C. Has the athletic trainer stabilized the posterior thigh with one hand?

Yes ___ No ___

D. Has the athletic trainer placed his or her hand on the posterior aspect of the distal lower leg?

Yes ___ No ___

E. Was the proper force applied to resist knee flexion (in neutral)?

Yes ___ No ___

F. Did the athletic trainer position the lower leg in internal rotation to resist the medial hamstrings?

Yes ___ No ___

G. Did the athletic trainer position the lower leg in external rotation to resist the lateral hamstrings?

Yes ___ No ___

Passing score = 6 questions correctly answered

PROBLEM VI

This task will require you to properly fit a football helmet on a player. Proceed through all the steps, verbalizing each step to the examiner until the fitting process is complete. Inform the examiner when you are done. You have 3 minutes to perform this task.

A. Did the athletic trainer verbalize he or she would wet the player's hair to simulate playing conditions and ensure a proper fit?

Yes ___ No ___

B. Did the athletic trainer apply the helmet from the back to the front and check to make sure the helmet fits snugly with no gaps between the pads and the head or face?

Yes ___ No ___

C. Did the athletic trainer check to see if the helmet covers the base of the skull?

Yes ___ No ___

D. With the chinstrap in place, did the athletic trainer pull down on the facemask to make sure the helmet did not move?

Yes ___ No ___

E. Did the athletic trainer push down on the helmet to make sure there is no movement?

Yes ___ No ___

F. Did the athletic trainer attempt to rock the helmet back and forth to check for any movement?

Yes ___ No ___

G. Did the athletic trainer attempt to rotate the helmet to check for any movement?

Yes ___ No ___

H. Did the athletic trainer check to see if the front edge of the helmet is no less than 2 finger widths above the eyebrows?

Yes ___ No ___

I. Did the athletic trainer check to see if the jaw pads fit snugly against the face?

Yes ___ No ___

J. Did the athletic trainer check to see if the facemask was 3 finger widths from the nose?

Yes ___ No ___

K. Did the athletic trainer check to see that the ear holes were aligned?

Yes ___ No ___

L. Did the athletic trainer check to make sure the chinstrap was properly adjusted?

Yes ___ No ___

Passing score = 11 questions correctly answered

PROBLEM VII

A lacrosse player is recovering from Achilles tendinitis of the right lower leg. This patient will need to be taped to prevent aggravating the area during play. Demonstrate the proper technique to tape the Achilles tendon. You have 3 minutes to perform this task.

A. Is the patient positioned in prone with the ankle in slight plantar flexion over the edge of the table?

Yes ___ No ___

B. Did the athletic trainer verbalize that tape adherent would be applied to the lower leg (after shaving it if necessary)?

Yes ___ No ___

C. Has the athletic trainer applied underwrap to the lower third of the calf area?

Yes ___ No ___

D. Has the athletic trainer applied anchor strips one-third of the way up the calf and around the forefoot?

Yes ___ No ___

E. Has the athletic trainer applied a 3-inch elastic strip from forefoot to the anchor strip on the calf?

Yes ___ No ___

F. Has the athletic trainer applied a second 3-inch elastic strip on top of the first, splitting it down the middle lengthwise and wrapping the 2 pieces anteriorly around the leg?

Yes ____   No ____

G. Did the athletic trainer close the tape job with elastic strips around the calf and the ball of the foot?

Yes ____   No ____

H. Does the tape job adequately prevent excessive dorsiflexion of the foot?

Yes ____   No ____

Passing score = 7 questions correctly answered

PROBLEM VIII

A football player has injured his ankle during a game. After having the ankle wrapped for support, crutches are issued. Demonstrate how to properly fit and walk with crutches in nonweightbearing. You have 3 minutes to perform this task.

A. Are the tips of the crutches approximately 6 inches from the lateral aspect of the shoe and approximately 2 inches in front of the toe during fitting?

Yes ____   No ____

B. Are the crutch handles in a position so the elbows are bent to approximately 30 degrees?

Yes ____   No ____

C. Are the tops of the crutches approximately 2 finger widths from the top of the axilla?

Yes ____   No ____

D. Did the athletic trainer review a tripod gait in which both crutches are moved forward approximately 12 inches and the athlete swings through the stationary crutches with the affected foot elevated?

Yes ____   No ____

Passing score = 3 questions correctly answered

PROBLEM IX

A football player comes to the sidelines after making a tackle. He is complaining of some neck discomfort and tingling sensations down his left arm. As part of the athletic trainer's initial assessment, an upper quarter screen is performed. Please demonstrate how to assess the motor function of the upper quarter and verbalize each level as it is evaluated. You have 2 minutes to perform this task.

A. (C3,4) Did the athletic trainer resist shoulder shrugs?

Yes ____   No ____

B. (C4,5) Did the athletic trainer resist shoulder abduction?

Yes ____   No ____

C. (C5,6) Did the athletic trainer resist elbow flexion and wrist extension?

Yes ____   No ____

D. (C6,7) Did the athletic trainer resist elbow extension and wrist flexion?

Yes ____   No ____

E. (C8,T1) Did the athletic trainer resist finger adduction and grip strength?

Yes ____   No ____

Passing score = 4 questions correctly answered

PROBLEM X

A baseball player comes into the athletic training facility following a practice complaining that his shoulder clicks and occasionally feels like it is slipping when he throws hard. To test the integrity of the glenohumeral joint, the athletic trainer performs an apprehension test. Demonstrate this test just as you would on an injured patient. You have 2 minutes to perform this task.

A. Has the athletic trainer placed the patient in sitting or supine?

Yes ____   No ____

B. Did the athletic trainer position the shoulder in 90 degrees of abduction with the elbow flexed to 90 degrees?

Yes ____   No ____

C. Did the athletic trainer gently externally rotate the shoulder until the patient demonstrates apprehension (facial grimace or the patient requests the athletic trainer to stop the motion)?

Yes ____   No ____

Passing score = 3 questions correctly answered

PROBLEM XI

A gymnast has a subacute left biceps strain. This athlete will need to be taped before participating in her next meet. Demonstrate the proper technique to tape the elbow to prevent hyperextension. You have 3 minutes to perform this task.

A. Did the athletic trainer verbalize that tape adherent would be applied to the elbow area?

Yes ____   No ____

B. Has the athletic trainer positioned the athlete with the elbow in 90 degrees of flexion?

Yes ___   No ___

C. Has the athletic trainer applied underwrap to the affected area?

Yes ___   No ___

D. Has the athletic trainer placed anchor strips with elastic tape at the mid-upper arm and mid-forearm areas?

Yes ___   No ___

E. Did the athletic trainer apply a check-rein made out of fanned 1.5-inch white tape or 2- or 3-inch elastic tape vertically down the anterior portion of the arm?

Yes ___   No ___

F. Did the athletic trainer apply additional anchor strips above and below the check-rein to secure it?

Yes ___   No ___

G. Did the athletic trainer apply a final wrap with elastic tape to close the tape job?

Yes ___   No ___

Passing score = 6 questions correctly answered

PROBLEM XII

A field hockey player comes into the athletic training facility with a large abrasion (4 × 4 inches) on the lateral side of her thigh. Demonstrate the proper procedure to care for this wound. You have 3 minutes to perform this task.

A. Did the athletic trainer verbalize or demonstrate good hand washing techniques?

Yes ___   No ___

B. Did the athletic trainer don protective gloves?

Yes ___   No ___

C. Has the athletic trainer cleansed the wound thoroughly with soap and water or hydrogen peroxide?

Yes ___   No ___

D. Has the athletic trainer applied an antiseptic to the wound?

Yes ___   No ___

E. If medication is applied, has the athletic trainer placed the ointment or cream on the pad or dressing (ie, not directly on the wound)?

Yes ___   No ___

F. Has the athletic trainer secured the dressing in place with an elastic wrap or tape?

Yes ___   No ___

G. Did the athletic trainer verbalize that the contaminated gloves would be disposed of in a biohazard bag?

Yes ___   No ___

Passing score = 6 questions correctly answered

PROBLEM XIII

A volleyball player limps into the athletic training facility after twisting her ankle on the court during a practice drill. An inversion sprain is suspected. To test the integrity of the ankle joint, an anterior drawer test is performed. Please demonstrate this test just as you would on an injured patient. You have 2 minutes to perform this task.

A. Is the patient positioned in supine or sitting on the edge of a treatment table with the feet relaxed and hanging freely over the edge of the table?

Yes ___   No ___

B. Has the athletic trainer stabilized the lower tibia with one hand?

Yes ___   No ___

C. Did the athletic trainer grasp the calcaneus with the other hand?

Yes ___   No ___

D. Did the athletic trainer attempt to move the calcaneus anteriorly with adequate force?

Yes ___   No ___

E. Did the athletic trainer verbalize that a clunking feeling at the endpoint of the movement is a positive finding?

Yes ___   No ___

Passing score = 4 questions correctly answered

PROBLEM XIV

A baseball player reports having pain along the ball of his right foot while walking and running. It has now progressed to the point where he is limping slightly. To decrease his pain while he is being treated for the inflammation, a metatarsal pad is applied for use during activity. Please demonstrate the proper technique to apply a metatarsal pad to this patient's foot. You have 2 minutes to perform this task.

A. Is the patient positioned in supine or sitting with the plantar surface of the affected foot turned upward?

Yes ___   No ___

B. Has the athletic trainer placed a 2- to 2.5-inch oval approximately 0.125- to 0.25-inch thick felt metatarsal pad just behind the metatarsal heads?

Yes ___   No ___

C. Did the athletic trainer secure the pad with loosely applied elastic tape?

Yes ___   No ___

Passing score = 3 questions correctly answered

PROBLEM XV

During a poorly executed dismount, a gymnast lands on his shoulder. After an initial assessment of the injury, the athletic trainer suspects a potentially serious shoulder injury. To make the patient more comfortable and for protection, the athletic trainer applies a cloth triangular bandage as a cervical arm sling. Please demonstrate how a cervical arm sling is properly applied. You have 2 minutes to perform this task.

A.   Is the patient positioned in standing with his arm in approximately 70 degrees of elbow flexion?

Yes ___   No ___

B.   Has the athletic trainer positioned the triangular bandage under the injured arm so that the apex is facing the elbow joint?

Yes ___   No ___

C.   Has the athletic trainer brought the superior corner up over the shoulder of the injured arm?

Yes ___   No ___

D.   Has the athletic trainer brought the inferior corner up over the shoulder of the uninjured side, tying it in a knot to the opposite corner behind the neck?

Yes ___   No ___

E.   Has the athletic trainer brought the apex of the triangle forward and secured it with a safety pin?

Yes ___   No ___

Passing score = 4 questions correctly answered

PROBLEM XVI

A baseball player mildly sprains his left ankle during a game. Following treatment, he is able to return to the next scheduled game but requires his ankle to be taped prior to playing. Please demonstrate the proper technique to tape an ankle to prevent a second inversion sprain. You have 3 minutes to perform this task.

A.   Are the patient's foot and ankle positioned in maximal dorsiflexion and eversion?

Yes ___   No ___

B.   Did the athletic trainer verbalize that he or she would apply tape adherent and underwrap prior to taping?

Yes ___   No ___

C.   Has the athletic trainer applied anchor strips around the lower third of the calf at the musculotendinous junction of the gastrocnemius?

Yes ___   No ___

D.   Has the athletic trainer applied anchor strips loosely around the foot over the base of the fifth metatarsal?

Yes ___   No ___

E.   Has the athletic trainer applied stirrup strips?

Yes ___   No ___

F.   Has the athletic trainer applied horizontal strips continually up the leg in either a basket weave form or as continual support?

Yes ___   No ___

G.   Has the athletic trainer applied double heel locks (with a figure-8 strip) for additional support?

Yes ___   No ___

H.   Upon inspecting the tape job, are there any gaps visible?

Yes ___   No ___

I.   Does the model feel the tape prevents active inversion of the ankle?

Yes ___   No ___

J.   Upon removing the tape, are there any noticeable wrinkles that could cause blisters?

Yes ___   No ___

Passing score = 9 questions correctly answered

PROBLEM XVII

Two football players collide on the field while scrambling for a fumble. One player appears dazed as he walks off the field to the sideline. During the athletic trainer's assessment, the cranial nerves are checked. Please demonstrate how each nerve, numbers I through XII, are evaluated. You have 3 minutes to perform this task.

A.   (CN I—olfactory) Did the athletic trainer ask the patient to smell something with his eyes closed?

Yes ___   No ___

B.   (CN II—optic) Did the athletic trainer ask the patient if he can see the athletic trainer's fingers in his periphery?

Yes ___   No ___

C.   (CN III—oculomotor) Did the athletic trainer ask the patient to track his or her finger up and down and side to side?

Yes ___   No ___

D.   (CN IV—trochlear) Did the athletic trainer ask the patient to track his or her finger up and down and side to side (same test as CN III)?

Yes ___   No ___

E.   (CN V—trigeminal) Did the athletic trainer check the sensation of the face (bilaterally)?

Yes ___   No ___

F.   (CN VI—abducens) Did the athletic trainer ask the patient to track his or her finger side to side (similar test as CN III)?

Yes ___   No ___

G.   (CN VII—facial) Did the athletic trainer ask the patient to frown or smile?

Yes ___   No ___

H. (CN VIII—acoustic) Did the athletic trainer check the patient's hearing (eg, with a watch or a tuning fork)?

Yes ___ No ___

I. (CN IX—glossopharyngeal) Did the athletic trainer ask the patient to swallow?

Yes ___ No ___

J. (CN X—vagus) Did the athletic trainer ask the patient to say "ah"?

Yes ___ No ___

K. (CN XI—spinal accessory) Did the athletic trainer ask the patient to shrug his shoulders?

Yes ___ No ___

L. (CN XII—hypoglossal) Did the athletic trainer ask the patient to stick his tongue out?

Yes ___ No ___

Passing score = 11 questions correctly answered

Problem XVIII

A patient is brought to the athletic training facility by his coach and a teammate. His right knee is positioned in slight flexion, and a small effusion is noted. To test the integrity of the anterior cruciate ligament, a Lachman's test is performed. Please demonstrate this test as you would on an injured patient. You have 2 minutes to perform this test.

A. Is the patient positioned in supine?

Yes ___ No ___

B. Is the patient's knee positioned in 30 degrees or less of flexion?

Yes ___ No ___

C. Has the athletic trainer stabilized the distal femur with one hand?

Yes ___ No ___

D. Has the athletic trainer grasped the proximal tibia with the other hand, attempting to move the tibia anteriorly on the femur?

Yes ___ No ___

E. Has the athletic trainer applied adequate force in the appropriate direction?

Yes ___ No ___

Passing score = 4 questions correctly answered

Problem XIX

A patient has been undergoing therapy after a significant ankle sprain. Using a goniometer, measure the range of motion of plantar flexion of the ankle (normal active range of motion is 0 to 40 degrees). Please verbalize your measurement to the examiner. The examiner should take the initial reading. You have 2 minutes to complete this task.

A. Is the patient positioned in sitting with his or her foot hanging freely?

Yes ___ No ___

B. Is the axis of the goniometer centered over the lateral malleolus?

Yes ___ No ___

C. Is the stationary arm of the goniometer aligned with the fibular shaft, siting the fibular head?

Yes ___ No ___

D. Is the movable arm of the goniometer aligned parallel to the plantar aspect of the calcaneus?

Yes ___ No ___

E. Is the athletic trainer's recording within 5 degrees of the examiner's reading?

Yes ___ No ___

Passing score = 4 questions correctly answered

Problem XX

This task will require you to properly fit football shoulder pads on a player. Proceed through all the steps, verbalizing each step to the examiner until the fitting process is complete. Inform the examiner when you are done. You have 3 minutes to perform this task.

A. Did the athletic trainer verbalize he or she would measure the width of the shoulders to determine the proper size of the shoulder pads?

Yes ___ No ___

B. Did the athletic trainer check to make sure that the inside shoulder pad covers the tip of the shoulder and is in line with the lateral aspect of the shoulder?

Yes ___ No ___

C. Did the athletic trainer check to make sure that the epaulets and cups cover the deltoid muscle(s)?

Yes ___ No ___

D. Did the athletic trainer check to make sure that the player can raise his or her arms overhead without the pads sliding back and forth?

Yes ___ No ___

E. Did the athletic trainer check the straps located under the arms to make sure the pads are not free to move?

Yes ___ No ___

Passing score = 4 questions correctly answered

PROBLEM XXI

You are covering an ice hockey game when a player comes to you complaining that he "pulled a muscle in his inner thigh" as he was skating. Once you have gotten him into the locker room, you find that he has the most discomfort when he tries to cross his leg over the other one at the knee. You suspect an injury to the sartorious muscle. Demonstrate a manual muscle test for the sartorious muscle as you would on a patient. You have 2 minutes to perform this task.

A.   Is the patient positioned in sitting?

Yes ___   No ___

B.   Did the athletic trainer have the patient first move the limb actively into full hip flexion, abduction, and external rotation with the knee in a flexed position?

Yes ___   No ___

C.   Has the athletic trainer placed his or her hand on the distal/lateral aspect of the thigh just above the knee joint?

Yes ___   No ___

D.   Has the athletic trainer placed his or her other hand on the posterior/medial aspect of the lower leg just above the ankle joint?

Yes ___   No ___

E.   Has the athletic trainer applied adequate force on the distal/lateral thigh to resist hip flexion and abduction?

Yes ___   No ___

F.   Has the athletic trainer applied adequate force on the posterior/medial aspect of the lower leg to resist hip external rotation and knee flexion?

Yes ___   No ___

G.   Did the athletic trainer perform this manual muscle test bilaterally?

Yes ___   No ___

Passing score = 6 questions correctly answered

PROBLEM XXII

A rower reports to his athletic trainer that during practice he felt a sharp pain on the left side of his lower back that is now radiating into his left buttock and posterior thigh to just above the knee. To test for possible neurological involvement, a Slump test should be performed. Demonstrate this test just as you would on an injured patient. You have 3 minutes to perform this test.

A.   Is the patient positioned in sitting with the legs supported, hips in neutral (ie, no rotation, abduction/adduction), and with his hands behind his back?

Yes ___   No ___

B.   Did the athletic trainer ask the patient to slump back into full thoracic/lumbar flexion while keeping the chin in neutral?

Yes ___   No ___

C.   Has the athletic trainer then applied overpressure while maintaining thoracic and lumbar flexion?

Yes ___   No ___

D.   Has the athletic trainer asked the patient to fully flex his cervical spine (ie, chin to chest)?

Yes ___   No ___

E.   While maintaining this position with overpressure, has the athletic trainer asked the patient to actively extend his knee while dorsiflexion of the foot is maintained?

Yes ___   No ___

F.   Has the athletic trainer repeated the test with the other leg and with both legs together?

Yes ___   No ___

G.   If the patient reported that he was unable to fully extend his knee because of pain, did the athletic trainer release the overpressure to the cervical spine and have the patient extend his neck to see if the symptoms were relieved?

Yes ___   No ___

Passing score = 6 questions correctly answered

PROBLEM XXIII

A patient comes to the athletic training facility 8 weeks post Colles' fracture of the left wrist. His wrist movements continue to appear somewhat limited because of the immobilization. Using a goniometer, measure the range of motion of wrist radial deviation (normal active range of motion is 15 degrees). Please report your measurement to the examiner. (Note: The examiner should take the initial reading.) You have 2 minutes to perform this task.

A.   Is the patient positioned in sitting with the left forearm pronated and resting on a tabletop with the elbow flexed to 90 degrees?

Yes ___   No ___

B.   Is the wrist neutrally positioned among radial deviation/ulnar deviation, flexion, and extension, and are the fingers loosely extended?

Yes ___   No ___

C.   Is the axis of the goniometer positioned over the capitate bone?

Yes ___   No ___

D.   Is the stationary arm of the goniometer aligned along the forearm siting the lateral epicondyle of the elbow?

Yes ___   No ___

E. Is the movable arm aligned along the shaft of the third metacarpal?

Yes ___ No ___

F. Is the wrist in the correct position of radial deviation at the end of the movement?

Yes ___ No ___

G. Is the athletic trainer's recording within 5 degrees of the examiner's reading?

Yes ___ No ___

Passing score = 6 questions correctly answered

PROBLEM XXIV

A lacrosse player has been participating in a rehabilitation program for an injury to the gluteus minimus and/ or the tensor fasciae latae muscle(s). Using a goniometer, measure the range of motion of hip internal rotation (normal active range of motion is 0 to 45 degrees). Please report your reading to the examiner. (Note: The examiner should take the initial reading.) You have 2 minutes to perform this task.

A. Is the patient positioned in sitting at the edge of a tabletop?

Yes ___ No ___

B. Is the axis of the goniometer aligned over the midpatellar surface?

Yes ___ No ___

C. Is the stationary arm of the goniometer aligned perpendicular to the floor?

Yes ___ No ___

D. Did the athletic trainer palpate a point midway between the 2 malleoli of the ankle as the site for the movable arm?

Yes ___ No ___

E. Is the hip in the correct position of internal rotation at the end of the movement?

Yes ___ No ___

F. Is the athletic trainer's recording within 5 degrees of the examiner's reading?

Yes ___ No ___

Passing score = 5 questions correctly answered

PROBLEM XXV

A baseball pitcher complains he is having diffuse left elbow pain after prolonged periods of throwing. While evaluating his elbow, the athletic trainer notices that the patient is not able to actively fully extend his left elbow because of a tight bicep muscle. Demonstrate how to stretch the bicep using a PNF stretching technique known as "hold-relax." You have 2 minutes to perform this task.

A. Is the patient positioned in a seated or supine position?

Yes ___ No ___

B. Has the athletic trainer asked the patient to actively move the elbow into maximal extension and hold this position?

Yes ___ No ___

C. Did the athletic trainer isometrically resist elbow flexion for 10 seconds?

Yes ___ No ___

D. Did the athletic trainer ask the patient to relax for 10 seconds and then move the elbow into the new range of extension?

Yes ___ No ___

Passing score = 3 questions correctly answered

PROBLEM XXVI

A tennis player reports that he has "lost power" while hitting overhead shots. When observing his thoracic area, the athletic trainer notices that his right scapula is "winging" (movement of the vertebral border of the scapula away from the thorax). Demonstrate a manual muscle test for the serratus anterior as you would perform on a patient. You have 2 minutes to perform this task.

A. Is the patient positioned in supine?

Yes ___ No ___

B. Is the upper extremity positioned in 90 degrees of shoulder flexion and slight abduction?

Yes ___ No ___

C. Does the athletic trainer have one hand on the patient's forearm and the other on his elbow?

Yes ___ No ___

D. Has the athletic trainer applied adequate force in a downward/inward direction toward the table?

Yes ___ No ___

Passing score = 3 questions correctly answered

Critical Thinking

In an attempt to bring you the most current information and allow you to prepare for the BOC exam, a chapter has been updated in this text for students to apply their critical thinking skills. Every day as an athletic trainer, we are charged with making a quick decision based on our ability to draw a conclusion from the subjective and objective information that is presented to us. These scenario-based problems will allow you to sharpen your diagnostic skills and/or choose a treatment path that is appropriate for a given scenario.

The scenario-based question format requires that a specific number of answers be chosen from a list of possible options that are offered. This type of question requires the candidate to read a short vignette that describes a patient with various risk factors/signs and symptoms and then select specific diagnoses, lab studies, or procedures that would be appropriate for the scenario that is described. Although a specific number of answers will be selected from the list, there is one **best** answer that will be described in the answer key unless otherwise indicated.

This is the basis of the development of a differential diagnosis or the algorithms that are used by medical professionals when trying to identify the disease/condition causing a patient's symptoms or when trying to prescribe a treatment for a particular problem.

NEUROLOGY (DIFFERENTIAL DIAGNOSIS)

A. Multiple sclerosis
B. Huntington's chorea
C. Myasthenia gravis
D. Guillain-Barré syndrome
E. Duchenne's muscular dystrophy
F. Cerebral palsy
G. Polio
H. Hemorrhagic stroke
I. Parkinson's disease
J. Bell's palsy
K. Brain tumor
L. Amyotrophic lateral sclerosis

1. A 64-year-old male has a gradual onset of bradykinesia, intentional tremors, dysphagia, and gait disturbances.
   Select the 2 most likely diagnoses from the set above.

2. A 50-year-old female presents with sudden dysarthria, hemianopia, and weakness of the left arm and face.
   Select the 2 most likely diagnoses from the set above.

Van Ost L, Lew Feirman K, Manfré K. *Athletic Training Exam Review: A Student Guide to Success, Sixth Edition* (pp 163-169).
© 2017 SLACK Incorporated.

3. A 46-year-old male experiences "glove and stocking" paresthesias with bilateral upper and lower extremity progressive weakness that takes a rapid course to respiratory distress.

    Select the 3 most likely diagnoses from the set above.

4. A 25-year-old female presents with ptosis of the right eye, dysphagia, and generalized muscle weakness (including respiratory muscle weakness). Her symptoms are more pronounced at the end of the day.

    Select the 2 most likely diagnoses from the set above.

RESPIRATORY (DIFFERENTIAL DIAGNOSIS)

A. Emphysema
B. Chronic bronchitis
C. Asthma
D. Rhinosinusitis
E. Viral pneumonia
F. Cystic fibrosis
G. Pneumothorax
H. Pleurisy
I. Viral upper respiratory tract infection

1. A 16-year-old female presents with complaints of chest tightness, slightly increased respiratory rate, and a cough with mild to moderate wheezing. She is afebrile.

    Select the 2 most likely diagnoses from the set above.

2. A 40-year-old male presents with a history of a chronic, productive cough lasting for more than 3 months over the past 2 to 3 years. He appears short of breath and does not tolerate moderately long periods of exercise. He is a smoker.

    Select the 2 most likely diagnoses from the set above.

3. A 25-year-old female presents with rhinorrhea, nasal congestion, sore throat, a nonproductive cough, and headache.

    Select the 2 most likely diagnoses from the set above.

4. A 30-year-old male presents with fever, headache, and tracheobronchitis.

    Select the 3 most likely diagnoses from the set above.

CARDIOVASCULAR (EVALUATIVE TESTS)

A. Echocardiography
B. Electrocardiogram
C. Ultrasonography
D. Nuclear scanning
E. Cardiac catherization
F. CT scans
G. MRI
H. Cardiac stress testing
I. Venography
J. Arterial Doppler

1. A 48-year-old male complains of a "constricting, suffocating" sensation over the substernal area of the chest when he walks uphill or climbs a flight of stairs. The pain radiates to his jaw and is alleviated after 2 minutes of rest.

    Select the 3 most appropriate evaluative tests for these symptoms from the set above.

2. A 21-year-old female complains of fatigue, mild chest pain, palpations, and dyspnea, and she has a systolic "click" with a murmur on auscultation. She is exercise intolerant.

    Select the 2 most appropriate evaluative tests for these symptoms from the set above.

3. A 70-year-old male presents to outpatient physical therapy 4 days postoperative right total knee reconstruction. He complains of right calf tenderness and the lower limb is edematous. There is a positive Homan's sign.

    Select the 2 most appropriate evaluative tests for these symptoms from the set above.

4. A 60-year-old male presents with consistent intermittent claudication of the lower extremities after walking 5 to 10 minutes. The pain is relieved with rest, and there are atrophic skin changes of the skin of both lower legs. He is diabetic and a smoker.

    Select the 4 most appropriate evaluative tests for these symptoms from the set above.

ORTHOPEDIC (DIFFERENTIAL DIAGNOSIS)

A. Lumbar degenerative joint disease
B. Lumbar muscle strain
C. Lumbar herniated nucleus propulsus
D. Piriformis syndrome
E. Hip osteoarthritis
F. Sacroiliac rotation
G. Femoral nerve entrapment
H. Scoliosis
I. Osgood-Schlatter disease
J. Slipped capital femoral epiphysis
K. Iliopsoas strain
L. Legg-Calvé-Perthes disease
M. Osteomyelitis
N. Osteonecrosis

1. After moving some heavy furniture, a 45-year-old male has an acute onset of lumbar spasms that he describes as "sharp, knife-like" pain radiating down the posterior aspect of his right thigh to the level of his knee. He has pain while forward flexing and when he coughs and sneezes. There is a positive straight leg raise on the right and you note some quadriceps weakness of the right lower extremity.
   Select the 2 most likely diagnoses from the set above.

2. A 5-year-old male presents with an acute onset of anterior groin, thigh, and knee pain. He has difficulty ambulating. A limp is noted with limited hip abduction and stiffness when moving into internal rotation. There is also a flexion contracture of the hip.
   Select the 2 most likely diagnoses from the set above.

3. A 65-year-old male presents with left groin and medial thigh pain with activity that radiates to the left buttock and knee with activity. The left hip joint is slightly flexed and adducted and there is a positive Patrick's sign of the left hip. The Slump test is negative.
   Select the 2 most likely diagnoses from the set above.

4. A 22-year-old female is 3 days postoperative open reduction internal fixation of the left tibia. She presents with a fever and pain at the operative site, and there is purulent drainage from the wound.
   Select the 2 most likely diagnoses from the set above.

GYNECOLOGY (EVALUATIVE TESTS)

A. Mammography
B. Needle biopsy
C. Complete blood count
D. Pap smear
E. Ultrasonography
F. Colposcopy
G. Bone scan
H. PET scan
I. Urinalysis
J. Cervicography
K. Laparoscopy
L. Internal pelvic examination
M. Microscopic sample examination

1. A 43-year-old female discovers a nodular, granular breast mass while in the shower that is very tender to palpation.
   Select all the appropriate diagnostic tests for this situation from the set above.

2. An 18-year-old female presents with lower abdominal pain after her menstrual period, purulent cervical discharge, and a painful cervix.
   Select all the appropriate diagnostic tests for this situation from the set above.

3. A 20-year-old female complains of dysmenorrhea, dyspareunia, and infertility.
   Select all the appropriate diagnostic tests for this situation from the set above.

4. A 25-year-old female complains of vaginal discharge and burning, itching, redness, and swelling of the vaginal tissue. She also has pain with urination.
   Select all the appropriate diagnostic tests for this situation.

GASTROINTESTINAL (TREATMENT)

A. Antibiotic (amoxicillin, tetracycline, clarithromycin)
B. Anti-inflammatory (NSAIDs, aspirin)
C. Laxatives (Metamucil, Dulcolax, milk of magnesia)
D. Antidiarrheal (Lomotil, Pepto-Bismol, Kapectolin, Imodium)
E. Antacids (Maalox, Tums, Mylanta)
F. Stool softeners (Colace, Fleet, mineral oil)
G. H2-receptor antagonist (Tagamet, Pepcid, Zantac)

H. Proton pump inhibitors (Nexium, Prevacid, Prilosec, Protonix)

I. Topical anesthetics (benzocaine, tetracaine)

J. Corticosteriods (hydrocortisone 1%)

K. Protectants (cocoa butter, lanolin, petrolatum)

1. A 53-year-old male complains of itching, burning, and pain at the anal opening and has a mild amount of bleeding if he strains during a bowel movement. He has been diagnosed with hemorrhoids.

    Select all the appropriate pharmacological agents used to treat this condition from the set above.

2. A 27-year-old female complains of diarrhea that is alternating with bouts of constipation and abdominal pain. She is afebrile. She has recently been diagnosed with irritable bowel syndrome.

    Select all the appropriate pharmacological agents used to treat this condition from the set above.

3. A 40-year-old male reports symptoms of dyspepsia, gastric regurgitation, feelings of abdominal distention, and "burning" epigastric pain that is brought on after eating spicy or fatty food. He has been diagnosed with gastroesophageal reflux disease.

    Select all the appropriate pharmacological agents used to treat this condition from the set above.

4. A 45-year-old male reports symptoms of a rhythmic, gnawing, cramping pain over the midline of the epigastrium near the xyphiod that occurs between meals. The pain occurs every few weeks. He has been recently diagnosed with peptic ulcer disease.

    Select all the appropriate pharmacological agents used to treat this condition from the set above.

DERMATOLOGY
(DIFFERENTIAL DIAGNOSIS)

A. Impetigo

B. Systemic lupus erythematosus

C. Psoriasis

D. Eczema

E. Scleroderma

F. Dermatitis herpetiformis

G. Epidermolysis bullosa

H. Hyperhidrosis

I. Seborrheic dermatitis

J. Herpes simplex

K. Tinea corporis

L. Tinea pedis

1. A 17-year-old wrestler reports to the athletic training facility with a few small pustules around his nose and chin that appears to be draining a honey-colored serous liquid that has hardened. The athlete is complaining of significant pruritus of the lesions, but he has no pain.

    Select the 2 most likely diagnoses from the set above.

2. A 15-year-old field hockey player reports to the athletic training facility with dry, leathery hyperpigmented areas at the base of her neck, behind her right knee, and behind her ears. She complains of severe pruritus of the lesions. She also tells you she has asthma.

    Select the 2 most likely diagnoses from the set above.

3. A 15-year-old basketball player reports to the athletic training facility complaining of a mildly scaly lesion between his toes. He reports severe pruritus with pain, and there is a foul odor noted when he removes his sock.

    Select the 2 most likely diagnoses from the set above.

4. An 18-year-old baseball player reports to the athletic training facility complaining of a "tingling" sensation of his lower lip that developed into a painful pustule after 2 days. You notice the lesion now looks "crusty," and the athlete is still complaining of pain with palpation of the area. As you speak with him, you find out his girlfriend had broken up with him 2 weeks ago.

    Select the 2 most likely diagnoses from the set above.

ORTHOPEDIC (EVALUATIVE TESTS)

A. MRI

B. Bone scan

C. Electromyography

D. Chest x-ray

E. CT scan

F. Ultrasonography

G. Aspiration

H. Complete blood count

I. Nerve conduction velocity test

J. Conventional radiology

K. Blood culture

L. Nuclear imaging

M. Bone biopsy

1. It is suspected that a 12-year-old male has Ewing's sarcoma of the femur.

    Select all the appropriate diagnostic tests for this condition.

2. It is suspected that a 17-year-old male has a meniscus tear of the right knee.

    Select all the appropriate diagnostic tests for this condition.

3. It is suspected that a 25-year-old male has osteomyelitis of the left lower extremity 1 week status post anterior cruciate ligament reconstruction.

    Select all the appropriate diagnostic tests for this condition.

4. It is suspected that a 50-year-old female has a fractured right humerus after falling on a patch of ice.

    Select all the appropriate diagnostic tests for this condition.

MUSCULOSKELETAL (TREATMENT)

A. Ultrasound
B. Phonophoresis
C. Iontophoresis
D. TENS
E. Electric muscle stimulation
F. Ice packs
G. Moist heat packs
H. Mechanical traction
I. Warm whirlpool
J. Paraffin bath
K. Cold whirlpool
L. Massage
M. Taping/splinting

1. A 23-year-old basketball player has an acute supraspinatus tendinitis of the left shoulder.

    Select all the appropriate modalities that can be used with this condition.

2. A 30-year-old construction worker presents with a subacute lumbar muscle strain and spasms.

    Select all the appropriate modalities that can be used with this condition.

3. A 60-year-old woman presents with arthritis of the hand and fingers.

    Select all the appropriate modalities that can be used with this condition.

4. A 32-year-old woman presents with acute cervical radiculopathy to the right upper extremity.

    Select all the appropriate modalities that can be used with this condition.

VISCERAL (SIGNS AND SYMPTOMS)

A. Cyanosis
B. Dyspnea
C. Deviated trachea
D. Absent bowel sounds
E. Referred pain—right scapula/shoulder, substernal area
F. Jaundice
G. Diarrhea
H. Low-grade fever (99°F to 100°F)
I. Abdominal rigidity/cramping
J. Rebound pain
K. Kehr's sign
L. Nausea/vomiting
M. Constipation
N. Hematuria
O. Gastrointestinal bleeding
P. Tachypnea
Q. Coffee-ground emesis
R. Increased white blood cell count
S. Metabolic acidosis
T. Respiratory alkalosis
U. Anorexia

1. A 24-year-old runner has been diagnosed with a spontaneous pneumothorax.

    Select all the appropriate signs and symptoms that correlate with the above diagnosis.

2. An 18-year-old baseball player has been diagnosed with acute appendicitis.

    Select all the appropriate signs and symptoms that correlate with the above diagnosis.

3. A 21-year-old field hockey player is diagnosed with gastroenteritis after eating in a restaurant while traveling.

    Select all the appropriate signs and symptoms that correlate with the above diagnosis.

4. A 16-year-old soccer player is diagnosed with spleen injury after colliding with an opponent.

    Select all the appropriate signs and symptoms that correlate with the above diagnosis.

PSYCHOLOGY (DIFFERENTIAL DIAGNOSIS)

A. Denial
B. Depression
C. Bargaining
D. Projection
E. Dissociation
F. Acceptance
G. Anger
H. Regression
I. Somatization
J. Suppression
K. Passive aggression
L. Compensation

1. During the final quarter of a college basketball game, the starting point guard severely injures his knee. He tries to convince the doctor, as well as himself, that he is able to play and spends the rest of the game begging the athletic trainer to allow him to return to the game.

    Select the 2 most appropriate descriptors from the set above that describes this athlete's behavior.

2. A 14-year-old gymnast has lost all interest in gymnastics following anterior cruciate ligament reconstruction surgery. She sulks, weeps intermittently, and spends a lot of time at home playing video games.

    Select the 2 most appropriate descriptors from the set above to describe this athlete's behavior.

3. The starting pitcher for a high school baseball team injures his elbow during the first inning of the state finals. He spends the remainder of the game throwing things, kicking the dirt, disrespecting those around him, and throws his glove in the trash. He tells the team that he "knows" he is going back in the game and pouts while sitting on the bench.

    Select the 2 most appropriate descriptors from the set above to describe this athlete's behavior.

4. A 22-year-old volleyball player had rotator cuff surgery on her left shoulder during the summer. When cleared from her doctor to begin exercising, she becomes lazy. She never shows up on time for her treatments with the athletic trainer. One day after receiving a stern talk from her coach and athletic trainer she begins to take responsibility for her rehabilitation.

    Select the 2 most appropriate descriptors from the set above to describe this athlete's behavior.

5. During a high school football game a 17-year-old senior starter sustains a concussion. This was his third concussion within the past year. The team physician deems him ineligible to play football or any other contact sport. He rages out of control when told the discouraging news. Six weeks later he was seen coaching a boy's flag football team for his local recreational playground.

    Select the 2 most appropriate descriptors from the set above to describe this athlete's behavior.

DOCUMENTATION/ MANAGEMENT STRATEGIES

A. SOAP notes
B. Focus charting
C. Charting by exception
D. Computerized information systems
E. WOTS UP
F. HOPS
G. CPT
H. ICD-10
I. HCFA 1500
J. UB–92 (HCFA 1450) claim form
K. UCR fee
L. Mission statement
M. Needs assessment
N. Market analysis
O. Cost-benefit analysis
P. Computer resources needs assessment

1. An athlete was seen by his orthopedic physician for a suspected ankle fracture. The physician performed a full evaluation and ordered x-rays and refers the athlete to physical therapy at a local sports medicine clinic.

    Select the 2 most appropriate diagnostic coding procedures from the set above.

2. Following a hockey game, the goalie complains of severe shoulder pain. Upon observation, the athlete's humerus appears to be subluxed. The athletic trainer immobilizes his shoulder and immediately refers him to the team physician.

    Select the 2 most likely types of documentation in which observation of the shoulder deformity would be recorded from the set above.

3. The Feirman State University athletic training program is going through their accreditation process. The final task is the determination of the program's strengths and weaknesses.

   Select the 2 most likely types of documentation/critique that this process may be recorded in from the set above.

4. A soccer player enters the athletic training facility to receive treatment and rehabilitation on her knee. The athletic training student, not knowing the history of the injury or the treatment protocol that has been implemented, looks up her medical record. Her records reflected treatments and protocols, but no particular information about the injury. One of the documents also included an unusual response to an ultrasound treatment.

   Select the 2 most likely types of documentation that would be used to record these findings from the set above.

5. The Wilson College athletic training department has determined that a computerized information management system would improve their record-keeping ability. They are in the process of deciding which types of hardware and software would be most beneficial for the department.

   Select the 2 most likely types of analyses utilized to make these decisions from the set above.

6. Eastern Oaks Physical Therapy Clinic received a referral to treat an athlete from the local high school. Eastern Oaks has to document each treatment performed during the athlete's rehabilitation.

   Select the 2 most likely types of insurance documentation needed in order to receive payment for the services given from the set above.

BUDGETING

A. Fixed budgeting
B. Variable budgeting
C. Laissez-faire budgeting
D. Lump-sum budgeting
E. Line-item budgeting
F. Zero-based budgeting
G. Spending ceiling
H. Spending reduction

1. The head athletic trainer for Manfré State University is given a fixed sum of money to use for the school year and is allowed to spend it any way he wants to without justification. He decides to purchase a new ice machine and treadmill.

   Select the 2 most appropriate types of budgeting models that might be applied from the set above.

2. The athletic trainer in the Southern Pines Sports Medicine Clinic is required to send a projected monthly list of expenditures to the accounts payable department.

   Select the 2 most appropriate types of budgeting models that might be applied from the set above.

3. An athletic training program submitted their budget in the beginning of the year for their anticipated expenditures for specific categories of their program. Seven months later, there was a small issue with much needed money to repair the modalities equipment. In order to receive the money from another category, it would have to be approved by higher management.

   Select the 2 most appropriate types of budgeting models that might be applied from the set above.

4. Rochester Sports Medicine Clinic has budgeted $30,000 for expenses in May, anticipating a monthly revenue of $65,000. The actual income for the clinic in May is $55,000. As a result, the clinical director is required to decrease spending by 20% the following month.

   Select the 2 most appropriate types of budgeting models that might be applied from the set above.

What to Do if
You Do Not Pass the First Time

There will always be a few candidates who do not pass the examination. If you find yourself in this position, do not panic. It is important to identify factors that may have led to mistakes.

Although it is understandable to feel sad, frustrated, or angry, it is best not to dwell too long on what cannot be changed; focus your energy on the next examination being offered. The BOC exam is offered up to 5 times a year at various testing centers across the country. You should allow yourself another 3 to 6 months (depending on your employment situation) to prepare for and pass the next exam. You may retake the exam as many times as you want as long as it is within 1 year of the date of your last attempt at passing the examination.

It is very important that you reregister as soon as you are ready. Your Emergency Cardiac Care CPR certification must be current and all of your academic coursework within the semester must be completed when you send in your application. Do not forget to pay the application fee online when you are registering on the BOC website. When the site selection window opens, you are allowed to select the site where you would prefer to take the exam provided spots are available. Be sure you are aware of the registration deadline; do not forget to mark your calendar!

If you fail the certification examination, the BOC recommends that you review your results with your endorsing athletic trainer so that he or she can counsel you regarding taking additional coursework or participating in further fieldwork to help you build your skills. This is a good piece of advice, given your supervising athletic trainer should know you the best and can provide valuable guidance. In addition, a list of references that are used to develop the BOC exam can be found on the BOC website at www.bocatc.org. These references may help you with your studies for your next attempt.

If for any reason you feel that you may have a disability or handicap that may have affected your performance during the examination, you may request that the BOC modify the certification procedures to accommodate your disability. Make sure that you send your request for this accommodation in writing to the BOC well in advance of the application deadline so special arrangements can be made.

It might benefit you to take a course on stress management techniques (eg, meditation or visualization) to help you reduce your anxiety while studying. It helps to talk things out with friends, coworkers, or your professors, but they may be limited in their ability to provide you with the tools needed to improve your coping skills. If you are finding you are having significant difficulty dealing with not passing the examination or your anxiety level is not manageable, we suggest you seek professional counseling. In general, try to maintain a positive attitude as you study and get yourself reorganized. Keep in mind that you will have a better idea of how the examination is presented because you have already been through it once.

It is also important to notify your employer (if it is relevant) of the status of your examination results. If you are honest and up front, he or she may be more understanding of your situation. Remember that you may not practice as a certified athletic trainer or refer to yourself as an athletic

Van Ost L, Lew Feirman K, Manfré K. *Athletic Training Exam Review: A Student Guide to Success, Sixth Edition* (pp 171-172).
© 2017 SLACK Incorporated.

trainer until you pass the certification examination and follow the laws in the state in which you plan to practice. To do so will put both you and your employer in jeopardy of a malpractice suit.

If you are very determined to be a certified athletic trainer, you will pass this examination. As mentioned before, give yourself the appropriate time to heal and then pull yourself up by the bootstraps and reorganize your approach. Critically examine your strengths and weaknesses and dig in for the long haul. Remember, the word *quit* is never in a true athletic trainer's vocabulary.

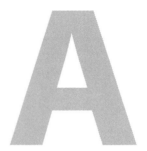

Sample Study Calendar and Daily Log

SUNDAY	MONDAY	TUESDAY	WEDNESDAY	THURSDAY	FRIDAY	SATURDAY
	1 *Register*	2 *Make a composite review*	3	4 *Anatomy*	5	6
7 *Immediate Care*	8	9 *Rehabilitation*	10	11 *Schedule exam*	12 *Critical Thinking*	13 *Take online practice exam*
14	15 *Organization and Administration*	16 *Review BOC Candidate Handbook*	17 *Professional Development*	18 *AT skills review*	19 *Print registration info*	20 *Take online practice exam*
21 *Check route to site*	22	23	24 *Exam day!*	25	26	27
28	29	30	31			

Figure A-1. Sample study calendar.

Van Ost L, Lew Feirman K, Manfré K. *Athletic Training Exam Review:*
A Student Guide to Success, Sixth Edition (pp 173-174).
© 2017 SLACK Incorporated.

HOUR	THURSDAY, APRIL 7	FRIDAY, APRIL 8	SATURDAY, APRIL 9
6:00 to 7:00 am			
7:00 to 8:00 am	Breakfast	Breakfast	Breakfast
8:00 to 9:00 am	Anatomy (UE)	Practice emergency procedures with Tim, Mike, Bob	Practice evaluations
9:00 to 10:00 am	Anatomy (UE)		Therapeutic modalities
10:00 to 11:00 am	Ankle/UE taping	Practice emergency procedures with Tim, Mike, Bob	Shoulder, knee, ankle
11:00 am to 12:00 pm	Knee taping		Shoulder, knee, ankle
12:00 to 1:00 pm	Lunch	Lunch	Lunch
1:00 to 2:00 pm	Nutrition	Anatomy (LE)	Anatomy (back/neck)
2:00 to 3:00 pm	Run	Anatomy (LE)	Anatomy (back/neck)
3:00 to 4:00 pm	Kinesiology/biomechanics	Health care administration	Psychology
4:00 to 5:00 pm	Kinesiology/biomechanics	Professional responsibility/ development	Human physiology
5:00 to 6:00 pm	Physics	Swim at pool	Biking with Sue
6:00 to 7:00 pm	Dinner	Dinner	Dinner
7:00 to 8:00 pm	Rehabilitation/therapeutic exercise	Athletic training evaluation	Exercise physiology
8:00 to 9:00 pm	Rehabilitation/therapeutic exercise	Athletic training evaluation	Movie
9:00 to 10:00 pm	Rehabilitation/therapeutic exercise	Athletic training evaluation	Movie
10:00 to 11:00 pm			

Figure A-2. Sample daily log.

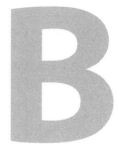

Answer Key
Knowledge Assessment

ATHLETIC TRAINING DOMAINS

Injury/Illness Prevention and Wellness Protection

1. D) A sphygmomanometer is an instrument used to indirectly determine arterial blood pressure.

2. B) The Q-angle is taken by first drawing an imaginary line from the anterior superior iliac spine, down the thigh, and through the midpoint of the patella. A second line is drawn down the midline of the anterior thigh to the tibial tubercle. The angle created by the intersection of the 2 lines is then recorded. An angle greater than 20 degrees is abnormal, causing excessive genu valgus. Excessive genu valgus may lead to patellar problems in the patient.

3. D) Shortening the stride during running may actually decrease the incidence of an overuse syndrome. Overstriding may result in a hamstring pull or knee pain.

4. C) Numbness or tingling in either or both hands in cold weather is symptomatic of Raynaud's syndrome, which is bilateral episodic spasms of the digital blood vessels. The cause is usually idiopathic.

5. E) Significant height, an arm span that is greater than the individual's height, pectus carinatum or excavatum, a high-arched palate, and myopia are all signs of Marfan syndrome.

6. C) Vital capacity is defined as the maximum amount of air that can be expired after a maximum inspiration.

7. D) Myopia is nearsightedness.

8. D) The liver participates in the metabolism of carbohydrates, detoxifies the blood of metabolic byproducts, and produces albumin, clotting factors, and plasma transport proteins.

9. D) Measuring the maximal O_2 consumption during exercise is a good way to determine the patient's ability to adapt to increased metabolic demands. Adequate pulmonary diffusion, appropriate vascular adaptation, and good physical condition of the active musculature all contribute to the patient's ability to maintain homeostasis during exercise.

10. D) Skin-fold measurements for estimating body fat are routinely taken from the biceps, triceps, suprailiac, and subscapular areas.

11. E) The ability to dissipate heat by evaporation is severely limited in a hot, humid environment because evaporation cannot occur unless volumes of dry air are available to absorb the water vapor given off.

12. E) Running short distances stimulates the breakdown of phosphocreatine into phosphorus and creatine in the muscle and glycogen and glucose to breakdown into lactic acid, allowing the muscles to work for short durations of time.

13. C) Power = force x distance. It is the intensity at which a muscle is able to perform work.

14. C) As a result of prolonged training and conditioning, the heart may increase in size to meet the increased demands.

Van Ost L, Lew Feirman K, Manfré K. *Athletic Training Exam Review: A Student Guide to Success, Sixth Edition* (pp 175-220).
© 2017 SLACK Incorporated.

15. B) The formula for calculating target heart rate is 220 – 25 (patient's age) = 195 x 80% = 156 BPM.

16. D) It takes between 10 and 15 minutes of a warm-up period to prepare the body for athletic competition. This warm-up period varies with each patient and may have to be extended with an older patient.

17. D) The average amount of calories a college athlete expends in a day is between 2200 and 4400 calories.

18. A) These percentages are according to USDA guidelines.

19. E) Because specific types of food and timing of the pre-event meal are significant to performance, it is important that the coach, athlete, and athletic trainer are all involved in its proper planning.

20. B) It takes a minimum of 3 to 4 hours for food to digest. Fats take as long as 5 hours to leave the stomach. Proteins take as long as 3 hours, and carbohydrates take approximately 2 hours to pass into the upper small intestine.

21. C) It is crucial that an athlete stay properly hydrated to maintain homeostasis and proper cardiac function. Average water needs for an adult are approximately 1 mL/Kcal burned. This equals approximately 2.4 liters for a 2400 Kcal energy output. Since the body does not conserve water well, it must be frequently replenished, especially while competing.

22. D) Female patients who do not menstruate on a regular basis or those who vigorously exercise may eventually sustain severe bone loss, and osteoporosis may result. A calcium supplement of 1500 mg/day may effectively reduce the bone loss in the total skeleton and reduce the need for estrogen therapy.

23. A) The idea behind a carbohydrate-loading program is to increase the storage of glycogen in the muscles to improve performance in the endurance athlete. The athlete should consume a meal that is high in carbohydrates, such as pasta, and only lightly exercise the day before competition.

24. C) As per universal precautions, the athletic trainer should always wear gloves when treating a bleeding patient.

25. A) To avoid the effects of jet lag, athletes should adjust all training, eating, and sleeping schedules to the local time in which they are competing.

26. E) The NATA's position statement on exertional heat illness includes, but is not limited to, recommendations on appropriate medical care and personnel who are familiar with heat illness prevention, recognition and treatment, proper weigh-in protocols to estimate body water loss during and after activity and ensure prepractice weight before the next practice, and steps to prevent heat-related illnesses.

27. C) Pediculosis is an infestation of body lice and is usually spread by close sexual contact.

28. E) When selecting and fitting an athlete for protective gear or sports equipment, the athletic trainer should make sure he or she buys the protective gear or equipment from a reputable manufacturer; ensure that the individual who assembles the equipment is competent to do so; that the cast, brace, or immobilizer does not violate the rules of the sport; and make sure that the equipment is not defective.

29. A) The helmet should not move if tilted, rotated, or turned side to side. The athletic trainer should push down on the crown of the helmet and check to see that the jaw pads and chin strap fit correctly.

30. D) A patient with renal disease, uncontrolled hypertension, or an acute infection would be disqualified from athletic competition.

31. B) The coach, equipment manager, athlete, and athletic trainer should all be involved in the selection and maintenance of the athlete's protective equipment.

32. E) NOCSAE stands for the National Operating Committee on Standards for Athletic Equipment.

33. A) The 2 major categories that football helmets may fall into are the air- or fluid-filled helmet and the padded helmet.

34. A) Maximum protection is provided by a mouthpiece when it is made of a flexible, resilient material and is form fitted to the teeth and upper jaw.

35. B) The epaulets and cups of properly fitting shoulder pads should cover the deltoids.

36. D) A flak jacket is a piece of protective equipment designed to protect the thoracic area after a rib injury.

37. D) The ASTM is responsible for setting the standards for eye protection for racquet sports.

38. D) Palm protectors for gymnastics are not considered an NCAA-mandated piece of equipment.

39. A) Research has shown that increasing vitamin B_6 intake may increase the synthesis of serotonin, thus decreasing the emotional disturbances related to premenstrual syndrome.

40. B) Red meat and pork are the best sources of dietary iron.

41. B) Sodas contain caffeine, which is a dehydrating substance. This would not be an appropriate drink when trying to maintain adequate hydration during exercise.

42. E) Vitamin A in large doses consumed over a prolonged period of time may lead to toxic symptoms and death in extreme cases.

43. A) A patient may sustain a stress fracture of the bone if he or she is subjected to a few high loads (eg, jumping on a hard floor) or many small loads (eg, jogging long distances).

44. C) Most schools are not prepared to have a blood-work station at a preparticipation examination, nor is it necessary or cost effective for most schools to do so.

45. E) The most common cause of an indirect sports death is heat stroke (ie, no direct trauma is sustained by the patient).

46. B) It is the responsibility of the manufacturers or distributors of recreational sports equipment to report any defective or potentially dangerous products to the Consumer Product Safety Commission.

47. A) Tanner's 5 stages of assessment is an assessment tool used to document the maturity of a patient's secondary sexual characteristics.

48. C) During the final checkout following a preparticipation physical examination, the athletic trainer and team physician should review each examination for final approval to participate.

49. C) According to the NATA position statement published in 2014, the team physician and institution have the legal right to restrict an individual from participating in athletics as long as the decision is individualized, reasonably made, and based on competent medical evidence.

50. E) Significantly overweight individuals who have large muscle mass are much more susceptible to heat stroke than small-framed, lightweight individuals.

51. C) It is prudent to advise the patient to place a damp towel between his or her skin and the ice pack to prevent a cryotherapy injury.

52. D) The spread of impetigo can be decreased by having the patient avoid sharing towels and clothing with other individuals.

53. A) Furosemide (Lasix) is a potent diuretic and is banned by the International Olympic Committee.

54. D) It is wise to suggest to this patient that he trim his toenails by cutting them straight across. He should do this on a weekly basis.

55. A) When advising an athlete about the proper construction of a running shoe, the athlete should make sure that the midsole is somewhat soft but does not flatten out easily under pressure, the forefoot area has good flexibility, the shoe is of good quality, and the heel counter is strong and fits well around the foot.

56. B) Antihistamines have a sedative side effect; therefore, it is advisable that the patient avoid taking them during the day.

57. D) The Dietary Guidelines for America provide authoritative advice for Americans ages 2 years and older about consuming fewer calories, making informed food choices, and being physically active to gain and maintain a healthy weight, reducing the risk of chronic disease and promoting overall health.

58. E) Shin guards are a necessary piece of protective equipment to dissipate the force from a direct blow to the anterior leg.

59. B) Wind and wet weather may increase the possibility of hypothermia while exercising in very cold weather conditions.

60. C) Cooper's ligaments are the suspensory ligaments of the breast and should be supported during exercise.

61. E) A fleshy, pink hue of the distal extremity is a normal finding.

62. C) Abuse of anabolic steroids will cause a reduction in body fat in the female.

63. A) It is important to maintain good hydration on long flights that cross numerous time zones.

64. A) Chronic use of chewing tobacco can cause leukoplakia (ie, the development of white patches on the mucous membranes of the mouth and cheek); mouth and throat cancer; bad breath; gum disease; tooth, bone, and enamel loss; cavities; and stained teeth.

65. C) The patient should be advised to concentrate on strengthening his ankles rather than relying on prophylactic taping.

66. A) An antioxidant is a nutrient that may be found in high amounts in fruits and vegetables and may protect the cells in the body from the detrimental effects of naturally occurring agents, such as oxygen.

67. C) Hyperextension of the wrist when hitting a backhand shot in tennis is a primary cause of lateral epicondylitis.

68. A) Those patients who weigh more than 220 pounds should avoid high-volume, high-intensity plyometric exercises because greater weight increases the compressive forces on joints during plyometric exercises, predisposing these joints to injury.

69. C) Free-weight exercises requiring the bar to pass over the face, move over the head, be positioned on the back, or racked at the front of the shoulders require one or more spotters.

70. C) Keratoderma is the hypertrophy of the stratum corneum of the epidermis, which occurs most frequently on the palms of the hands and soles of the feet. Keratoderma is also known as a callus and can be prevented by wearing 2 pairs of socks and properly fitting shoes, applying a lubricant to the skin to prevent friction, and protecting the palms of the hands with special gloves, tape, or moleskin.

71. B) Urinary tract infections may be avoided with adequate hydration, practicing sanitary bowel and bladder habits, washing the genital area before intercourse, emptying the bladder after intercourse, and removing contraceptive devices after intercourse.

72. C) A torus fracture, otherwise known as a buckle fracture, is a fracture caused by a compressive force causing the bone to bow under the pressure. This is usually seen in the pediatric population.

73. E) The number of servings should be according to the patient's height and weight.

74. A) At the secondary school level, educational items that involve the athletic training student should include the education/training of the universal precautions and first aid for wounds, education regarding the risks of transmissions/infection from the patients for which they care, education on the availability of HIV testing, education on the availability of hepatitis B virus vaccinations and testing, and the education of parents/guardians regarding the students' risk of infection.

75. B) The American College of Sports Medicine recommends that when performing flexibility exercises, a stretch should be held 10 to 30 seconds—only as long as it is comfortable—to obtain optimal results.

76. D) To rectify low blood glucose levels, more free fatty acids are mobilized from adipose tissue than the liver can metabolize, resulting in ketosis. These excess ketone bodies are released into the urine and during respiration, resulting in low blood pH levels.

77. C) Increased muscle capillary density is a morphological change that occurs during resistance training. It is not a neural change.

78. C) Storage and the inventory of athletic uniforms/equipment are not a facilities maintenance task.

79. A) The use of multiple adapters and extension cords may cause a serious electrical hazard in the athletic training facility and should never be used.

80. B) The physician or physician's assistant are the only personnel qualified to examine the patient for adenopathy, abnormalities of the genitalia, and hernias.

81. C) The "flash-to-bang" method is a means by which an athletic trainer can estimate how far away lightning is occurring.

82. D) Patients who live/play in urban or industrial areas should practice in the late afternoon after rush hour when the pollution level is at its lowest point.

83. A) A rubberized, padded cup has an elevated heel, which can compress downward so that the heel never actually makes contact with the interior of the shoe. The other heel cup is a rigid plastic cup. It fits snugly and does not allow the fat tissue to flatten, thus protecting the heel.

84. D) The Achilles tendon tape job is used to restrict the amount of dorsiflexion at the ankle.

85. C) Wearing layers of lightweight clothing is recommended for the prevention of cold-related injuries.

86. B) The patient should alternate pairs of shoes every day to help prevent fungal skin infections.

87. D) Water alone cannot kill an infectious micro-organism. Water can be mixed with bleach (10:1), and this will disinfect soiled surfaces. There are also a number of commercial products that will disinfect soiled surfaces.

88. B) The secondary stage of disease prevention focuses on early detection of an illness or disease and preventing or reversing progression of the disease.

89. E) Medications, age, conditioning level, and hydration status of the patient are all predisposing conditions to heat illness.

90. E) Persistent headaches, constant pain, insomnia, and malaise and fatigue are all considered red flags that should alert the athletic trainer to certain pathologies.

91. B) Immobilization of muscles causes a decrease in muscle tension produced.

92. E) Malaria is transmitted through blood/body fluids.

93. A) Isokinetic exercise is a type of exercise that involves a muscle contraction in which the length of the muscle is changing while the contraction is performed at a constant velocity.

94. B) A shoe with shorter and more cleats is better because the foot does not become fixed to the surface and the shoe still allows controlled running and cutting.

95. A) Ballistic stretching is not recommended.

96. D) To prevent hypothermia, the patient should replace wet clothing with dry clothing, perform warm-up exercises, and wear warm clothing.

97. C) Sixty-five percent of heat produced by the body during exercise is lost by evaporation.

98. D) Heat is lost in the warm, vascular areas of the head and neck, which may account for 50% of heat loss from the body.

99. A) SPF 5 means an individual can be exposed to ultraviolet light 5 times longer than without having the sunscreen on before his or her skin turns red.

100. E) Seizures are not a primary sign of dehydration.

101. E) Shoe sharing between patients may spread tinea pedis.

102. D) A headband will not prevent internal ear damage from loud noises.

103. A) An athlete should have a spotter when lifting at all times to prevent weight-training injuries.

104. B) Weather is not an intrinsic factor of injury.

105. E) Russian stimulation prevents atrophy by contracting the muscles.

106. A) The D2 flexion pattern involves external rotation with flexion and abduction. The D2 extension pattern involves internal rotation with extension and adduction across the anterior aspect of the body.

107. C) Symptoms of bulimia include binge eating followed by self-induced vomiting.

108. E) Enlargement of the spleen is usually a complication caused by mononucleosis.

109. B) The entire sternum should be covered for the shoulder pads to be legal.

110. C) OSHA suggests that a barrier mask is used when performing CPR to minimize the risk of disease transmission.

111. E) Calcium increases the density of bone, which decreases the risk of osteoporosis.

112. E) An anorexic patient will not gain weight during the off-season because of abnormal eating habits.

113. A) Ballistic stretching involves a bouncing motion during stretching and should be discouraged in favor of a static stretch.

114. C) Stretching should be performed bilaterally.

115. E) Stretching, wearing proper footwear, and proprioceptive and strength training may prevent injuries to the lower leg.

116. D) Minimizing the effects of microtrauma; maintaining cardiovascular and lower extremity conditioning; and facilitating good communication among the patient, athletic trainer, coach, and physician will help a throwing patient prevent injuries while training.

117. C) Tertiary prevention is the prevention of a chronic or debilitating illness or injury through appropriate care and rehabilitation.

118. E) Periodization is the concept of dividing the annual training plan into smaller segments, phases, or cycles.

119. D) Extrinsic risk factors are those factors that are independent of the individual's physical makeup. Intrinsic risk factors are inherent in the physical makeup of the individual.

120. E) The overload principle states that muscle strength, power, endurance, and hypertrophy increase only when muscles perform workloads greater than those loads previously encountered.

121. A) A patient with mononucleosis will present with an enlarged spleen, which is susceptible to rupture while playing a sport.

122. B) A patient should return to physical activity only after being cleared by a physician or designee specifically trained and experienced in concussion evaluation and management.

123. E) When evaluating a cervical injury, the first thing the athletic trainer should do is assess the patient's level of consciousness.

124. D) If the athletic trainer suspects shoulder dislocation, it is important to check the neurovascular status of the upper extremity, including the dermatomes and myotomes.

125. A) Shoulder pads protect the superior and lateral aspect of the shoulder. This prevents injury to the acromioclavicular joint.

126. E) The signs and symptoms for sickle-cell anemia and the sickle-cell trait are more likely to present themselves in hot, humid environments or events that take place in high altitude. The patient may present with lumbar or lower quadrant cramping. Other symptoms to watch for are altered state of consciousness, hyperventilation, tachycardia, and hypotension. If the patient collapses, emergency transport to a hospital is required.

127. A) Approximately 17% of individuals with Down syndrome have atlantoaxial instability. This patient should have medical clearance before participating in a sport that might stress the muscles supporting the head and neck.

128. C) The hepatitis B vaccine also prevents hepatitis D.

129. E) The hepatitis B vaccine is given as a series of 3 shots over the course of 9 months.

130. E) Genital warts are caused by the human papillomavirus and are fibrous overgrowths of the dermis, which are acquired via sexual contact. The warts grow rapidly in moist areas of the body.

131. D) The MMR vaccine is given in protection against measles, mumps, and rubella.

132. B) The most common type of cerebral palsy is spastic cerebral palsy or hypertonia.

133. C) A patient who has been diagnosed with cardiac hypertrophy but chooses to ignore the risks associated with continued intense exercise may experience a fatal cardiac event.

134. A) The pituitary gland increases the release of estrogen in females and testosterone in males and stimulates thyroid function. It also produces antidiuretic hormone, causing an increase of water absorption in the kidneys.

135. B) An echocardiogram is a necessary diagnostic tool in the detection of Marfan syndrome. It is used to screen for abnormalities of the aorta.

136. D) Because pathological arrhythmias may compromise blood flow and blood pressure and cause sudden death, certain arrhythmic conditions require limitation of activity in asymptomatic patients without structural heart disease. These arrhythmias include atrial flutter and fibrillation, ventricular tachycardia and fibrillation, second-degree heart clock (Mobitz II), third-degree and acquired complete heart block, and long QT syndrome.

137. A) The incidence of sudden death from hypertrophic cardiomyopathy is 2 to 3 times higher in children and adolescents than in the adult population.

138. E) The label on a dietary supplement must contain all the following elements: the name and location of the manufacturer, the name of the packer or distributor, a complete list of ingredients, the content of the product, and identification of each dietary and nondietary ingredient.

139. C) Beta-blockers decrease blood supply to the skin and antihistamines decrease sweating, both of which affect the body's ability to cool itself in hot weather.

140. D) Bismuth subsalicylate should not be taken by a patient for whom use of aspirin is a precaution. When ingested, bismuth subsalicylate is converted into salicylic acid and bismuth oxychloride.

141. B) Beta-blockers decrease heart rate and the force of contraction of the heart, which prevents overexertion of the heart, but this also prevents an automatic increase in cardiac output, which results in exercise fatigue.

142. B) According to the NATA's position statement on the prevention of pediatric overuse injuries, full effort throwing limits for players 9 to 14 years old should be 75 pitches/game or 600 pitches/season.

143. A) According to the NATA's position statement on the prevention of pediatric overuse injuries, a pediatric athlete should have at least 1 to 2 days off a week from competitive practices, competitions, and sport-specific training.

144. E) According to the NATA's position statement regarding safe weight loss and maintenance practices in sport and exercise, body weight should be assessed relative to body composition.

145. B) According to the NATA's position statement on the management of the patient with type 1 diabetes mellitus, the patient's diabetes care plan should include blood glucose monitoring guidelines, insulin therapy guidelines, and guidelines for hypo- and hyperglycemia recognition and treatment.

146. E) According to the NATA's position statement on safe weight loss and maintenance practices in sport and exercise, a valid and reliable body composition assessment technique includes the use of the following methods: hydrodensitometry, air displacement plethysmography, skin-fold measurements, and bioelectric impedance.

147. D) According to the consensus statement between the Inter-Association Task Force for Preseason Secondary School Athletics and the NATA's Secondary School Athletic Trainer's Committee, *Preseason Heat Acclimatization Guidelines for Secondary School Athletics*, the recovery period between a practice session and walk through (or visa versa) should be 3 hours.

148. E) It is important not to compliment a patient on physical appearance or strength gains, as it may reinforce his or her abusive behavior.

149. A) *Stacking* is defined as simultaneously administering multiple anabolic-androgenic steroids.

150. A) Sex-specific, sport-centered, and coach-facilitated educational programs that promote performance-enhancing alternatives appear to be effective as AAS abuse deterrents for adolescent student-patients.

151. E) According to the NATA's position statement on lightning safety for athletics and recreation, aspects of an emergency action plan specific to lightning safety include the promotion of lightning safety slogans, establishing a chain of command, using a reliable means of monitoring the weather, and identifying locations that are safe from the lightning hazard.

152. C) The facemask should be located 3 finger widths from the nose for a correct fit.

153. C) Thermomoldable plastics, such as Orthoplast, may be used as a hard protective covering for an injured area of the body, such as a dome covering for a quadriceps contusion.

154. B) Assessing activity areas for safety, proper equipment maintenance, and documentation of treatments are all ways of reducing the risk of injury.

Clinical Evaluation and Diagnosis

1. E) Thompson's sign involves squeezing the gastrocnemius-soleus complex while the patient lies prone on a table. The foot should plantar flex when the common muscle belly of these muscles is squeezed. An absence of plantar flexion upon squeezing is a positive test, indicative of a possible Achilles tendon rupture.

2. B) The radial nerve innervates the extensor carpi radialis longus, extensor carpi radialis brevis, extensor carpi ulnaris, and extensor digitorum of the wrist, which when acting together, extend the wrist.

3. D) The most common type of ankle sprain is an inversion sprain. The primary mechanism of injury is a plantar flexion/inversion movement, which usually affects the anterior talofibular ligament first. As the sprain increases in severity, other ligaments around the ankle become involved, such as the calcaneofibular or tibiofibular ligaments.

4. C) A "burner" is a nerve injury commonly caused when the head is forced to one side while the opposite shoulder is depressed. It usually affects the upper trunk of the brachial plexus. A pinched nerve syndrome may also be caused by a nerve root entrapment, subluxed cervical facets, a bulging intervertebral disc, or a combination of lesions (nerve root entrapment and traction injury).

5. A) A sag sign is positive for a torn posterior cruciate ligament when the tibial plateau sags posteriorly as the patient is lying supine and the knee is flexed to 45 degrees, causing a sulcus just inferior to the inferior border of the patella of the affected leg.

6. A) An athletic trainer's initial evaluation of an injury should begin the moment the injury is witnessed or upon initial contact with the patient or another individual who might have witnessed the injury.

7. A) Panner's disease is an osteochondrosis of the capitellum of the elbow, which develops as a result of chronic repetitive trauma, congenital/hereditary factors, or endocrine disturbances. It is typically seen in children 5 to 10 years of age or in a throwing athlete. It must be distinguished from osteochondritis dissecans of the elbow, which also affects the capitellum and may result in intra-articular loose bodies. Panner's disease heals spontaneously with little or no deformity.

8. C) The L5 nerve root innervates the extensor hallucis longus muscle.

9. E) A positive Phalen's test is indicative of carpal tunnel syndrome. The patient is asked to stand with the dorsal aspect of both hands in full contact so both wrists are maximally flexed for 1 minute. A complaint of numbness and tingling in the medial nerve distribution of the fingers is a positive test.

10. C) Trendelenburg's test is used to test for gluteus medius weakness of the hip. The patient is asked to stand on one leg for approximately 10 seconds and then

switch to the other leg. If the pelvis on the unsupported side drops noticeably lower than the pelvis on the supported side, it is a positive finding (ie, weakness of the gluteus medius on the supported side).

11. D) The varus stress test is used to test the integrity of the lateral collateral ligament of the knee. The patient is asked to lie supine with the knee in full extension. The athletic trainer places his or her hand distally on the lateral ankle and the other hand proximally on the knee medially. With the ankle stabilized, a varus force is applied with the proximal hand. Lateral joint pain and/or increased varus movement with an absent or poor endpoint when compared to the uninvolved side are positive findings for a torn lateral collateral ligament.

12. B) A positive drop-arm sign is indicative of rotator cuff pathology. The patient is asked to stand as the athletic trainer passively abducts the patient's arm to 90 degrees and then instructs the patient to slowly lower his or her arm to the side. If the patient has significant pain with the movement or is unable to control the adduction of the arm during testing, the sign is positive.

13. B) The golfer's elbow test is used to identify inflammation in the area of the medial epicondyle. The patient is asked to flex both the elbow and wrist with the forearm fully supinated. The patient is then asked to fully extend the elbow. If the patient complains of pain over the medial epicondyle during testing, the findings are considered positive.

14. D) A sign is an objective entity, one that can be measured, felt, seen, smelled, or heard. A symptom, such as dizziness, is subjective in nature. Symptoms can only be experienced by the individual who is affected by the ailment or injury.

15. D) Tactile information alone will not provide the athletic trainer with enough information to adequately assess the patient's functional status. It is crucial that a well-planned, comprehensive evaluation is performed to assess all aspects of the patient's condition prior to treatment.

16. E) The extensor pollicis longus of the thumb is innervated by the C8 nerve root.

17. D) A positive clunk test is indicative of a possible glenoid labrum tear. The patient is asked to lie supine. The athletic trainer places his or her proximal hand on the posterior aspect of the involved shoulder and the other hand distally on the humerus. As the athletic trainer passively abducts and externally rotates the subject's arm overhead, an anterior force is applied to the humerus as he or she circumducts the humeral head in the glenoid fossa. A clunking or grinding sensation is a positive finding.

18. D) Recurrent anterior subluxation of the shoulder most frequently occurs with repetitive throwing motions, primarily during the cocking and follow-through phases. With constant repetition, the anterior capsule and labrum may stretch or tear, allowing the humeral head to slip anteriorly.

19. B) A pneumothorax occurs when there is the presence of air within the chest cavity in the pleural space but outside the lung. In an intact chest, a pneumothorax can occur if a fractured rib has lacerated a lung or spontaneously if the patient has a congenitally weakened area on the surface of the lung, which may rupture without antecedent trauma. Sudden chest pain and difficulty breathing as the lung collapses are major signs of a spontaneous pneumothorax.

20. A) The posterior tibial and dorsalis pedis pulses should always be palpated after an acute knee injury to ensure the peripheral circulation of the involved limb is intact.

21. E) An injury to the peroneal nerve of the lower leg will result in foot drop. The common peroneal nerve innervates the peroneus longus muscle, the superficial peroneal nerve innervates the peroneus brevis muscle, and the deep peroneal nerve innervates the peroneus tertius muscle of the lateral aspect of the lower leg and foot.

22. B) A Type V Salter-Harris epiphyseal fracture is a crush injury to the epiphysis.

23. C) Cranial nerve VII is the facial nerve. It supplies both sensation and motor control to the facial muscles.

24. B) The latissimus dorsi muscle is innervated by the thoracodorsal nerve.

25. D) A second-degree burn is also known as a partial-thickness burn and appears as a bright red area with blisters.

26. A) The medial and lateral pectoral nerves innervate the pectoralis major muscle, which flexes, adducts, and internally rotates the upper arm.

27. D) Spondylolysis occurs when there is a defect in the pars interarticularis. A "Scottie dog" sign is a radiographic finding of spondylolysis. On an oblique view of the lumbosacral spine, there is an outline that looks like a Scottish terrier. The defect in the pars interarticularis appears as the collar on the neck of the Scottie dog.

28. C) The levator palpebrae superioris muscle elevates the eyelid.

29. D) Vision is controlled by the occipital lobe of the brain.

30. E) Jaundice is a symptom of liver disease that causes the skin to appear yellow in color. It occurs when bile cannot be made or excreted normally.

31. A) A Bankart lesion is an injury to the anterior capsule of the shoulder with an associated tear of the glenoid labrum.

32. B) Pronation and supination of the forearm take place in the horizontal plane.

33. A) An aura is a sensation that occurs just prior to a seizure. It may last for a few seconds and appears as a smell, sound, or specific feeling. It acts as a warning

to the patient and generally takes the same form every time it occurs.

34. E) Signs of inflammation include redness (rubor), pain (dolor), warmth (calor), and swelling (tumor).

35. A) Exercise may cause a temporary increase in blood pressure, while a change in posture may raise or lower the pressure.

36. B) Type 1 diabetes is also known as juvenile-onset diabetes or insulin-dependent diabetes, and it usually has its onset prior to age 25. It is not usually associated with obesity.

37. C) Symptoms of mononucleosis include tender lymph nodes, fever, sore throat, and a stiff neck. Low back pain is not a characteristic symptom of this illness.

38. D) Candida is a yeast infection that causes vaginitis.

39. D) Osteoporosis rarely occurs in an obese individual. Obesity is not considered a risk factor for the disease.

40. C) The normal leukocyte (white blood cell) count is between 4000 and 10,000 cu mm.

41. C) The AIDS virus attacks the T-helper lymphocytes of the body's immune system, leaving the individual vulnerable to infection.

42. B) EIA stands for exercise-induced asthma.

43. C) The patient will hike the hip to allow his or her foot to clear the floor during the swing phase of gait.

44. E) Crutches widen the base of support. This allows for the line of gravity to fall within the base of support, increasing stability.

45. E) Anorexia nervosa is an eating disorder that is most commonly seen in adolescent females. The patient consumes a progressively diminishing amount of food until she is malnourished, and there is a weight loss of 25% of the original weight. Because of an intense fear of becoming obese, the patient will not maintain normal body weight for her height and age, even when emaciated. It is a sign of a significant underlying psychological problem.

46. E) There are 5 emotional phases a patient may experience after a significant injury or loss. These phases include denial, anger, bargaining, depression, and acceptance. These reactions are normal when faced with a serious injury or illness, and the athletic trainer should allow the patient a chance to work through each stage without interference.

47. D) Symptoms of overtraining include emotional lability, loss of appetite, decreased concentration, decreased motivation to participate in practices and competitions, chronic fatigue, indigestion, and changes in bowel and sleeping patterns. An athlete who experiences staleness should be temporarily removed from activity and allowed time to rest and relax to stimulate renewed interest and motivation to play.

48. E) Signs of depression include loss of appetite, insomnia, fatigue, and a feeling of hopelessness.

49. C) An obsessive-compulsive patient may perform ritualistic behaviors, such as cleaning his equipment after each game, and repeat specific behaviors obsessively, such as hand washing numerous times after touching a dirty uniform or money.

50. A) A patient might be prone to injury for a number of reasons, some of which are physical and some of which are psychological. Physical factors include poor strength and endurance, inflexibility or hypermobility, and poor coordination. Emotional factors include depression, family or school problems, or anxiety.

51. A) Dehydration causes a decrease in blood volume, which results in lowered cardiac filling pressure and stroke volume. The heart rate increases to compensate for these adverse effects.

52. B) This meal is high in fat and protein and will take a long time to pass through the digestive tract.

53. A) Consuming a simple sugar prior to an event will stimulate the pancreas to produce high levels of insulin, which in turn will cause a sudden reduction in blood glucose.

54. D) Vitamin C is found in high concentrations in green vegetables, fruits, and citrus.

55. C) Tetracycline should be taken 2 to 3 hours after meals to avoid the possibility of the drug binding to either iron or calcium.

56. D) Percent body fat in females should not go below 12% because the internal organs lose a protective layer of adipose tissue.

57. E) Water loss of 2% to 3% total body weight will begin to adversely affect athletic performance. Losses of 4% to 5% total body weight or greater are life-threatening percentages.

58. C) Tylenol (acetaminophen) has analgesic and antipyretic properties but is not an anti-inflammatory drug.

59. B) Ultram is a centrally acting analgesic drug used to control moderate to severe pain.

60. B) Tinactin is an antifungal medication that is supplied as an aerosol powder, cream, powder, or solution and is indicated for treatment of tinea pedis (patient's foot) or tinea cruris (jock itch).

61. B) To determine if there is a fracture of the jaw, it is appropriate for the athletic trainer to have the patient bite down and observe for any malocclusion, ask the patient to open and close his mouth and observe for movement asymmetry, and palpate the jaw for any deformities.

62. A) The liver is located in the upper right quadrant and may be injured with blunt trauma to that area of the abdomen.

63. C) According to the NATA position statement on Management of Sport Concussion, there should be a minimum of 24 hours between return to play progression stages following a concussion.

64. C) Cauliflower ear is an injury to the pinna of the ear caused by continuous friction or direct trauma to the

auricle, which results in bleeding into the soft tissue of the ear. It is characterized by localized perichondrial swelling, discomfort, and deformity of the outer ear.

65. C) If a patient has increased protein in the urine (most commonly diagnosed by urinalysis during a preparticipation medical exam), it may indicate renal or urinary tract pathology.

66. E) Because stress fractures of the bone can be so small, a typical x-ray will often miss the injury. A bone scan involves injection of a radioactive substance into a vein, which is absorbed by bone. A scanner is used to detect abnormal levels of uptake or hot spots in the bone, indicating a stress fracture or abnormal lesion.

67. D) The cornea, which is the clear surface covering the front of the eye, is most often injured by a foreign body, causing a corneal abrasion.

68. D) Measuring the amount of motion available at a joint will provide the athletic trainer with no significant information regarding the neurovascular status of the injured limb.

69. E) Anaphylactic shock is caused by a severe allergic reaction to a foreign protein or drug. There is a contraction of smooth muscle fibers and increased capillary permeability, causing dyspnea, cyanosis, convulsions, unconsciousness, and, if untreated, death.

70. C) Endorphins are polypeptides that are produced in the brain and produce analgesia by binding to the opiate receptor sites of pain perception in the body.

71. C) The classical mechanism of injury for an anterior shoulder dislocation is forceful shoulder abduction with external rotation.

72. B) Insomnia, shortness of breath with exertion, headache, fatigue, tachycardia, bradycardia, confusion, and edema are all symptoms of acute mountain sickness.

73. E) A manual muscle grade of 2/5 is also known as a poor muscle grade and is defined as completing full range of motion in a gravity-eliminated position. A grade of 3/5, or fair, is defined as completion of full range of motion against gravity, and a grade of 1/5 is a trace grade, in which the examiner observes or palpates contractile activity in the muscle, but no movement is present.

74. C) The scouring test is used to test for hip joint pathologies, such as arthritis, osteochondral defects, avascular necrosis, and acetabular defects.

75. A) To test the strength of the piriformis, the patient should be sitting. The lower leg is resisted as the patient attempts to externally rotate the hip.

76. B) Average range of motion for elbow flexion is 0 to 135 degrees.

77. B) The biceps femoris is tested with the patient lying in the prone position. Knee flexion is then resisted with the tibia in full external rotation.

78. A) The sacroiliac nerve root innervates the posterior tibialis, plantaris, peroneus longus, and peroneus brevis muscles, which act to plantar flex the ankle and foot.

79. A) To test the function of the rhomboid major, the athletic trainer should ask the patient to retract his or her scapula.

80. C) The biceps brachii muscle originates on the supraglenoid tubercle of the scapula (long head) and the apex of the coracoid process (short head). It inserts into the tuberosity of the radius. It functions to supinate the forearm, flex the elbow, and flex the shoulder.

81. A) Hip abduction occurs in the frontal plane.

82. E) The gastrocnemius muscle plantar flexes the foot and flexes the knee.

83. B) The flexor pollicis longus originates on the radius, adjacent interosseous membrane, and coronoid process of the ulna and inserts on the distal phalanx of the thumb. Its primary action is flexion of the thumb.

84. D) Movements of the eyes are controlled by the oculomotor nerve—cranial nerve III.

85. D) The rectus femoris muscle flexes the hip and extends the knee when it contracts.

86. B) The gluteus maximus externally rotates the hip.

87. B) Nerve roots C6, C7, and C8 represent the sensory dermatomes of the hand (from radial to thumb sides, respectively).

88. E) The serratus anterior muscle functions to protract the scapula and stabilize it against the rib cage.

89. C) The quadratus lumborum originates on the iliac crest, the lumbar vertebrae, and lumbodorsal fascia and inserts onto the 12th rib and the transverse processes of upper lumbar vertebrae. It functions to laterally flex the trunk.

90. C) The supinator muscle of the forearm is innervated by the radial nerve.

91. B) The extensor digitorum longus extends the toes.

92. E) Food passes from the stomach through the duodenum and mixes with the secretions from the pancreas and liver before continuing into the jejunum and ileum.

93. C) The median nerve passes though the carpal tunnel at the wrist.

94. C) The ileum is part of the lower small intestine.

95. C) The femoral nerve innervates the pectineus muscle, and the obturator innervates the adductor longus, magnus, brevis, and gracilis.

96. B) The abductor digiti minimi abducts the fifth finger.

97. D) The sternocleidomastoid flexes and rotates the head.

98. C) The tibial nerve innervates the gastrocnemius, flexor hallucis longus, and biceps femoris musculature.

99. D) Cranial nerve II is the optic nerve (vision), cranial nerve I is the olfactory nerve (smell), cranial nerve XII (hypoglossal) is the nerve responsible for movement

of the tongue, and cranial nerve VIII is responsible for hearing.

100. A) To test the gluteus medius in an antigravity position against resistance, the patient must be side-lying with the affected limb on top.

101. E) The average range of motion of the knee is 0 to 135 degrees.

102. D) True leg length discrepancy is measured between the anterior superior iliac spine to the medial malleolus of the ankle.

103. C) To test the hip flexor musculature, the patient should be sitting. The athletic trainer then applies a force down onto the anterior aspect of the thigh as the patient resists the movement.

104. B) To test the deltoids, the patient's shoulder should be positioned to 90 degrees.

105. C) Scoliosis is a lateral curvature of the spine with rotation of the vertebrae around its long axis. The ribs may become prominent on the convex side of the curve (rib hump) as the vertebral bodies rotate toward the convex side and the spinous processes rotate toward the concave side of the curve.

106. C) If there is an injury to the long thoracic nerve, which innervates the serratus anterior muscle, the scapula cannot be protracted, and it will result in winging, which is a prominence of the vertebral border of the scapula.

107. B) The average range of VO_2 max for the average college patient is 45 to 60 mL/kg/min.

108. E) Measuring the heart rate during submaximal stress testing is used to indirectly determine the VO_2 max. It is known that heart rate rises linearly with increasing workloads.

109. D) The oxygen consumed by the patient during the recovery phase of exercise replenishes the oxygen levels in the tissue fluids, increases the myoglobin in the muscles to preactivity levels, and restores the venous oxyhemoglobin to pre-exercise levels.

110. D) Progressive pulse rate test, the Harvard step test, and the Cooper 12-minute run-walk test are all classified as submaximal stress tests.

111. A) A goniometer is the instrument most commonly used for measuring joint range of motion in the clinical setting. A goniometer may come in a variety of shapes and sizes and may be made of metal or plastic.

112. C) Periostitis, myositis, tendinitis, or a combination of conditions may cause tenderness and pain with induration and swelling of the pretibial musculature of the patient's lower leg. They may be classified as anterior or posteromedial "shin splints," depending on which group of structures are involved.

113. C) A positive Speed's test may suggest bicipital tendinitis. The patient is asked to stand or sit with the involved shoulder flexed to 90 degrees and the elbow fully extended with the forearm supinated. The athletic trainer should have his or her distal hand on the volar aspect of the forearm and the proximal hand palpating the bicipital groove. As the athletic trainer resists shoulder flexion, it should be noted if there is tenderness or pain over the biceps tendon.

114. E) Sever's disease is most frequently seen in children 7 to 10 years of age. It is a calcaneal apophysitis, which is associated with growth spurts, decreased Achilles and hamstring flexibility, and biomechanical abnormalities, which contribute to poor foot shock absorption.

115. A) A positive talar tilt test is indicative of a torn calcaneofibular ligament. The patient is asked to lie on his or her uninvolved side with the involved foot and ankle over the edge of the table and the knee flexed to 90 degrees. The athletic trainer's proximal hand stabilizes the tibia as the distal hand grasps the talus. As the ankle is initially placed in neutral, the examiner then tilts the talus into an adducted position. If the range of motion in the adducted position of the involved ankle is greater than the uninvolved, the findings are considered positive.

116. D) Whether or not the patient has medical insurance should not be an immediate concern of the athletic trainer during the history-taking portion of the initial evaluation. Only those pieces of information that assist the athletic trainer in developing a course of action or treatment plan for the patient should be considered pertinent.

117. C) The L4 nerve root innervates the rectus femoris muscle and the vastus medialis, intermedius, and lateralis muscles, all of which extend the knee.

118. C) A positive Neer's test is indicative of shoulder impingement of the supraspinatus tendon or the tendon of the long head of the biceps.

119. A) A positive finding, such as a palpable clunk or shift with 20 to 30 degrees of knee flexion, is indicative of an anterolateral instability of the knee, secondary to a torn anterior cruciate ligament or torn posterolateral capsule of the knee.

120. B) Spearing occurs when a football player uses the top of his head as a ram, making contact with an opponent. The force is transmitted axially through the cervical spine, causing injury. Most cervical spine injuries result from forced hyperflexion, often with a combined rotation movement.

121. D) The most common mechanism of injury for an anterior shoulder dislocation is shoulder abduction and external rotation.

122. D) Glenohumeral instability allows increased movement of the humeral head within the glenoid fossa, which in turn may lead to microscopic damage to the tissues that lie beneath the coracoacromial arch. Resultant edema and microhemorrhage cause a reduction in the joint space and impingement, most commonly of the supraspinatus tendon.

123. C) Plantar fasciitis is an inflammation of the plantar fascia of the foot. It has a variety of possible causes but is commonly due to one or all of the following: pronated feet; poor footwear, leading to decreased shock absorption; and/or tight plantar fascia, Achilles, and hamstrings. A metatarsal pad would only be indicated if the patient also had a diagnosis of metatarsalgia (ie, inflammation in the area of the metatarsal heads).

124. A) Because of the constant purging, the patient is vulnerable to an electrolyte imbalance and dehydration. Hypokalemia (potassium deficiency) may result from chronic vomiting or laxative/diuretic abuse, causing muscle fatigue, weakness, kidney damage, or an arrhythmia.

125. B) Hypoesthesia is dulled sensation to touch.

126. A) Diabetic coma, which results from severely elevated blood sugar levels, results in the patient feeling drowsy and having acetone-smelling or fruity breath. The skin may be flushed and dry, the respirations deep, and the thirst intense. This is caused by inadequate insulin intake (ie, insulin-dependent patient). Although diabetic coma rarely occurs in an active patient, it can result from a mismanaged insulin schedule, severe infection, or poor diet.

127. E) McMurray's test is used to test the knee for a tear in the medial or lateral meniscus with the patient lying in supine. The knee is fully flexed, and the tibia is externally rotated with a valgus force and extended, or internally rotated with a varus force and extended. A palpable "click" is indicative of a positive test.

128. A) Impetigo is a skin infection caused by staphylococcal bacteria. It is prevalent in wrestlers because of their close contact with other athletes. The bacteria can be carried under the nails and in the nose, infecting open skin wounds or abrasions. The lesion looks similar to herpes simplex lesions—a superficial ulcer with a yellow crust. The skin around the lesion appears normal. Treatment consists of local cleansing with soap and water and oral antibiotics.

129. A) Altered vital signs, such as a rapid pulse; decreased blood pressure; ashen skin color; rapid, shallow respirations; and rebound tenderness are all signs of shock, indicating a significant internal injury.

130. D) The primary movements of the pectoralis major are shoulder adduction, flexion, and internal rotation. If the pectoralis muscle is torn, the patient will experience pain and weakness with resistance to these movements, as well as pain to palpation of the injured area.

131. D) Signs of pulmonary edema include acute dyspnea, cough, headache, and weakness. These symptoms can occur in athletes who train in high altitudes.

132. D) Most often a "pop" is associated with an anterior cruciate ligament injury and less frequently with a subluxed patella.

133. C) A Colles' fracture is a fracture of the distal radius and tip of the lunate. This usually occurs as a result of a fall on an outstretched arm and hand.

134. B) Allen's test is used to test the integrity of the radial and ulnar arteries of the hand. It is performed by first having the patient pump his or her hand by repetitively making a fist. The patient then maintains the fist while the examiner compresses the radial artery with his or her thumb and the ulnar artery with his or her finger. As the patient relaxes his or her hand, the radial artery is released, followed by the ulnar artery. If there is a delay in flushing of the radial or ulnar sides of the hand or fingers, there may be an occlusion of the radial or ulnar artery, respectively.

135. B) The lunate is the most frequently dislocated carpal bone, which occurs from a fall on an outstretched hand. This in turn opens the space between the proximal and distal carpal bones, and the lunate dislocates to the palmar side of the wrist.

136. A) When the tibia is stabilized in an externally rotated position and a strong valgus force is applied, the medial collateral ligament, medial meniscus, and anterior cruciate ligament are vulnerable to injury.

137. A) Nerve root compression is most appropriately evaluated by electromyography or by a nerve conduction velocity test.

138. B) A papule may be described as a solid, well-defined pink/red elevated area on the skin. A wart is an infection of the skin caused by the papillomavirus. The lesions are raised flesh-colored or pink papules with a rough surface that tend to grow inward into the foot, causing pain while walking.

139. E) The C5 dermatome is located over the area of the middle deltoid.

140. B) In order to expose the anterior deltoid to resistance in an antigravity position, the shoulder must be in 90 degrees abduction and in full external rotation. The forearm must be in full supination.

141. D) The most common symptom of lumbar discogenic injury is a sharp, radiating pain down one or both legs. This is caused by a bulging or herniated disc impinging on a nerve root in the lumbar spine.

142. D) An avulsion of the ischial tuberosity will cause local acute pain deep in the proximal thigh/distal buttock area.

143. D) The iliotibial band moves back and forth over the lateral epicondyle of the femur as the knee is flexed and extended. If the iliotibial band is too tight or it overrides and rubs on the lateral epicondyle during downhill running, the bursa between the iliotibial band and epicondyle becomes inflamed. Pain is elicited as the knee is brought into about 30 degrees of flexion. A popping sensation is not a consistent finding with this syndrome.

144. B) The contact phase of the running gait consists of foot strike, midsupport, and take-off. The swing phase includes the follow-through, forward swing, and foot descent. One foot is in contact with the ground during the contact phase, and the leg and foot freely move through the air during the swing phase.

145. B) The tibia internally rotates during midsupport, following pronation of the subtalar joint.

146. B) To check the vascular integrity of the hand after an acute elbow dislocation, it is important to assess the presence and quality of the radial pulse and check for good capillary refill of the nailbeds of the fingers.

147. B) The cardinal symptoms of an extradural hemorrhage include a lucid interval usually lasting for a few minutes up to a couple of hours, followed by a period of lethargy, which may precede a seizure and coma. This is a true medical emergency, and the patient must receive treatment immediately in order to survive.

148. E) Sinding-Larsen-Johansson disease is a result of excessive strain on the inferior patellar pole at the origin of the patellar tendon. It is commonly seen in children ages 8 to 13 who participate in running or jumping sports. It is often missed unless the athletic trainer palpates the inferior patellar pole with the patient's knee in extension and the patellar tendon relaxed.

149. B) Pain with resisted hip adduction and hip flexion with diffuse tenderness and ecchymosis of the medial thigh is indicative of a strain of the groin area.

150. C) With a rupture of the rectus femoris muscle, a large bulge is seen in the upper thigh, and there is pain along the entire muscle belly. Extension is limited because of the inability to contract the rest of the quadriceps musculature.

151. C) Burning pain with tenderness to palpation over the lateral epicondyle of the femur is associated with iliotibial band syndrome. If the iliotibial band is too tight, it will rub over this area during running, causing localized inflammation. Ober's test is appropriate for a tight iliotibial band.

152. E) The quadriceps musculature is innervated by the femoral nerve, which originates at the L2, L3, and L4 nerve levels.

153. A) The spinal accessory nerve innervates the upper trapezius muscle. If it is injured, the patient will not be able to perform a shoulder shrug.

154. A) The pes anserinus (sartorius, gracilis, semitendinosus) flexes the knee and will weakly internally rotate the tibia.

155. D) Heat exhaustion is characterized by profuse sweating, cool and clammy skin, rapid pulse, a mildly elevated rectal temperature (approximately 102°F), and hyperventilation.

156. C) A complete blood count is a test that assesses the red and white blood cell count, hemoglobin and hematocrit levels, and platelet count.

157. E) A -3/5 muscle denotes an incomplete movement against gravity.

158. D) Mallet finger is caused by a blow to the tip of the finger by a thrown ball, which jams the finger and results in an avulsion of the extensor tendon from its insertion.

159. E) Decreased sensation over the dorsum of the foot, inability to dorsiflex the great toe/ankle, and a diminished patellar reflex are suspect of L5 nerve root irritation or injury.

160. A) Active range of motion is used to determine the patient's willingness to move.

161. B) A cardinal sign of rhabdomyolysis is the presence of myoglobin in the urine.

162. D) The 3 most commonly affected organ systems in Marfan syndrome are the skeletal, ocular, and cardiovascular systems. Symptoms may include, but are not limited to, scoliosis, anterior chest deformity, tall height, various cardiac abnormalities, myopia, superior lens dislocation, retinal detachment, and eye shape irregularities.

163. A) Graves' disease is an autoimmune disorder that is also known as hyperthyroidism. Some of the signs and symptoms of this disease include, but are not limited to, an enlarged thyroid, heart palpitations, gastrointestinal irregularities, significant weight loss, anxiety, retracted eyelids, and exophthalmos (bulging of the eyes).

164. C) Guillain-Barré syndrome is an acute autoimmune syndrome manifesting as a rapid, diffuse, demyelinating disorder of the spinal roots and peripheral nerves. More than 50% of those individuals affected have a history of a viral respiratory or gastrointestinal infection from 1 to 3 weeks prior to the onset of neurological symptoms.

165. A) The most common complications of hepatitis C are cirrhosis of the liver and liver cancer.

166. B) The incubation period for HIV and human papillomavirus is 1 to 6 months.

167. A) Cystic fibrosis is the most commonly inherited disorder among White Americans. It is a genetic disorder that affects the exocrine glands and is most prevalent in the respiratory and digestive systems.

168. B) Amyotrophic lateral sclerosis is a peripheral nerve disease that primarily affects the motor neuron of a motor unit. It most commonly occurs during middle age and has an unknown etiology. This disease is manifested by a gradual weakness of the distal extremities and is progressive, ultimately affecting the ability to speak and swallow. It is a terminal disease in which 50% of the patients live for only 3 years after initial onset.

169. D) Reflex sympathetic dystrophy is a condition that affects a distal extremity after a significant traumatic injury. It occurs as a result of overactivity of small fiber pain receptors. The initial signs of reflex sympathetic dystrophy include range of motion limitations, swelling of the limb, an increased skin temperature, and atrophic changes. If the syndrome becomes chronic, atrophy of the limb may be evident and vascular changes may occur. If left untreated, the limb may potentially become completely dysfunctional.

170. E) Multiple sclerosis is caused by regions of intermittent inflammation, known as *plaques*, which result in demyelination of the neurons of the central nervous system.

171. A) Mumps is a contagious viral disease that is manifested by enlarged parotid glands (parotitis).

172. E) Spina bifida occulta is the incomplete formation of the posterior vertebral arch without herniation of the meninges or spinal cord. It is often detected by x-rays taken for symptoms of low back pain.

173. C) The biceps tendon reflex correlates to the C5 spinal level.

174. B) The patellar tendon reflex correlates to the L2-4 spinal level.

175. D) Romberg's test is used to evaluate for possible dysfunction of the cerebellum or basal ganglia. These areas of the brain control vestibular and postural control.

176. C) Cranial nerve VIII, the vestibulocochlear nerve, controls hearing and can be tested by crumpling paper or rubbing fingers together near the ear.

177. D) Cranial nerve XI, the spinal accessory nerve, is tested by resisting a shoulder shrug.

178. D) Cranial nerve IX, the glossopharyngeal nerve, controls the ability to swallow. Tracheal deviation or complaints of dysphagia are abnormal.

179. E) Changes in cognition and behavior and disorientation after a head injury are indicative of dysfunction of the cerebrum.

180. E) The adrenal glands release aldosterone, cortisol, epinephrine, and norepinephrine. Growth hormone is produced by the pituitary-hypothalamus.

181. E) Glucogen is a hormone produced by the pancreas, which stimulates the release of glucose from the liver into the blood.

182. D) Mast cells are specialized cells that are found in connective tissue throughout the body. They release histamine, which is one of the chemicals that initiate the inflammatory process.

183. E) Lysosomes function to digest material brought into the cytoplasm of the cells during phagocytosis.

184. C) Chemotaxis is the process by which leucocytes are drawn to the site of injury by chemical mediators during an inflammatory reaction.

185. A) Rhabdomyolysis is a fatal disease caused by renal failure. It is associated with the sickle-cell trait and intense levels of exercise.

186. A) Decortication may occur after a severe head injury and presents as extension of the lower limbs with flexion of the elbows, wrists, and fingers.

187. B) A peak flow meter is used to measure forced expiratory volume. A decreased forced expiratory volume is an indication of exercised-induced bronchospasm.

188. E) A goiter, which is an enlarged thyroid, is the primary symptom of Hashimoto's thyroiditis.

189. B) Wolff-Parkinson-White syndrome is characterized by ventricular tachycardia and is a result of a short PR interval, a prolonged QRS complex, and early depolarization of the heart.

190. B) The diagnostic tool that is considered the "gold standard" for detecting hypertrophic cardiomyopathy is echocardiography.

191. C) The Homan's sign is used to screen for suspected deep vein thrombosis. It is performed by passively dorsiflexing the ankle, stretching the gastrocnemius. The sign is positive if this maneuver causes leg pain.

192. D) The hallmark sign of peripheral vascular disease is intermittent claudication, which manifests as cramping, weakness, numbness, and pain of the lower extremities and is provoked by exercise of a given intensity and duration.

193. A) Caffeine withdrawal may cause fatigue, headache, irritability, restlessness, anxiety, yawning, and a runny nose.

194. D) When the biceps brachii reflex is tested, it correlates with the function of the C5 nerve root.

195. E) A positive cervical distraction test is indicative of a nerve root compression or facet dysfunction.

196. C) The T7 nerve root correlates to the dermatome at the level of the xyphoid process and costal margins.

197. A) A Brudzinski-Kernig test is performed if meningitis is suspected. As the patient lies in supine, the neck is passively flexed and the patient is asked to perform a straight leg raise on the tested side to end range or point of pain. Then the patient is asked to flex the knee to 90 degrees while maintaining the hip in flexion on the tested side. The opposite extremity stays in extension on the table. A positive finding is spine pain or lower extremity symptoms that increase with neck and hip flexion and are relieved with knee flexion. A positive test is indicative of nerve root impingement or meningeal/dural irritation.

Immediate and Emergency Care

1.   D) Naproxen is the generic form of the brand name drug Naprosyn, which is an NSAID. Naproxen does not come in a topical form and is delivered orally.

2. D) Aristocort, Kenalog, and Topicort are all corticosteroids that are used to treat the inflammation and pruritic manifestations of psoriasis. Betadine is a topical microbicide agent used for skin and wound infections.

3. E) Butisol is a barbiturate used as a sedative in the treatment of insomnia.

4. B) Xanax is a medication used to treat anxiety and panic disorders.

5. B) Penicillin inhibits the metabolism of bacteria.

6. A) Acute compartment syndrome is a condition in which soft tissue pressure is increased and the viability of the muscles and nerves of the anterior lower leg are jeopardized. This condition may progress from an initial hematoma, usually resulting from a blow to the anterolateral side of the leg, to total foot drop as a result of injury to the peroneal nerve.

7. D) It is appropriate during the acute stages of a quadriceps contusion to apply ice to the injured area and put the knee into a slight amount of passive flexion to maintain the flexibility of the quadriceps muscle.

8. C) With deep frostbite, there should be rapid rewarming of the body part in warm water between 100°F to 110°F. Rewarming of the body part should continue until it is deep red/bluish in color.

9. A) An athlete should be immediately referred to a dentist if a tooth has been knocked out, if a tooth has been displaced 2 mm or more, or when a crown is fractured and the tooth is still alive.

10. C) When a male athlete sustains a direct blow to the genitalia, the testicular area may go into spasm. It is best to have the athlete lie supine and flex his knees to his chest until the pain subsides and then apply an ice pack to the scrotal area.

11. B) When performing 2-person adult CPR, the correct compression-to-breath ratio is 30 compressions to 2 breaths (30:2).

12. D) Shock after a severe injury can result from hemorrhage or stagnation of blood.

13. B) A patient who has a known diagnosis of mononucleosis is vulnerable to a possible spleen injury/rupture if the patient returns to a sport too soon. The patient may resume light activity after 3 weeks from the onset of the illness if the spleen is not enlarged or painful, the patient's liver function studies are normal, no fever is present, and any other complications are resolved.

14. D) Romberg's sign is the inability to balance the body when the eyes are shut and the feet are together. It is a sign of sensory ataxia.

15. D) In this case, it is known the patient is unconscious from a blow to the head and neck, not from aspirating an object or debris. It is only necessary to perform a finger sweep if the athletic trainer cannot ventilate the patient and an object that is blocking the passage of air is visible in the mouth.

16. A) The proper position for the fist that is resting on the patient's body is on the abdomen between the xyphoid process and the umbilicus.

17. A) When treating for an impaled object, always leave the object in place and apply a bulky bandage around it to control bleeding and to stabilize the object.

18. B) During a seizure, it is best to keep the area around the patient clear of objects or spectators and protect the patient's head and body from further injury. It is important to turn the patient on his or her side so if he or she vomits, he or she will not aspirate. A prolonged seizure is a serious medical situation, and it is prudent to call for additional medical support.

19. C) Brain damage is most likely to occur if the brain is deprived of oxygen for approximately 4 to 6 minutes.

20. A) The carotid pulse is palpated in the groove between the larynx and sternocleidomastoid muscle.

21. C) The sternum must be depressed at least 2 inches, but not more than 2.4 inches for compressions to be effective in an average-sized adult during CPR.

22. C) Heat stroke is considered a medical emergency. Heat stroke results in severe hyperthermia with the failure of the thermoregulatory system and dysfunction of the central nervous system. This condition does not spontaneously reverse its course, and the patient may die without immediate medical attention.

23. D) Signs of an acute tension pneumothorax include tracheal deviation, distended neck veins, unilateral absence of breath sounds, and cyanosis.

24. E) Flank pain, difficulty/inability to void, and hematuria are all signs of kidney, bladder, or urethra injury.

25. E) During emergency care of the unconscious patient, the athletic trainer should make sure the patient's airway is clear and he or she is breathing normally.

26. D) The most devastating cervical injuries sustained in athletic participation occur from cervical hyperflexion and axial compression.

27. A) The patient will complain of severe lower right abdominal pain with acute appendicitis and will complain of tenderness to the same area with palpation.

28. D) When transporting a patient with a suspected spinal cord injury, a spine board should be used to stabilize the patient during transport and additional medical support should be employed.

29. E) The elbow should be slightly flexed to approximately 30 degrees, which places the hand at hip level.

30. D) CPR should not be stopped until the athletic trainer is too exhausted to continue, spontaneous breathing and circulation have resumed, or another responsible party continues CPR in place of the athletic trainer.

31. C) Reflex pain experienced in the left shoulder and upper arm after a severe blow to the abdomen, resulting in a ruptured spleen, is known as Kehr's sign.

32. A) Although total immobilization of the ribs is not possible, a rib belt or rib taping may help minimize movement and make the patient more comfortable.

33. C) Athletic taping and bandaging serves many functions, including supporting or immobilizing an injured body part, protecting wounds from further injury or infection, holding protective equipment in place, and controlling hemorrhage.

34. C) Continuous taping around a limb may result in compromised circulation.

35. B) The compression to breath ratio during one-person CPR is 30:2.

36. A) Applying pressure will minimize the bleeding. Keep the area clean with sterile saline or hydrogen peroxide, apply butterfly strips for temporary closure, and use ice and a compressive dressing to minimize further bleeding. Refer the patient to the physician for sutures, if necessary.

37. D) Placing the tooth in a moist cloth and encouraging immediate implantation is the only means by which to save the tooth. Tooth reimplantation after 24 hours has a poor success rate.

38. E) During an emergency, important information the athletic trainer should provide to the emergency personnel includes the type of emergency, the type of injury that is suspected, the current status of the patient, the type of care currently being given to the patient, and the exact location of the emergency (including landmarks).

39. D) With a suspected fracture of the knee joint or of the surrounding area, the splint should stabilize all the lower limb joints and one side of the trunk.

40. E) Mast cells and platelets release histamine and serotonin during the reaction phase of an acute injury.

41. C) During the initial phases following a soft tissue injury, there is transitory vasoconstriction followed by vasodilatation and increased permeability, causing redness and swelling of the area.

42. D) The bone marrow contains immature stem cells that differentiate into red and white blood cells and platelets.

43. C) When an athlete is injured, he or she may react strongly to pain and become very fearful of the possibility of being disabled. During this time, the athlete may display signs of overreacting by becoming argumentative or sarcastic. It is important that the athletic trainer provides emotional support and allows the athlete to express his or her emotions. It is best to be reassuring and divert the athlete's attention away from the injury.

44. E) Vitamin K contributes to blood clotting because it imparts a calcium binding ability to certain blood proteins, such as prothrombin.

45. A) RICE stands for rest, ice, compression, and elevation.

46. D) A potentiating drug is one that is used to increase the effect of another drug.

47. B) Athletes should avoid standing near tall objects, such as trees or telephone poles, which may attract a lightning strike.

48. A) Tinea pedis (patient's foot) is caused by a fungus infection. The athletic trainer should advise the patient to keep his or her feet clean and dry and wear clean socks on a daily basis.

49. B) Pulling the tick off the skin can leave the tick's head still embedded in the skin. Covering the tick's body with mineral oil or nail polish remover will cause the tick to remove its head from the skin.

50. E) The primary adverse side effect of the NSAID group is gastrointestinal discomfort.

51. B) Common side effects of antibiotic therapy are abdominal cramping, diarrhea, nausea, and vomiting.

52. E) Aspirin is administered in 325-mg tablets.

53. B) Side effects of oral contraceptives include nausea and vomiting, fluid retention, amenorrhea, and a feeling of sluggishness.

54. C) A female may develop a condition known as hirsutism, which is the excessive growth of hair in unusual places, with the ingestion of testosterone.

55. C) Otitis externa is a bacterial or fungal infection of the outer ear canal that is characterized by severe ear pain, hearing difficulty, drainage from the ear canal, swelling of the canal, and occasional dizziness. Prevention includes avoiding prolonged exposure to water (eg, swimming/showering) and keeping the ear dry after water activities with acetic acid or a similar drying agent.

56. B) The helmet should be left in place unless the facemask cannot be removed to gain access to the airway, OR if with the facemask is removed, ventilation still cannot be provided, OR if the helmet and chin straps do not hold the head secure, OR if the helmet prevents immobilization for transport in an appropriate position.

57. C) A flathead screwdriver is not an appropriate tool to remove a loop strap on a helmet.

58. D) A patient with congenital or acquired spinal stenosis is more likely to develop paralysis after a fracture-dislocation because the spinal canal is already too small for the spinal cord.

59. C) The patient may be immobilized on a standard spine board, a vacuum mattress, a scoop stretcher (otherwise known as a split litter), or the Miller full-body splint.

60. D) Histamine is given off by blood platelets, basophilic leukocytes, and mast cells during the beginning of the inflammatory process, causing arterial dilation and capillary permeability.

61. B) Dysplasia is the abnormal development of tissue.

62. A) Poor blood supply and poor immobilization are 2 conditions that interfere with fracture healing.

63. A) Epinephrine is a sympathomimetic drug that may be delivered via an injective device, such as an EpiPen, to halt an anaphylactic reaction.

64. D) Tagamet (cimetidine) and Zantac (ranitidine) are both examples of histamine-2 blockers, which reduce stomach acid output by blocking the action of histamine cells in the stomach.

65. E) Before administering a NSAID, the athletic trainer must determine if the patient is allergic to aspirin because a cross reaction may occur in patients allergic to aspirin.

66. E) Manual conveyance is a method by which an injured patient is transported a greater distance than he or she is able to walk with ease. The most convenient carry is performed by 2 athletic trainers.

67. C) The average respiratory rate for an adult is 12 to 15 breaths/min.

68. A) The bell of the stethoscope should be placed over the brachial artery during auscultation.

69. B) During orthostatic syncope, the rapid perfusion of the limbs decreases the blood supply to the brain, which will cause a loss of consciousness. Orthostatic syncope occurs during a rapid change in postural positioning.

70. C) Fatty foods may exacerbate gallbladder pathology.

71. D) A seizure that lasts over 5 minutes, a primary seizure, and a seizure that does not fit into the patient's pattern of previous seizures are all indications for physician referral.

72. E) TID means 3 times a day.

73. A) When there is a suspected spinal cord injury and the decision is made to remove the helmet and shoulder pads, they should be removed simultaneously to avoid cervical hyperextension.

74. A) The Inter-Association Task Force recommends that no fewer than 4-plus persons lift a patient suspected of having a spinal cord injury.

75. E) An otoscope is an instrument used to visually examine the ear canal and tympanic membrane.

76. B) The primary reason an athletic trainer would perform pulmonary auscultation is to identify potential abnormal breath sounds that would indicate a pathological condition.

77. E) Dysuria, an urgency to urinate, decreased urine volume, nocturia, back pain, pyuria, or hematuria all indicate the patient has cystitis, which is a bladder infection.

78. C) These are symptoms of a rhinovirus infection, which causes the common cold. Supporting the immune system with fluids, rest, and good nutrition will help to limit the duration of the infection. It is best to limit the patient's activities until the fever subsides and slowly increase exercise as tolerated.

79. A) Itchy skin on the feet and toes is not a medical emergency requiring immediate referral to a physician.

80. C) A hard-shell pad would be an appropriate choice when the goal is to completely cover an injured area (such as a contusion) and prevent further harm.

81. A) The brace should be adaptable to a variety of anatomic shapes and sizes. Not all prophylactic braces need to be custom molded to achieve this goal.

82. C) The athletic trainer should recommend an athletic shoe with a sole that has good shock absorption and is durable.

83. E) The most common types of soft materials utilized by athletic trainers to make pads or protective devices include gauze, cotton, felt, adhesive-backed felt, sponge rubber, or foam.

84. E) An AED, or automated external defibrillator, is used when an unconscious victim has no pulse.

85. D) Avoidance is one of the most frequent methods utilized by managers, but it resolves nothing. The conflict will occur again if the athletic trainer is not proactive in seeking a resolution.

86. E) Abnormal pain associated with a burning sensation that gets worse when the patient lies supine or consumes caffeine, spicy food, or alcohol is highly indicative of esophageal reflux or peptic ulcer.

87. A) A sudden onset of chest pain, dyspnea, hemoptysis, and cyanosis is highly suspect for a pneumothorax.

88. E) Diarrhea, vomiting, and abdominal cramping that occurs within 6 hours of eating is highly indicative of food poisoning.

89. B) Each quadrant of the abdomen should be auscultated for at least 2 to 3 minutes before deciding bowel sounds are absent.

90. C) Cold urticaria is an allergic reaction to cold exposure. If left unrecognized, it may lead to a systemic anaphylactic response.

91. D) The athletic trainer should not provide psychological counseling unless he or she is qualified to do so.

92. C) When using iontophoresis, the athletic trainer should be aware of possible skin irritation and chemical burns caused by ion flux during treatment.

93. A) A patient with an abdominal injury should never be given anything to eat or drink because it increases the risks of surgery if an operative procedure becomes necessary, and it may make the patient's symptoms worse.

94. B) Confusion, dizziness, apprehension, and diaphoresis are all signs of insulin shock. Any diabetic patient who does not respond favorably within 2 to 3 minutes of receiving sugar should be transported immediately to the hospital.

95. B) The point at which the first sounds of the pulse are heard through the stethoscope is the systolic pressure.

96. D) A relationship between the athletic trainer and the patient built on trust and mutual respect is essential to the patient's psychological and physical well-being.

97. A) A patient who shows undue concern over minor injuries, but the concern is self-limiting, should not be referred for professional psychological counseling.

98. E) Deficits such as tinnitus, decreased hearing, or deafness may suggest involvement of the vestibulocochlear nerve.

99. C) The initial dose of Tylenol (acetaminophen) is 2 tablets, 325 mg each. The dose may be repeated every 4 to 6 hours, PRN.

100. A) The initial dose of Advil (ibuprofen) is 1 to 2 tablets, 200 mg each. The dose may be repeated every 6 hours, PRN. Do not exceed 6 tablets in a 24-hour period without consulting with a physician. (Note: This medication should not be administered to a patient who is less than 12 years old regardless of parental consent.)

101. B) The initial dose of Pepcid AC (famotidine) is one 10-mg tablet to be taken with water up to 2 times a day. Do not administer more than 2 tablets in a 24-hour period.

102. B) Constipation may occur secondary to poor hydration or decreased fiber intake. It is recommended that the patient increase his or her fluid intake and increase his or her consumption of foods high in fiber.

103. C) Nonsteroidal anti-inflammatory analgesics, skeletal muscle relaxants, and anti-inflammatory steroids (glucocorticoids) all have complementary/synergistic effects to cryotherapy treatments.

104. D) Systemic vasoconstrictors may decrease perfusion of the peripheral tissues.

105. A) The 3 most common sites for avulsion fractures and apophysitis in the pelvic region are the ischial tuberosity and the hamstring attachment, the anterior inferior iliac spine and rectus femoris attachment, and the anterior superior iliac spine and the attachment of the sartorius.

106. D) A shin contusion that is poorly managed can lead to osteomyelitis, which results in the destruction and deterioration of the bone.

107. E) A metatarsal bar is used for the treatment of metatarsalgia and sesamoiditis.

108. E) The median, radial, and ulnar nerves and the neurovascular status of the brachial artery should be evaluated pre- and post-reduction of a dislocated elbow.

109. B) A Bennett's fracture occurs at the carpometacarpal joint of the thumb. It is structurally unstable and the patient should be referred to an orthopedic surgeon.

110. E) Anxiety caused by fear may in turn lead to hyperventilation. An increased breathing rate results in the patient rapidly blowing off carbon dioxide, which causes respiratory alkalosis, which is manifested by peripheral numbness, tingling, and light-headedness.

111. D) The muscle spasm has an end feel that is an abrupt, firm, springy resistance to motion. This is caused by the protective muscle spasm.

112. A) Checking for sensations of numbness, tingling, or burning is a component of a secondary survey.

113. C) Immediately transport the patient to an emergency care facility for intravenous glucose administration. This is necessary to avoid possible brain damage or death.

114. A) Referred symptoms occur distally from the site of injury.

115. B) Restlessness is not a sign/symptom of postconcussion syndrome. The patient will show signs of fatigue.

116. D) Tinel's sign identifies ulnar nerve compression or transmission interference at the elbow.

117. C) During anaphylactic shock, blood pressure drops very quickly as the blood pools into the expanded capillaries.

118. B) A contusion is a closed wound (ie, an injury of the soft tissue beneath the skin).

119. C) Heat stroke is a condition of rapidly rising internal body temperature that occurs when the body's mechanisms for the release of heat are overwhelmed.

120. E) The dorsal pedal pulse should always be assessed when dealing with injuries to the lower extremity.

121. E) Psychogenic shock is commonly referred to as fainting and is caused by a temporary dilation of blood vessels that reduces the normal amount of blood in the brain.

122. B) When a minor is injured and it is a life-threatening situation, the athletic trainer may provide emergency care even if the parents have not given written consent. This is known as implied consent.

123. C) A sign of heat stroke is hot and relatively dry skin.

124. D) Slow and weak pulse is not a sign of a diabetic coma.

125. A) The brachial and femoral arteries are the 2 most common sites to apply direct pressure to control severe bleeding of an upper or lower extremity.

126. B) Septic shock is the result of a widely disseminated infection of the body.

127. D) Slow and weak pulse is not a sign of hypovolemic shock.

128. C) Brain cells begin to die after the brain has been deprived of oxygen between 4 to 6 minutes.

129. D) Noisy respiration, such as wheezing or gurgling, is a sign of inadequate ventilation.

130. C) Gaining access to the airway is the only reason a football helmet should be removed before a spinal injury has been ruled out.

131. E) The xyphoid process is the bony prominence most commonly chipped during CPR.

132. B) Heat exhaustion causes a person to sweat profusely and become dizzy and nauseated. Also, his or her blood pressure drops during heat exhaustion.

133. D) It is not wise to give food or fluids to a patient who is in shock because of the possibility of aspiration.

134. D) A patient with a skull fracture may have a bony deformity, Battle's sign, "raccoon" eyes, and tenderness of the hard palate.

135. A) Apply direct pressure to the wound.

136. B) Hold in-line stabilization decreases any chance of increasing the severity of the injury.

137. D) Immobilization is initiated before rehabilitation begins.

138. A) When ice is applied during the initial care of an acute injury, there is a decrease in local metabolism.

139. B) Afferent pathways carry impulses toward the central nervous system.

140. E) Friction massage is a type of deep massage.

141. D) To determine if a patient is breathing, the athletic trainer should LOOK for the rise and fall of the chest, LISTEN for the breath sounds, and FEEL for breathing.

142. C) Dilated pupils are a sign of shock, hemorrhage, or cardiac arrest.

143. B) A patient's blood pressure will be low if he or she is in shock.

144. A) Signs of frostbite include blotchy white to yellow-gray skin.

145. D) A patient suspected of having heat exhaustion should be administered cool fluids, unnecessary clothing should be removed, and he or she should be moved to a cool place.

146. E) According to the NATA's position statement on the management of sports-related concussion, transport to a medical facility for a concussion may be necessary if the patient is unconscious for a prolonged period of time, shows declining mental status during or after the injury evaluation, or demonstrates signs and symptoms of an injury more severe than a concussion.

147. B) Cranial nerve disorder or altered breathing patterns caused by trauma or disease are indicative of midbrain or medulla dysfunction.

148. C) A fatal ventricular arrhythmia, known as *commotio cordis*, can occur as the result of a blunt force trauma to the chest.

149. D) Diabetic ketoacidosis occurs when the blood glucose levels are too high. It is a metabolic state caused by excess accumulation of keto acids in the body and a decreased pH of the blood. This can result in a diabetic coma.

150. E) Wolff-Parkinson-White syndrome is associated with an accessory electrical pathway in the heart proximal to the ventricles which can lead to supraventricular tachycardia.

151. C) If the core body temperature falls below 90°F, the muscles become cold and stiff and blood is shunted away from the periphery to the core to maintain vascular volume. This is known as *cold diuresis* or *polyuria*.

152. A) The normal oxygen saturation level is between 95% to 100%.

153. B) The normal systolic blood pressure reading for a child between 6 to 10 years of age is 80 to 122 mm Hg.

154. E) When assessing the venue prior to an event, the athletic trainer should consider the condition of the court or field of play to identify any potential hazards, the location of emergency exits, location of the ambulance or entrances where EMS personnel will arrive, and the location of emergency equipment.

155. A) The correct size of an oropharyngeal airway is selected by measuring the distance between the tip of the ear and the corner of the mouth.

156. D) Suctioning of a patient is indicated to clear the airway when he or she is unresponsive and vomits.

157. B) A posterior elbow dislocation is considered a medical emergency. It occurs as a result of a violent impact causing the elbow to move into severe hyperextension or valgus, causing the ulna to be driven in a posterior or posterolateral direction. Because it is likely there might be both circulatory and nerve impairments of the upper extremity, the radial pulse and motor and sensory function should be assessed and then the patient's arm should be immobilized. The patient should be treated for shock and transported to the nearest medical facility.

158. E) Turf toe is caused by extreme hyperextension or hyperflexion of the great toe. It is a sprain of the plantar capsular ligament of the first metatarsophalangeal joint. Treatment includes ice, rest, NSAIDs, taping to limit motion at the first metatarsophalangeal joint, and shoe modification.

159. D) The Food and Drug Administration classifies oxygen as a drug. Therapeutic oxygen systems are different than emergency oxygen systems in that they may be operated only by allied health professionals or medical personnel licensed to do so and require a prescription from a physician to be used. Emergency oxygen systems do not require a prescription for use.

160. A) Prior to transferring and securing a patient with protective equipment (as in football or ice hockey), the facemask should be removed and the straps and laces on the shoulder pads must be cut to provide the EMS team with adequate access to the patient as necessary without causing excessive movement.

161. E) The first step in treating an abrasion or laceration is to reduce the wound contamination by removing large pieces of debris with a sterile dressing and cleaning the wound surfaces.

162. D) If a bronchodilator is used more often than recommended it may cause tachycardia.

163. E) Portable radios and land-line telephones are preferred over personal cell phones during an emergency primarily because a cell phone may be unreliable in some areas due to weak cellular signals.

164. E) A capillary refill time of greater than 2.0 seconds indicates inadequate perfusion and may be an indication of shock, dehydration, hypothermia, or peripheral vascular disease.

Treatment and Rehabilitation

1. D) An extension lag exists when the patient cannot fully extend his or her knee.

2. D) A hand dynamometer is a simple tool used to objectively assess the functional strength of the hand and forearm.

3. A) Tissue healing begins with a cellular response, which is associated with vascular changes, followed by phase II, or regeneration, of both soft tissue and bone. The third phase is known as remodeling, in which there is an increased organization of extracellular matrix and decreased synthetic activity.

4. E) It may take up to 1 year before soft tissue remodeling is complete.

5. A) The primary location of adenosine triphosphate in skeletal muscle is the sarcomere.

6. C) Golgi tendon organs are sensory receptors found in the muscle tendons that monitor the tension generated in a muscle during contraction.

7. A) A neurapraxia is the demyelination of the axon sheath of a nerve fiber. This condition will cause a failure of the nerve to conduct impulses, causing a conduction block. It is usually reversible.

8. D) Osteoclasts are cells that reabsorb bone during growth.

9. A) Cell division for new cartilage growth does not occur in the adult.

10. D) The patient will experience the feelings of cold, followed by burning, then aching, and finally numbness.

11. D) A warm whirlpool is a superficial heater. It will only heat the superficial tissues.

12. E) Fibroblasts become active during the regeneration phase of the inflammatory response to begin building collagen.

13. A) Shivering is a method by which the body generates heat.

14. B) External force created by a muscle depends on the velocity of the muscle shortening (as the speed of shortening increases, the force decreases), the angle of the pull of the muscle (ie, when the muscle pulls at right angles to the bone it is moving, the muscular force will be optimal), and the length of the muscle (the tension developed with a contraction is greatest if the muscle is at its maximum resting length to start).

15. D) Proprioception is the awareness of movement, changes of equilibrium, and posture of the body and its segments. The "control center" for proprioceptive awareness in the brain is located in the cerebellum.

16. A) A static stretch requires that the patient stretch the muscle and hold the position to prevent a muscle injury, which may occur with ballistic stretching.

17. A) The cardiovascular and respiratory systems must work together to meet the oxygen demands of the skeletal musculature during exercise. If the demand is not met by increasing the respiratory rate, the cardiac output must increase to increase the delivery of the red blood cells from the lungs to the heart to the muscles.

18. E) Visualization, also known as *therapeutic imagery*, incorporates the mental rehearsal of a positive rehabilitative experience followed by full recovery. It is a psychological tool used to enhance physical healing after an injury.

19. A) For rehabilitation of an injury to be successful, the athletic trainer must establish a good rapport with the patient so that the patient is comfortable and there is a mutual environment of trust.

20. C) An attention-seeking patient generally will not accept responsibility for him- or herself and enjoys being dependent upon other individuals. As a result, the patient is demanding and is not satisfied with the amount of time other patients receive, always wanting more time and attention by the athletic trainer taking care of him or her. This type of patient is very draining to the health care staff and requires specific boundaries so the staff is not burned out by the patient.

21. D) In order to lose 1 to 2 pounds a week, an athlete must reduce his or her daily caloric intake by 500 to 1000 calories a day.

22. E) Cryotherapy is used as an anesthetic and to prevent or decrease the inflammatory process.

23. C) Eddy currents are heat-producing currents that are administered by means of an induction coil or condenser plate of a short-wave diathermy unit. It uses a magnetic field to create these currents within the tissues.

24. D) A monophasic spike waveform delivered in pairs is used with high-voltage pulsed generators.

25. B) Because a moist heat pack is a form of superficial heat, it does not increase the muscle tissue temperature.

26. A) The negative pole or cathode will cause local vasodilatation under the pad, tissue softening, irritation, and edema reduction.

27. B) Inflammation of a body part is an indication for the use of cryotherapy.

28. B) Single-leg hopping would be an appropriate functional skill in assessing the patient's readiness for play after an ankle injury. Lifting tolerance is not a skill.

29. A) Normal range of motion of a joint must be restored before and concurrently with strengthening exercises during rehabilitation. Limb endurance and proprioception follow in the later phases of treatment.

30. C) Slow-reversal-hold-relax is a PNF stretching technique.

31. D) The hip is moving into a pattern of flexion, adduction, and external rotation during a Dl flexion pattern.

32. A) The proper timing sequence for a D2 extension pattern of the upper extremity is shoulder extension followed by forearm pronation and finger flexion.

33. A) Grade I joint mobilization is appropriate for decreasing pain and spasm.

34. A) An inferior humeral glide is the proper glide to employ when trying to restore or increase shoulder abduction.

35. B) Isokinetic training is generation of a muscular force with observable joint movement that occurs at a constant speed with variable external resistance.

36. D) Cupping, hacking, and pinching are all methods of tapotement.

37. E) Effleurage is a superficial or deep stroking technique used to produce relaxation.

38. C) Proprioception is the awareness of posture, positioning, and movement as the limb is moved through space.

39. E) The quadriceps must contract eccentrically to allow for deceleration of the body in downhill running.

40. D) Postseason conditioning should focus on identifying and emphasizing specific areas of the conditioning components the patient needs to improve upon.

41. B) During the acute phase of an ankle injury, some form of cryotherapy should be initiated. The water temperature should be set at 55°F to 65°F (cold) to prevent swelling.

42. B) The girth measurements of the involved leg do not have to be exactly equal before returning the patient to full activity, as slight differences are normal.

43. C) Restoration of normal proprioception of the affected limb is the most commonly forgotten component of the rehabilitation program.

44. C) Isometric strengthening exercises are the safest exercises to initiate immediately postoperatively, as there is no joint movement initiated during muscular contraction.

45. B) Jumper's knee is an overuse syndrome of the extensor mechanism of the knee. There is injury to the proximal pole of the patella, as it is subjected to the repetitive traction pull of the quadriceps musculature. The quadriceps muscle should be strengthened during rehabilitation to prevent further injury.

46. B) Trochanteric bursitis can be caused or aggravated by a tight tensor fasciae latae muscle.

47. D) A tight Achilles tendon can cause early heel-off or excessive pronation in order to allow the lower leg to move over the foot during running.

48. D) The coach's opinion concerning when the athlete should return to play should not influence the athletic trainer's professional judgment in designing a rehabilitation program and following prudent guidelines for care.

49. A) Range of motion and strength of the shoulder girdle is intimately related to the function of the cervical area.

50. A) The proper sequence for rehabilitating a grade II ankle sprain includes RICE (rest, ice, compression, elevation), stretching exercises, isometric exercises, proprioceptive exercises, and isotonic strengthening exercises.

51. A) Rehabilitation should begin as soon as possible after an injury with the initiation of modalities for pain relief (ie, RICE).

52. E) The first set of 10 repetitions is with a weight that is 50% of the weight that will be lifted in set 3 when utilizing the DAPRE technique of progressive resistive exercise.

53. C) With a diagnosis of patellofemoral pain syndrome, chondromalacia patellae, or subluxing patella, it is important to strengthen the quadriceps with an emphasis on the vastus medialis obliquus muscle and the hip adductors in order to improve the tracking of the patella.

54. D) Stretching the anterior chest wall (especially the pectoralis muscles) and strengthening the midthoracic musculature (especially the rhomboids and middle trapezius) improve posture and decrease pressure on the structures of the thoracic outlet.

55. E) Williams' flexion exercises encourage a position of lumbar flexion, which opens the vertebral foramina, taking the pressure off the nerve root.

56. A) The patient's body is in a stable, static position while using a recumbent stationary bicycle and does not need to rely on proprioception to perform this activity.

57. C) Scapular musculature should be strengthened first to promote stability before the distal musculature is strengthened to provide mobility.

58. E) Hamstring strengthening should be initiated early in anterior cruciate reconstruction rehabilitation because the hamstrings are the main secondary stabilizers for the anterior cruciate ligament.

59. D) An isotonic knee extension machine is not a closed-chain exercise because the feet are not in contact with any surface.

60. B) Lateral epicondylitis is an overuse syndrome of the wrist extensors. Once the inflammatory process is under control, strengthening the wrist extensors will help prevent a reoccurrence of the problem.

61. B) McKenzie extension exercises are appropriate for treating a lumbar herniated disc, as they encourage the mechanical movement of the disc anteriorly away from the nerve root.

62. B) When performing an abdominal crunch (sit-up), the patient should cross his arms across his chest, tuck in his chin, bend his knees, inhale, and then exhale as he pulls his torso up toward his knees.

63. C) A rehabilitative brace might be used postoperatively or during rehabilitation after an acute injury.

64. E) Running on a treadmill would most closely relate to the type of activity a soccer player would participate in during his or her sport.

65. A) Mechanical traction is not indicated for treatment of acute sprains and strains.

66. C) The anterior deltoid, triceps, pectoralis major, and latissimus dorsi are all active while performing a bench press.

67. C) The quadriceps, hamstrings, the erector spinae, and the gluteus maximus are all active when performing a full squat with weights.

68. D) The trapezius, pectoralis major, serratus anterior, and triceps musculature are all active when performing a seated military press.

69. B) A grade III joint mobilization is a large amplitude movement throughout the full available range of motion of the joint.

70. A) The SAID principle stands for Specific Adaptation to Imposed Demands.

71. E) A wall is an immovable object and may be used for an isometric exercise. During isotonic exercise, there is a fixed resistance with variable speed of movement.

72. A) Ballistic stretching places high, intermittent demands on the muscle, possibly exceeding its physiological limitations, leading to a muscle tear.

73. C) Plyometric training involves loading a muscle eccentrically prior to performing a powerful concentric contraction. This places the muscle in a fully stretched position just prior to contraction-enhancing explosiveness, which is important in a sport such as volleyball.

74. B) Having the patient stand on the injured limb on a mini-trampoline enhances proprioception by making the patient react to a slightly unleveled surface. The goal is to have the patient maintain this position without wobbling or losing his or her balance.

75. D) Because eccentric muscle strengthening requires high muscle tension to be generated, exercising the quadriceps eccentrically is initiated in the later stages of the rehabilitation.

76. A) Full knee extension exercises (from 90-degree knee flexion to 0-degree extension) should be avoided in the early stages of anterior cruciate reconstruction rehabilitation because of the high shearing forces placed on the tibia by the contracting quadriceps.

77. C) Partial sit-ups assist in strengthening the abdominals, and trunk extension exercises (with or without resistance) strengthen the erector spinae musculature.

78. B) Any finding that the athletic trainer observes, palpates, or measures is recorded under the objective (O) section of a SOAP note.

79. C) Bracing for structural scoliosis may be effective up to approximately age 18. After this age, the epiphyseal plates close and external devices for correction do not work well.

80. E) Ultrasound is based on the reverse piezoelectric effect.

81. E) Ultrasound waves cannot be transmitted through air. Ultrasound energy must be transmitted through a coupling medium, such as water or a lotion.

82. B) Convection is a method of heating by which heat is transferred from the source to the recipient by means of movement of the heating medium (eg, air or water).

83. D) The duty cycle is that time in which sound waves are being emitted during one pulse period.

84. A) A moist heat pack is considered a superficial heater.

85. B) Conventional TENS uses a frequency in the 50 to 100 pulses per second range with a phase duration of 2 to 50 µseconds.

86. A) Galvanic burns are the most serious adverse reaction to iontophoresis and are caused by the galvanic current itself.

87. C) The temperature of a paraffin bath should be maintained between 126°F and 130°F to keep it in a molten state.

88. B) Ultrasound converts high-frequency sound energy into heat energy as it penetrates the tissue.

89. D) Ultrasound waves are reflected by bone and absorbed by muscle.

90. B) Inflammation, hemorrhage, infection, and phlebitis are all contraindications for massage.

91. D) Diathermy is used to increase local circulation, reduce spasms, decrease pain after a musculotendinous injury, and with patients with osteoarthritis.

92. A) Scar tissue may be reduced with the use of pulsed ultrasound.

93. B) The inverse square law states that the intensity of radiation from a light source varies inversely to the square of the distance from the source.

94. D) Phonophoresis is the delivery of medication via sound waves, and iontophoresis is the delivery of medication via direct electric current.

95. A) The primary indication for cervical traction is to reduce muscle pain and spasm.

96. E) The proper referral for a patient with an eating disorder would be to a psychologist or psychiatrist because of the complex nature of the condition. It should be recognized by the athletic trainer that anorexia nervosa or bulimia is not just a simple nutritional problem but an underlying psychological problem.

97. D) Symptoms of gonorrhea in a male include a tingling sensation in the urethra followed by a greenish-yellow discharge of pus with painful urination. The patient should be instructed to refrain from all sexual activity until he is treated.

98. C) It is important that the athletic trainer educate the patient about the treatment process, as it will decrease his anxiety.

99. A) It is proper to have the patient breathe in deeply at the beginning of the lift and forcefully exhale at the end of the lift.

100. B) Constant pressure on the axilla may cause crutch or "Saturday night" palsy, which is temporary or permanent numbness in the upper extremities and hands.

101. C) It is important to assess the athlete's training schedule and diet to make sure he or she is not overtraining and eating a poor diet. Both may affect an athlete's performance level.

102. E) To prevent reinjury during the rehabilitation of a soft tissue injury, it is important that the patient not experience pain during active movement.

103. A) Sinding-Larsen-Johansson disease is an apophysitis at the inferior pole of the patella and is characterized by swelling, pain, and point tenderness at the site. It usually occurs during adolescence. Isotonic exercise is not appropriate for this particular condition, as it may increase the symptoms by causing too much stress on the affected area.

104. D) It is important that the patient be advised as to when to take his or her medication and with which foods/drugs it should not be combined.

105. B) It is appropriate for the athletic trainer to encourage the patient to express her feelings and needs.

106. D) Heavy strength training workouts should be limited to off-season and preseason periods.

107. B) Scheuermann's disease is a degeneration of the vertebral epiphyseal endplates, which may cause the intervertebral disc to herniate. An increased kyphotic curve is seen in a patient with this condition. Extension and postural exercises may help reduce the symptoms of backache in the early phases of the disease.

108. A) It is important to emphasize the importance of good hip flexor, lumbar paraspinal, and hamstring flexibility during the rehabilitation of a lumbar strain to prevent reinjury.

109. B) It is best to sleep in a side-lying position with the knees bent slightly to avoid pressure on the low back area.

110. E) It is wise for the athletic trainer to advise and consult with the team strength and conditioning coach regarding the development of a reconditioning program postinjury.

111. A) Honesty and respect are important qualities that an athletic trainer should possess when counseling a patient who is in a state of distress.

112. C) The patient may feel a burning sensation during an ultrasound treatment if the intensity is set too high, not enough coupling medium is being used, or if the transducer head is moving too slow.

113. B) Pain that occurs at a site distant to damaged tissue and does not follow the course of a nerve is known as referred pain.

114. B) Continuous and pulsed diathermy are used to decrease pain and muscle spasm. Diathermy is contraindicated for use with acute inflammation and joint effusion, pregnancy, and open wounds.

115. A) When a convex surface moves on a concave surface during joint mobilization, the roll and glide occur in opposite directions.

116. C) Cervical traction is indicated with a cervical disc herniation.

117. B) Muscle energy techniques are methods used to stretch tight muscles by having the patient contract a muscle against a counterforce in a specific position.

118. C) Delayed-onset muscle soreness normally occurs 24 to 72 hours postexercise.

119. A) Reduced submaximal heart rate does occur as a result of aerobic endurance training, but it is a cardiovascular adaptation, not a respiratory adaptation.

120. D) The latissimus dorsi, teres major, middle trapezius, and rhomboids are all involved when performing a seated row exercise.

121. D) The flexor carpi radialis and flexor carpi ulnaris are the primary muscles involved in performing a wrist curl.

122. B) Proprioceptors are specialized sensory receptors that are sensitive to changes in pressure or tension within a joint, muscle, or tendon. They are responsible for relaying information regarding muscle dynamics to the central nervous system.

123. E) Goal setting is the most effective motivator for compliance to rehabilitation of an athletic injury.

124. A) A major disadvantage of isometric exercise is that it can produce a spike in systolic blood pressure, which can lead to a potentially life-threatening cardiovascular accident.

125. C) The knee-jerk reflex (which is a monosynaptic stretch reflex) is a simple example of muscle spindle activity.

126. B) Passive insufficiency of a muscle occurs when the length of a muscle prevents full range of motion at the joint or joints over which the muscle crosses.

127. C) An exercise designed to improve balance must incorporate a multisensory approach.

128. C) A patient who presents with posterior instability of the glenohumeral joint should avoid a combined position of internal rotation, horizontal adduction, and flexion.

129. D) The length of a rehabilitation program is irrelevant in regard to the development of a functional progression sequence.

130. A) Closed kinetic chain exercises of the upper extremity are used primarily for strengthening and improving proprioception and neuromuscular control of the muscles that stabilize the shoulder girdle.

131. B) The general adaptation syndrome consists of 3 stages: the alarm stage, the resistance stage, and the exhaustion stage.

132. D) An ice bath (or ice immersion) is a mixture of ice and water with a temperature range of 50°F to 60°F in which a body part, most typically the fingers or toes, is immersed. It is used to decrease pain and edema.

133. A) One method of decreasing skin-electrode resistance when performing an electrotherapy treatment is to moisten the electrodes with water.

134. D) When it is met with air, 99.9% of ultrasound energy is reflected.

135. C) The stimulation point placement of electrodes is most commonly used with brief-intense TENS.

136. A) Goal setting is important when developing a treatment program because it identifies outcomes, establishes timeliness of the treatment program, measures the effectiveness of the treatment protocol, and allows the patient to be part of the treatment.

137. E) There should be no metal in the immediate treatment area when using short-wave diathermy.

138. B) Dexamethasone and lidocaine are commonly combined when utilizing iontophoresis.

139. E) Ultrasound units should be calibrated at least once a year to ensure their safe use.

140. E) The patient is presenting with a carbuncle, which is a bacterial (staphylococci) infection often resulting as a complication of folliculitis.

141. A) Herpes simplex is caused by a viral strain that is associated with skin and mucous membrane infection. Herpes simplex labialis is most commonly known as a cold sore.

142. E) Pediculosis (ie, lice) is an infestation by the louse and is most effectively treated with a parasiticide.

143. A) An infection caused by tetanus bacillus may occur secondary to a deep puncture wound.

144. C) Adaptations in skeletal muscle that occur as a result of resistance training, such as increases in strength and muscle mass, may begin to reverse in 48 hours.

145. B) Circuit training is an effective technique for improving strength and flexibility.

146. D) Computerized parts will significantly drive up the cost of the bike and do not ensure superior results.

147. C) Treading water is not a necessary skill for participating in an aquatic therapy program. Many types of buoyant devices may be used to keep the patient afloat.

148. D) Decongestants are vasoconstrictors increasing the possibility of heatstroke. Antihistamines decrease the peripheral sweating, and diuretics limit cutaneous vasodilatation. Beta-adrenergic blockers decrease the blood supply to the skin, which minimizes the cooling mechanism.

149. E) A patient's heart rate will gradually rise as the intensity of the exercise rises and will plateau at a given level in approximately 2 to 3 minutes.

150. B) The efferent/motor response to neural/sensory information is known as *neuromuscular control*.

151. D) A fracture that fails to heal spontaneously within a normal time frame is known as a nonunion fracture.

152. D) The thermal effects of ultrasound may increase edema.

153. A) Iontophoresis results in the movement of ions into the body through the use of an electrical current.

154. E) Pétrissage is the method of massage that involves lifting and kneading the skin, subcutaneous tissue, and muscle with the fingers or hand.

155. B) Loss of function is a cardinal sign of inflammation.

156. C) Raynaud's phenomenon is a vascular reaction to cold that results in a white, red, or blue discoloration of the extremities. The fingers and toes are the first to be affected.

157. C) The heat of the water causes vasodilatation and creates an outward filtration of fluid into the tissues. When combined with the dependent position of the body part, a warm whirlpool will cause an increase in edema.

158. A) Graves' disease is the most common form of hyperthyroidism.

159. E) Dyspnea is air hunger marked by labored or difficult breathing.

160. B) Neurapraxia is a stretch injury to a nerve resulting in transient symptoms of paresthesia and weakness.

161. A) The pes anserinus muscle group is formed by the semitendinosus, gracilis, and sartorius muscles.

162. C) Stress is the internal reaction or resistance of tissue to an external load.

163. D) Clonic cramps/spasms are an involuntary muscle contraction characterized by alternate contraction and relaxation in rapid succession.

164. C) *Myofascial release* is a term that refers to a group of techniques used for the purpose of relieving soft tissue from the abnormal grip of tight fascia.

165. B) Half-life is the rate at which a drug disappears from the body through metabolism, excretion, or both.

166. B) Circuit training is a type of training that employs a series of stations consisting of various combinations of weight training, flexibility, calisthenics, and brief aerobic exercise.

167. E) Diaphoresis means sweating.

168. B) Mechanoreceptors are found in ligaments, musculotendinous junctions, capsules, menisci, and fat pads. They are not found in the brain.

169. D) Cognitive function may be affected by dehydration, malnutrition, abnormal body temperature, or medication.

170. E) Polydipsia means excessive thirst.

171. D) Strengthening exercises generally follow a progression from isometric, to isotonic, to isokinetic, to plyometric.

172. D) Isotonic exercises for external rotation of the glenohumeral joint focus on the infraspinatus, teres minor, and posterior deltoid muscles.

173. C) Injury or disease of the pancreas creates pain in the upper left quadrant of the abdomen.

174. B) A Morton's neuroma is most commonly located between the third and fourth metatarsals.

175. B) An excessive valgus force would cause tension on the medial collateral ligament, resulting in a sprain or tear.

176. A) The female athletic triad describes the simultaneous presence of an eating disorder, amenorrhea, and osteoporosis.

177. E) Neer's test is performed to assess for shoulder impingement.

178. B) Cryostretch involves the use of ice or a cold spray prior to stretching a body part.

179. C) Ultrasound would increase blood flow to the area and should not be used when an acute hemorrhage is present.

180. A) Functional braces are used after rehabilitation to prevent recurrent injury but maintain range of motion.

181. B) Russian stimulation deeply penetrates the muscle and causes an intense contraction of the muscle.

182. B) Protective spasm of the muscular abdominal wall is known as rigidity.

183. A) Black, tar-like stools are indicative of upper gastrointestinal bleeding.

184. D) An ice pack can decrease the mean skin temperature 3.4°C during a 15-minute application.

185. C) A dry, nonproductive cough is most often caused by allergies to environmental irritants.

186. B) Rehabilitation or a reconditioning program is developed with the main goal of returning the patient to his or her previous functional level.

187. D) Archimedes discovered the principle of buoyancy, which states that when a body is wholly or partially immersed in a fluid at rest, the body experiences an upward thrust equal to that of the fluid it displaced.

188. A) Interferential current is not a classification of electric stimulation.

189. C) Electrical stimulation (ie, TENS) is used to control labor pains.

190. B) Coulomb's law states that like charges repel each other, but unlike charges attract to each other.

191. C) Ice massage should never be applied to anesthetized skin because of the loss of sensation to the area.

192. B) Low-intensity stimulators deliver current at very low frequencies (1 PPS) and are of subsensory intensity.

193. C) Galvanic current is uninterrupted direct current.

194. D) Intensity is the amount of power given off by the ultrasound unit during treatment.

195. C) Treatment temperature ranges of fluidotherapy are usually between 100°F to 113°F.

196. B) The D2 flexion pattern works the abductors, flexors, and external rotators of the hip.

197. E) The rhomboids retract, rotate, and stabilize the scapula during the throwing motion.

198. D) McKenzie extension exercises are used for degenerative disk disease and postural dysfunction.

199. D) The biceps and triceps stabilize the rotator cuff. The rotator cuff consists of the supraspinatus, infraspinatus, teres minor, and subscapularis muscles, which all must be strengthened during rehabilitation.

200. C) During static stretching, the muscle is placed in a position of maximum stretch and held without bouncing or movement.

201. E) Plyometric exercise helps develop eccentric control during dynamic movements.

202. D) An evaluation of the injured area should be performed before proceeding with any treatment.

203. E) A positive posterior drawer test is indicative of a posterior cruciate ligament tear.

204. C) The medial condyle of the femur is one structure of the knee that should be palpated during the evaluation of a knee injury.

205. B) The athletic trainer should take a thorough history of the injury prior to proceeding with the rest of the evaluation.

206. B) Cartilage has limited ability to heal because it has limited or no direct blood supply.

207. A) The shoulder rarely dislocates in the superior direction because the acromion process is in the way.

208. D) "Snapping hip" syndrome is a condition that may lead to chronic bursitis. It is prevalent in patients such as runners, dancers, gymnasts, and cheerleaders. It may be caused by the iliotibial band or gluteus maximus snapping over the greater trochanter during hip flexion; the iliopsoas snapping over structures deep to it such as the iliopsoas bursa, femoral head, or lesser trochanter; or it can be caused by intra-articular lesions such as a labral tear. It is typically treated conservatively with ice and NSAIDS, biomechanical corrections, flexibility exercises, and proper training techniques.

209. A) Treatment for cystic fibrosis includes nutritional support, pulmonary therapy to clear thick secretions, and a course of antibiotics to prevent infection.

210. E) Modalities that produce heat should be avoided when treating a patient with multiple sclerosis as there is evidence that heat may exacerbate the symptoms.

211. A) Myasthenia gravis is an autoimmune disorder affecting the neuromuscular junction causing fatigue, diplopia, and ptosis. Corticosteroids or medications that act at the neuromuscular junction may help to improve functional activity in a patient diagnosed with this disease.

212. A) Tranquilizers and sedatives are the most commonly prescribed medications used in the treatment of epilepsy.

213. A) Salicylate is the only NSAID used topically in the United States. It is usually found in the form of methyl salicylate (as in Ben-Gay or Icy Hot products) and trolamine salicylate (as in Sportscreme and Aspercreme).

214. C) Dexamethasone is the generic name for the corticosteroid Decadron.

215. B) Tagament is the trade name of the chemical (generic) cimetidine. It is a H2 receptor antagonist used for the treatment of heartburn, peptic ulcer disease, and gastroesophageal reflux disease.

216. E) Vicodin is the trade name of the drug hydrocodone.

217. A) Constipation is a common adverse reaction to opiod analgesics.

218. E) The half-life of a drug refers to the time required for the amount of drug in the blood to be reduced by one-half.

219. E) Routes of drug administration include oral, topical, parenteral, sublingual (and buccal), inhalation, and rectal.

220. E) Four types of goals have been identified in the goal-setting literature: subjective goals, which lack an objective measuring system; general objective or outcome goals, which set a performance standard focusing on the results of a contest; specific objective/performance goals, which are goals indicating improvement relative to one's past performance; and process goals, which specify the procedures the performer will use during the performance.

221. E) Aspirin and ibuprofen are the most commonly prescribed NSAIDs to reduce fever. Tylenol (acetaminophen) is the most commonly prescribed antipyretic that is not a NSAID.

222. B) Prilosec, which is an over-the-counter proton pump inhibitor, is available as a delayed-release, once-a-day medication for the treatment of frequent (2 or more days a week) heartburn and is to be taken for a course of 14 days.

223. B) Over-the-counter topical hydrocortisone is available in 0.25% and 1% concentrations.

224. E) A reusable cold pack may lower the skin temperature below the freezing point because it uses a combination of silica, water, and a form of antifreeze instead of frozen water as its medium.

225. C) The drawback to the use of ice bags is that the ice machines are expensive and their cost may be prohibitive.

226. D) Massage stimulates the autonomic nervous system and pacinian receptors, which decrease nociceptive impulses.

227. E) Joint mobilization should not be employed as a treatment technique if there is acute inflammation present, the patient has osteoporosis, or a malignancy or an infection is present. Other contraindications include fractures, advanced osteoarthritis, congenital bone deformities, hypermobility, neurologic pathology, vascular disease, rheumatoid arthritis, or the presence of new surgical sutures.

228. C) Open-chain kinetic exercises, not closed-chain kinetic exercises, isolate a specific muscle group for strength and endurance training.

229. E) Rehabilitation includes assessment of the level of function/dysfunction of a patient, organization and interpretation of the results of the assessment, formation of a problem list, establishment of goals, development of a treatment plan, and implementation of a supervised program with periodic reassessment.

230. A) High-voltage pulsed stimulation may be used as an adjunct treatment in controlling acute and chronic pain through the gate control mechanism and the stimulation of the body to release opiates.

231. B) When massaging an extremity to reduce edema in an extremity, the athletic trainer should first begin proximally and move distally. This procedure is known as *uncorking the bottle.*

232. E) Intertrigo is also known as chafing of the skin. Chafing is a superficial dermatitis caused by friction of a fabric against moist, warm skin. It often occurs in the creases of the skin as in the neck, axilla, buttocks, breast, or groin areas. It is treated with the application of a cold compress, which is followed by cleaning the area with mild soap and water and the application of a soothing ointment.

233. E) Ultrasound energy is reflected off metal, increasing the intensity in various areas near the metal.

Organizational and Professional Health and Well-Being

1. D) Permission-to-treat forms, preparticipation physical examination forms, release forms for patients with increased risks, and medical history forms should be completed and given to the athletic trainer prior to the first team practice.

2. B) A policy is a broad statement of intended action developed by those who are empowered to govern the operation of an organization. A procedure outlines a specific strategy for members of an organization to follow when following a policy.

3. E) The following topics should be addressed in an athletic training program policies and procedures manual: who the athletic training program will serve, facility use and maintenance, risk management plans, and chains of command and supervision.

4. C) It is prudent for the athletic trainer to maintain some form of documentation on a daily basis.

5. D) A patient's medical records may not be released to any individual or organization without written permission from the patient or his or her guardian or parent.

6. C) The athletic trainer is legally responsible for the patient's health care. The athletic trainer is acting in place of the team physician in making decisions for the patient's physical health unless there is a situation that is out of the boundaries of the athletic training practice act.

7. B) Focus charting is a method of documentation that lists information about a patient's injury, the actions taken by the athletic trainer, and the response to the athletic trainer's action in column form instead of a narrative or SOAP note format.

8. D) A physician's letter of agreement is an informal legal contract that outlines the physician's duties and responsibilities. This type of contract should specifically identify the physician as the individual who is ultimately responsible for the patient's health care.

9. E) An athletic trainer in the nontraditional setting can be considered a manager. A manager functions as an organizer, director, and controller.

10. D) The athletic trainer should follow OSHA guidelines in maintaining proper hygiene and sanitation in the athletic training facility.

11. E) The Commission on Accreditation of Rehabilitation Facilities establishes standards of quality for organizations that provide rehabilitation services.

12. D) A well-written SOAP note should be legible and concise, include many objective measurements, express progress in terms of functional achievements, and it should describe a clear plan of treatment.

13. B) Documentation such as the athletic trainer's treatment log or SOAP notes could be subpoenaed during a civil litigation suit.

14. D) Capitation is a fixed method of payment made to a provider per member over a specific period of time, regardless of the amount of services provided.

15. A) A HCFA-1500 form is a standard insurance claim form that is accepted by most insurance carriers. It must be filled out thoroughly for quick reimbursement to be obtained.

16. A) It is illegal for an athletic trainer to dispense a prescription drug to a patient. Only those individuals who are legally licensed to prescribe or dispense prescription drugs may give a patient a prescribed medication.

17. D) Maintaining accurate records for a high school patient is the responsibility of the athletic trainer, school nurse, and team physician.

18. C) The WOTS UP analysis (weaknesses, opportunities, threats, and strengths) is a technique that looks at the strengths and weaknesses of an athletic training program.

19. A) A gatekeeper is appointed by an insurance company to oversee the medical care given to a patient and is usually a primary care physician.

20. E) The UCR (usual, customary, and reasonable) is a charge that represents the maximum amount of money that an insurance company will pay for a service.

21. A) The National Safety Council is responsible for drawing sports injuries data from numerous sources.

22. B) The Hockey Equipment Certification Council sets standards to certify facemasks that are used in ice hockey helmets.

23. E) Expendable supplies include items such as adhesive tape, gauze pads, adhesive bandages, and items that cannot be used again.

24. B) Security, fire safety, and management of emergency injuries must be taken into consideration when developing a risk management plan.

25. D) Bidding is a process in which competing vendors quote prices on specific pieces of equipment, and orders by the purchasing institution are usually placed with the lowest bidder.

26. D) A copayment is a percentage of the total amount the policyholder is required to pay for medical services rendered.

27. E) Any athletic trainer who is in the position to hire a new staff member is governed by federal laws that require all applicants receive equal consideration regardless of race, gender, nationality, or religion.

28. D) The athletic trainer's daily documentation should include any treatments administered and how they were implemented, rehabilitation progression, the patient's current playing status, and a daily injury log.

29. D) Only the team physician has the authority to clear an injured patient so he or she can return to play.

30. B) Only a licensed physician may diagnose an illness and is in charge of overseeing the treatment administered by the athletic trainer.

31. C) The fee-for-service model is a traditional reimbursement model by which the provider is paid on the amount of service provided to a patient, often leading to a higher total reimbursement for the provider.

32. D) The goals must be written in functional terms to ensure proper reimbursement.

33. A) The ICD-10 codes are used to identify a patient's diagnosis and are employed by private insurance companies as a method of standardizing the classification of an injury.

34. D) It would be unethical for the athletic trainer to manipulate his or her documentation for any form of personal financial gain.

35. B) Space requirements and traffic flow patterns must be addressed in the schematic drawings to ensure adequate space to function, grow, and enhance the movement of people from one section of the athletic training facility to another.

36. A) If the equipment is based on complex technology, the department may be able to replace it before it becomes obsolete.

37. C) Only confidential information relating to a staff member's employment should be included in the personnel file. This would include performance evaluations, salary and promotion records, employee application information, and employee contracts.

38. C) Database software allows the athletic trainer to input, store, manipulate, and retrieve information with regard to athletic injury and treatment.

39. A) A "rider" is a supplementary clause to an insurance contract that covers the cost of conditions that extend beyond those associated with the standard policy.

40. C) Consulting a certified public accountant or professional financial advisor would not be appropriate in this situation.

41. D) A qualified individual, such as another certified athletic trainer or coach, should accompany an injured patient to the hospital if it becomes necessary. It would be inappropriate to give a student athletic trainer this responsibility.

42. A) It is critical that the athletic trainer meet at least once a year with the local rescue squad and any individuals who may be involved in the event of an emergency to establish and practice procedures that will be utilized.

43. A) The biggest budgetary obstacle a high school athletic trainer faces is the lack of a room and special facilities to operate his or her program.

44. E) There are 4 types of supervisory models commonly used by athletic trainers: clinical, developmental, inspection, and production. Inspection and production are usually combined because they have very few differences. Clinical supervision involves direct observation of the employee's work and the subsequent development of an action plan to improve any deficiencies in his or her performance. Developmental supervision involves participative management, in which the employees discuss common problems and develop solutions with their supervisors. Inspection-production supervision was originally developed and implemented in industrial settings. It emphasizes authoritative managerial efficiency. It relies on the strict observance of program policies and procedures and measures success through the measurement of input and output, which is not easily accomplished in the sports medicine setting. This model is the least utilized in athletic training.

45. C) Negotiation is one of the 6 steps in the purchasing process and is not a phase of budget planning.

46. C) Third-party reimbursement is the process by which health care practitioners are reimbursed by a policyholder's insurance company.

47. E) Managed care is a system that has set forth coordinated efforts to help reduce the costs of medical coverage. The goal of managed care is to provide appropriate service with cost control in mind.

48. A) The athletic trainer who is designing a new sports medicine facility should always be concerned with function/economy of space instead of aesthetics.

49. E) Capitation is not a type of insurance. Capitation refers to a form of reimbursement used by managed care organizations to determine the amount of money that is going to be paid to a provider for services for a member in a predetermined period of time.

50. A) Establishing an emergency plan should be one of the first tasks that an athletic trainer should perform when developing a new high school program.

51. B) Developing a mission statement is a priority when developing any place of business, such as a sports medicine center. A mission statement is a written expression of an organization's philosophy, purpose, and characteristics.

52. E) CPT stands for Current Procedural Terminology.

53. C) Personalistic culture is a type of organizational culture characterized by autonomy in decision making and problem solving, allowing an individual to make decisions with little consultation of others.

54. E) Quality control is a negotiable point in sports medicine purchasing that should be done prior to the purchasing process to ensure you will be receiving the appropriate items.

55. D) An ICD-10 code identifies a specific diagnosis.

56. A) The athletic trainer is not required to have a treatment consent form signed by the patient's parent or guardian if the patient is 18 years of age or older.

57. E) Ideally, the athletic trainer, physician, and local EMTs and/or paramedics should be involved in the development and implementation of the emergency action plan including decisions regarding the transport of an injured patient.

58. C) The statute of limitations set forth by each individual state gives the athletic trainer the time frame in which one can file a claim.

59. C) The primary care physician makes the decision that a referral to a specialist is needed. The primary care physician acts as the gatekeeper.

60. C) Planning is defined as a decision-making process in which a course of action is determined in order to bring about a future state of affairs.

61. E) Bedfellows support a plan but are not trustworthy and may be manipulative in their dealings.

62. A) A procedure is an operational plan that provides specific guidelines and directions for an individual of the company or organization to follow.

63. B) An insurance "carrier" is a charge-based provider contracted by the federal government charged with reviewing Medicare claims made by physicians or other health care providers.

64. E) Personal power is the potential to influence others by virtue of personal characteristics and personality attributes.

65. C) There is no such thing as laissez-faire budgeting.

66. B) Primary coverage is defined as a type of health, medical, or accident insurance that begins to pay for covered expenses immediately after a deductible has been paid.

67. A) Medical records provide an accurate account of ongoing treatment, history, and background information pertinent to the patient. They are valuable tools in providing health care to a patient.

68. E) The P in SOAP means "plan of action." In this section one should incorporate long-term goals, short-term goals, and the plan of care.

69. B) The athletic trainer should adopt and communicate policies that limit the institution's financial obligations to those injuries that are covered by the school's insurance policy.

70. D) Medical insurance is a contract between a policyholder and an insurance company to reimburse a percentage of the cost of the policyholder's medical bills.

71. A) Confidentiality between the patient and the athletic trainer cannot be broken by pressure from the media.

72. C) There is a lower initial cost with leasing equipment.

73. E) Collegial culture is a type of organizational culture characterized by consensus, teamwork, and participatory decision making.

74. C) There are 10 steps for recruiting and hiring sports medicine personnel. The following is the most common order:
    1. Request for position
    2. Position request approval
    3. Position vacancy notice
    4. Application collection
    5. Telephone interviews
    6. Reference checks
    7. On-site interview
    8. Recommendation and approval for hiring
    9. Offer of contract
    10. Hiring

75. A) Lump-sum budgeting is a method that allocates a fixed amount of money for an entire program without specifying how the money will be spent.

76. C) Zero-based budgeting is a model that requires justification for every budget line item without reference to previous spending patterns.

77. D) Negligence is a type of tort in which an athletic trainer fails to act as a reasonably prudent athletic trainer would act under the same circumstances.

78. B) Feasibility standards are performance evaluation standards intended to help foster practicality in the employee appraisal process.

79. B) The correct order in the staff selection process should be hiring, promotion, retention, performance evaluation, and demotion.

80. C) Program goals are procedures carried out in the inspection-production supervision.

81. E) An organization plan is ideally used in short periods of times. This allows the organizational plan to change as needed.

82. D) The equal employment operating chief deals with all employees regarding any concerns that they may have. Any issue or problems related to employment or employees should be dealt with by the equal employment operating chief.

83. B) The individual must provide you with some type of medical documentation from a physician or state agency. The record should state the disability and any accommodations that may be necessary.

84. C) The design/build concept allows the firm to make adjustments and decisions regarding the building. They are able to work within their own firm rather than having to deal with any other outside groups or entities.

85. B) Developing a traffic pattern chart is a vital step in determining space needs when designing a new facility.

86. C) Endowments are usually used for scholarly endeavors in the educational field. These endowments are to ensure the continuation of the program. Endowments can be used to create or support a professorship or provide scholarships for students.

87. B) Chronic overuse injuries can be included in a rider. This may cause the cost of the premium to go up, but the injury will be covered.

88. A) A deductible is the amount of money that a patient would pay before the insurance company begins paying.

89. C) Secondary coverage begins when the individual's personal insurance or any other primary policy that may be in use has already paid.

90. A) The AMA, the American Medical Association, set forth codes to help standardize the language used by medical professionals when billing. This made it easier for insurance companies to reimburse correctly. Most of the Current Procedural Terminology codes that would be used by athletic trainers can be found under the physical medicine codes.

91. D) Capital expenses include major costs, such as buildings and land. Small supplies, such as tape, ultrasound

gel, and others used for treatment purposes, are direct costs, while office supplies are indirect costs. Staff salaries are not capital costs.

92. D) Changing/locker rooms for the patients should not be included as a section of the athletic training facility.

93. E) Factors that influence space requirements when designing a sports medicine facility include number of clients to be served, types of clients to be served, amount and kinds of equipment needed, and the projected growth of the program.

94. B) The electrical outlets should be approximately 4 to 5 feet above the floor of the training facility with spring-loaded covers to prevent the possibility of electrical shock.

95. A) The athletic trainer should utilize a password to maintain confidentiality and security and to prevent unwanted individuals from gaining access to the database.

96. D) The Board of Certification requires all certified athletic trainers to earn 10 hours of evidence based practice CEUS every two years.

97. E) The BOC Standards of Professional Practice consists of 2 sections: Practice Standards and Code of Professional Responsibility

98. C) The BOC identified the domains of athletic training as defined by the *Role Delineation Study*.

99. D) The athletic trainer should keep accurate and up-to-date records in the athletic training facility. This information should include items such as injury reports, injury evaluations and progress notes, daily treatment logs, and medical records.

100. E) Line-item budgeting is a method in which the athletic trainer must anticipate the expenditures for specific program functions, such as team physician services, supplies, and equipment repair.

101. D) Licensure is the most restrictive form of regulation for athletic training. Licensure limits the practice of athletic training to those individuals who have successfully met the minimal requirements set by a state licensing board.

102. C) A successful athletic trainer must be an individual who has a love for athletics and competition. He or she must be able to adapt to a variety of environments and deal with diverse personalities of those he or she comes into contact with on a daily basis. The athletic trainer must have a sense of humor and be able to empathize with a patient who has been injured or is ill. Most importantly, the athletic trainer must be of the highest morals and integrity.

103. D) The school nurse's function in a high school sports medicine program is to act as a liaison between the athletic trainer and the school's health services program.

104. D) The NATA was developed in 1950 to establish practice guidelines and a code of ethics for the athletic training profession.

105. E) This behavior violates the NATA *Code of Ethics* Principle 4.3, which states, "Members shall not place financial gain above the patient's welfare and shall not participate in any arrangement that exploits the patient."

106. C) Physical therapists are trained in the rehabilitation of a diverse patient population. The athletic trainer has expertise in the prevention, treatment, and rehabilitation of the athletic and physically active populations.

107. A) Difficulty sleeping, feelings of anger or guilt, self-preoccupation, and constantly feeling tired are all signs of job burnout.

108. D) Organizing professional seminars and conferences, providing high-quality care to the patient, and publishing articles in professional journals are among the best means of educating the general public and other health care workers regarding the role of the athletic trainer.

109. A) The most important thing an athletic trainer should do is listen carefully to what the patient has to say relating to the injury or problem.

110. E) According to the definition developed by the American College of Sports Medicine, *sports medicine* is a generic term that is multidisciplinary in nature.

111. A) The athletic trainer must be competent in classroom teaching methods and should incorporate multimedia and visual aids.

112. C) A tort may be a direct result of an act of omission or commission.

113. B) The athletic trainer should carry professional liability insurance and be familiar with the details of the policy.

114. A) Developmental supervision could be considered a "mentoring" approach in which the head athletic trainer facilitates his or her assistant's professional development while overseeing the day-to-day operations of the athletic training facility.

115. D) AIDS is not a bacterial infection.

116. A) It is crucial that any infected individual, including an infected health care worker, not deny his or her condition and seek the proper medical care when it is appropriate.

117. E) In general, a plaintiff has between 1 and 3 years to file a negligence suit. This can vary from state to state.

118. D) The athletic trainer should carry professional liability insurance in case of a criminal suit.

119. A) Principle I (1.2) states, "Member's duty to the patient is the first concern and therefore members are obligated to place the welfare and long-term well-being of their patient above other groups and their own self-interest to provide competent care in all decisions and advocate for the best medical interest and safety of their patient at all times as delineated by professional statements and best practices."

120. C) The 3 types of state regulations that govern athletic training are certification, licensing, and registration.

121. D) It is illegal for an athletic trainer to prescribe and dispense prescription medications.

122. E) The athletic trainer working in a clinical setting is best suited to treat the physically active patient.

123. D) It is not a violation for a certified athletic trainer to function as a clinical athletic trainer in a sports medicine clinic as long as he or she practices within the confines of the individual state's practice acts.

124. E) Liability is the state of being legally responsible for the harm one causes another person.

125. A) The athletic trainer may be considered negligent if he or she failed to dry the floor if it was wet or warn the patient that the floor was wet prior to him stepping out of the whirlpool.

126. D) Keeping an updated résumé on file with the athletic director will have no impact on avoiding litigation. However, it is important for the athletic trainer to have a written job description on file.

127. B) Principle II (2.6) states, "Members shall refrain from substance and alcohol abuse. For any member involved in an ethics proceeding with NATA and who, as part of that proceeding is seeking rehabilitation must be provided to the NATA Committee on Professional Ethics as a requisite to complete a NATA membership reinstatement or suspension process."

128. A) Principle I (1.1) states, "Members shall render quality patient care regardless of the patient's race, religion, age, sex, ethnic or national origin, disability, health status, socioeconomic status, sexual orientation or gender identity."

129. E) Recreational therapy is not a field that is related to sport and injury.

130. E) In June 1990, the AMA recognized certified athletic trainers as "allied health care professionals."

131. C) Athletic training scope of practice parameters set by legislation fall into the following areas: definition of athletic training or athletic trainer, site of practice restrictions, modality use restrictions, definition of patient restrictions/physically active individual, and the supervision of athletic trainers.

132. E) A primary care provider is an individual who is the direct provider of care. He or she is usually a physician specializing in internal medicine, pediatrics, or general practice. A physical therapist, orthopedic technician, and nurse are all secondary providers (ie, those who render services, equipment, or testing procedures that enable the physician to care for his or her patient).

133. A) A group of 5 components that athletic trainers should adhere to when using evidence-based practice have been developed. Those 5 components include defining a critically relevant question, search for the best evidence, appraise the quality of the evidence, apply the evidence to clinical practice, and evaluate the outcomes of the applied evidence.

134. E) When taking a history during an initial evaluation, the athletic trainer should be functioning at the "analytical" level of listening. The analytical level of listening involves listening for very specific kinds of information.

135. A) Commitment to the job and a state of openmindedness and professional growth are key elements of professionalism.

136. D) Continuing education units would not be awarded by the BOC for writing a medical or health-related column in a local newspaper or popular magazine.

137. A) The athletic trainer and team physician should be the only individuals with access to databases containing a patient's medical records.

138. A) Occupational "burnout" is demonstrated by physical and emotional exhaustion and a negative attitude toward work. Signs of burnout include anger, guilt, insomnia, and self-preoccupation.

139. D) A biomechanist is an expert in analyzing human movement through the use of video and computer-enhanced digital analysis equipment.

140. C) A hallux valgus deformity is also known as a bunion. A podiatrist would be the most appropriate individual for the athletic trainer to consult with in the care of this patient.

141. C) The medical practice act of each state is what governs the athletic trainer and makes him or her aware of what is permissible practice of a certified/licensed athletic trainer within that particular state.

142. E) Malpractice occurs when an athletic trainer has an adverse outcome from a patient treatment. An athletic trainer can be sued for malpractice when he or she is not in full compliance with protocols set forth by state law and practice acts.

143. D) The athletic trainer is not allowed to provide anyone, aside from the parent, with any information regarding the patient. Keeping in mind that the patient is still a minor, the parents/guardians must be consulted first regarding any information that is given out about the patient's status.

144. D) Random selection provides for an equal probability that any subject within a given group or population will be chosen for testing.

145. B) By signing the assumption of risk form the patient is made aware of the risks of athletic participation and the activities that he or she engages in freely without being forced to do so. These activities include competition, practice, and conditioning.

146. D) A medical condition not covered by an insurance policy is an exclusion.

147. C) Ethics are defined as the rules, standards, and principles that dictate right conduct among members of a society or profession. Ethics are based on moral values.

148. A) Good documentation is a way for the athletic trainer to protect him- or herself from litigation.

149. A) Licensure is a form of state credentialing, established by statute and intended to protect the public, that regulates the practice by specifying who may practice and what duties he or she may perform.

150. D) Principle IV states, "Members Shall Not Engage in Conduct That Could be Construed as a Conflict of Interest, Reflects Negatively on the Athletic Training Profession, or Jeopardizes a Patient's Health and Well-Being."

151. C) Assumption of risk is a legal defense that attempts to claim that an injured plaintiff understood the risk of an activity and freely chose to undertake the activity regardless of the hazards associated with it.

152. B) The insured's mother's maiden name is not necessary when obtaining insurance information for a patient's medical records.

153. D) Socialism is not an approach to ethical decision making. Egoism involves athletic trainers making decisions that result in the greatest benefit to themselves. Utilitarianism involves choosing a course of action that benefits the greatest number of people. Formalism is most likely to be followed by athletic trainers who see a clear professional duty that they believe should be implemented universally.

154. E) Sports medicine encompasses the fields of biomechanics, massage therapy, sports nutrition, and sports psychology.

155. D) Nurses, sports psychologists, and social workers all work with the athletic trainer to ensure the health and safety of the patients.

156. C) NATA does not have a guideline or position statement regarding eye safety in sports.

157. C) The physical therapist is not considered a member of the primary sports medicine team.

158. E) The NATA was formed in 1950.

159. B) The team physician is responsible for compiling medical histories and conducting physical examinations for each patient on a team.

160. E) An athletic trainer may be employed in an industrial, high school, college/university, or hospital setting.

161. C) Delegation is not a form of state regulation.

162. A) CAATE is the accrediting body for athletic training programs.

163. B) Diagnosis of athletic injuries is not a domain of athletic training.

164. B) Athletic trainers are secondary decision makers, which are professionals responsible for delivering a program within an organization.

165. A) Negligence is defined as a situation in which an athletic trainer fails to act as a reasonably prudent athletic trainer would act under the same circumstances.

166. A) Going to meetings for athletic training is not only a great way to network, it is also required as part of the continuing education that helps athletic trainers stay up to date.

167. D) Documentation cannot protect an athletic trainer from an individual attempting to sue.

168. B) Licensure does prohibit anyone that is not licensed from performing the task of an athletic trainer under state law.

169. E) Ethics dictate the rules, principle of right, conduct, and standards to which members of a specific organization or society must adhere.

170. A) Principle I (1.3) states, "Members shall preserve the confidentiality of privileged information to a third party not involved in the patient's care without a release unless required by law."

171. B) Internal chart audits are a procedure during chart auditing; it is accomplished before the outcome assessment methods.

172. C) Input and output are not easily quantified in sports medicine clinics.

173. E) Omission is the failure to carry out your legal duty.

174. E) An ally is a person who is highly cooperative in a support plan.

175. C) Athletic directors, owners, staff, and coaches are all part of a major inside interest group.

176. D) A sports medicine program should provide the best possible health care, have good communication among members of its team, and have good communication between the athletic trainer and parents to be successful.

177. E) The physician has the final say regarding the patient's ability to play.

178. D) The athletic administrator's role should include the following: establish a positive chain of command for the sports medicine team and ensure that each member's credentials are proper and that the appropriate personnel are hired for specific positions.

RELATED ATHLETIC TRAINING SUBJECT MATTER

Human Anatomy

1. E) Golfer's elbow and Little League elbow are overuse syndromes of the medial forearm flexor musculature, resulting in medial epicondylitis. This group of muscles originates on the medial epicondyle and crosses the volar aspect of the wrist. Injury occurs with repetitive valgus stresses at the elbow.

2. A) The olecranon process is located on the proximal end of the ulna and extends posteriorly, preventing hyperextension of the elbow.

3. A) The peroneus tertius muscle originates on the lower two-thirds of the fibula and inserts on the tuberosity of the fifth metatarsal bone. It assists to dorsiflex the ankle.

4. A) The deltoid muscle of the upper arm is innervated by the axillary nerve.

5. C) The collateral ligaments are most taut in full knee extension and at 30-degree knee flexion.

6. E) Cranial nerve I is the olfactory nerve.

7. C) The muscles of the rotator cuff include the supraspinatus, infraspinatus, teres minor, and subscapularis.

8. A) The rectus femoris muscle originates on the anterior inferior iliac spine and inserts into the quadriceps tendon, which attaches to the upper border of the patella. The patella is attached to the tibial tuberosity by the patellar tendon. Therefore, the rectus femoris flexes the hip and extends the knee.

9. D) The pes anserinus is described as a goose foot-shaped expansion of the tendons of the sartorius, gracilis, and semitendinosus.

10. A) The subscapularis muscle of the rotator cuff originates on the subscapular fossa and inserts into the lesser tubercle of the humerus.

11. D) The gluteus maximus muscle originates on the upper portion of the ilium, sacrum, and coccyx and inserts on the gluteal tuberosity of the femur and the fasciae latae. Its primary actions are to extend and externally rotate the hip.

12. E) The C7 nerve root innervates the triceps muscle, which extends the elbow.

13. A) Cranial nerve VIII, the vestibulocochlear or acoustic nerve, is responsible for hearing and equilibrium.

14. B) Movements of the tongue are controlled by the hypoglossal nerve (ie, cranial nerve XII).

15. A) Continuous pressure on the palm that irritates the deep branch of the ulnar nerve just distal to the canal of Guyon will cause weakness in the muscles of the hand that are innervated by the ulnar nerve.

16. C) The scaphoid bone of the wrist is palpated just distal to the styloid process of the radius.

17. D) The extensor carpi ulnaris is innervated by the radial nerve.

18. D) The hip joint is a diarthrotic or ball and socket joint.

19. B) Knee flexion and extension occur in the sagittal plane around a coronal axis.

20. A) An impacted fracture is a fracture in which one part of the bone telescopes on the other part of the bone.

21. A) A uniaxial diarthrodial joint is a synovial joint that is characterized by hyaline cartilage that covers the articulating surfaces and a synovial membrane that lines the interior of the joint. It moves in one plane only around a single axis.

22. E) The biceps femoris is one of the hamstring muscles and is active in hip extension.

23. A) Because of the angulation of the articulating surfaces of the facets of the thoracic vertebrae, movement is greatest in lateral flexion.

24. B) The peroneal nerve, artery, and muscle groups compose the lateral compartment of the lower leg.

25. A) A Baker's cyst is a localized accumulation of fluid in the popliteal fossa of the knee. It may represent a true bursitis or synovial herniation through the posterior capsule.

26. B) The shoulder girdle is composed of the sternoclavicular, acromioclavicular, glenohumeral, and scapulothoracic joints.

27. A) The coracoclavicular ligaments consist of the trapezoid and conoid ligaments and connect the coracoid process of the scapula to the inferior surface of the clavicle.

28. E) A mortise joint is a joint in which there is a groove or slot into or through which another bone fits or passes (eg, the talus sits between the distal ends of the tibia and fibula).

29. A) The ulnar nerve and artery run through the tunnel of Guyon, which is located in the wrist. It is formed by the volar carpal ligament, the pisohamate ligament (which is an extension of the flexor carpi ulnaris), the hook of the hamate, the transverse carpal ligament laterally, and the pisohamate ligament and pisiform bone medially.

30. A) The muscle most prominently involved with lateral epicondylitis is the extensor carpi radialis brevis.

31. D) The multifidi are small muscles located in the back, which extend and rotate the vertebral column.

32. C) The psoas major originates on the transverse processes of the lumbar vertebrae and inserts on the lesser trochanter of the femur. It acts to flex and internally rotate the hip.

33. D) The vastus lateralis originates on the lateral aspect of the femur and inserts into the common tendon of the quadriceps muscle.

34. D) The anatomical snuff-box is located along the dorsoradial aspect of the thumb and is bordered by the extensor pollicis brevis, abductor pollicis longus, and extensor pollicis longus tendons.

35. B) The superior vena cava carries deoxygenated blood from the head and upper body back to the heart.

36. E) Gas exchange of oxygen and carbon dioxide occurs at the alveoli.

37. E) The peroneal artery originates off the posterior tibial artery below the popliteal fossa in the proximal posterior lower leg.

38. C) The odontoid process, or dens, is a projection off the second cervical vertebra that acts as a pivot point for rotation of the atlas.

39. B) The cuneiform is one of the tarsal bones of the foot.

40. D) The plantar fascia is located on the sole of the foot.

41. A) The origin of the sternocleidomastoid muscle is on the superior/medial portion of the clavicle and the manubrium and inserts into the mastoid process.

42. B) The erector spinae is a large muscle group, composed of the iliocostalis, longissimus, and the spinalis, that acts as the primary extensor of the trunk.

43. A) The femoral artery, vein, and nerve pass through the femoral triangle.

44. C) The axillary artery is a continuation of the subclavian artery beyond the first rib in the axilla.

45. D) The peroneus brevis assists to plantar flex and pronate the foot.

46. B) The cochlea is an osseous structure of the inner ear.

47. D) The dermatome for the C3,4 nerve roots is over the superior aspect of the shoulders and posterior neck area.

48. E) The spleen is located in the upper left abdominal quadrant below the diaphragm.

49. A) Little finger abduction is controlled by the abductor digiti minimi, which is innervated by the C8,T1 nerve root.

50. E) The liver and gallbladder are located in the upper right quadrant of the abdomen.

Human Physiology

1. E) The top number of a blood pressure reading is the systolic number, and the bottom number is the diastolic number. The systolic pressure is representative of the blood pressure during ventricular contraction. The diastolic pressure represents the blood pressure during ventricular filling between cardiac contractions.

2. E) The hunting response is a reactive vasodilatation of local blood vessels after initial vasoconstriction. This occurs with the application of cryotherapy to a body part.

3. D) Acetylcholine is a chemical found at the endplate of a motor neuron, which plays a significant role in the transmission of nerve impulses at synapses and myoneural junctions.

4. A) The average level of desirable total cholesterol is less than or equal to 200 mg/100 dL.

5. A) The separation of electrically charged particles causing a transmembrane electrical potential difference is known as the resting membrane potential.

6. A) The 2 phases of an action potential are known as depolarization and repolarization.

7. B) The primary component of striated muscle is the muscle fiber.

8. C) A motor unit is made up of a motor neuron and the muscle fibers it innervates.

9. E) Type II or "fast twitch" muscle is more prevalent in the sprinter, as this type of activity is more anaerobic in nature.

10. B) Calcium (Ca^{++}) is a mineral that is necessary for proper muscular contraction to occur. Ca^{++} is a necessary component in the activation of cross-bridging between actin and myosin to shorten the length of the sarcomere in the muscle myofibril.

11. C) During glycolysis, ATP is broken down to release energy. In addition to the release of energy, the by products ADP and PO_4 are released.

12. A) The Krebs cycle is a complex series of chemical reactions in which there is oxidative metabolism of pyruvic acid, carbohydrates, proteins, and fats.

13. A) Sclerotomic pain is a deep, diffuse, aching pain that arises from deep somatic tissues and is transmitted by unmyelinated C fibers.

14. A) Fusiform muscle fibers are arranged in a cord-like shape, while the pennate muscle fibers are arranged in a feather shape.

15. B) Amenorrhea is defined as an absence of flow during menses.

16. A) Laxatives and enemas can lead to dehydration and electrolyte imbalance, which can endanger the patient's health and impair performance.

17. E) Hemophilia is a disorder in which the plasma coagulation factor VIII is lacking, resulting in abnormal bleeding.

18. D) The rate of passive diffusion of oxygen from the alveoli depends on the partial pressure of oxygen, the thickness of the alveolar capillaries, and the amount of surface area available for diffusion to take place.

19. E) Vital capacity is the maximal amount of air that can be expired after maximal inspiration.

20. E) During the follicular phase of the menstrual cycle, which lasts from day 5 or 6 to day 13, the primary follicles grow. Toward the end of this phase, just prior to ovulation, one follicle reaches maturity and becomes a graafian follicle.

21. C) The 2 main phases of menstruation are the follicular or preovulatory phase and the luteal or postovulatory phase.

22. D) The pulp of a tooth is innervated, not the enamel.

23. D) By 4 weeks, a large laceration will heal by secondary healing. Areas of tissue loss are filled with scar tissue.

24. B) The stimulation of the periaqueductal gray area of the midbrain and raphe nucleus of the pons and medulla during injury will cause analgesia. Endorphins and enkephalins are produced in these 2 areas of the brain.

25. B) It may take up to 1 year for a ligament to completely heal with scar maturation.

26. C) To avoid hypoglycemia and insulin shock from taking too much insulin and metabolizing significant amounts of glycogen during exercise, the patient should consume a snack of a complex carbohydrate and protein prior to exercise.

27. A) Cold therapy used in an acute injury will decrease the local metabolic rate.

28. B) If a scaphoid fracture is not properly immobilized, aseptic necrosis may occur and the fracture will not heal.

29. E) Hematuria means blood in the urine.

30. E) The scalene muscles are striated and have an arrangement of contractible proteins in a cross-striated pattern.

31. D) Valsalva's effect occurs when the patient holds his or her breath during the contraction, which increases the intrathoracic pressure and causes a dramatic rise in blood pressure.

32. A) Ballistic stretching causes constant stimulation of the muscle spindles, which causes continuous resistance to further stretching. A muscle must be stretched a long enough time to stimulate the Golgi tendon organs.

33. B) The adrenal glands, which are part of the endocrine system, are responsible for secreting the hormones cortisol, epinephrine, aldosterone, estrogen, norepinephrine, and androgen.

34. B) The primary function of the testes is to produce spermatozoa and testosterone.

Exercise Physiology

1. A) The training effect during exercise is reflected by changes in cardiac output. Cardiac output in the trained patient is a product of an increased stroke volume and a decreased heart rate.

2. A) Three sessions a week is how often (frequency) the patient should exercise. Forty-five minutes is how long (duration) the exercise should continue, and 80% of VO_2 max is the intensity of exercise.

3. B) Total cholesterol is composed of low-density lipoproteins (LDL), high-density lipoproteins (HDL), and very-low-density lipoproteins (VLDL).

4. B) The sternocleidomastoid and scalenes assist during inspiration by lifting the ribs to allow for the intake of greater volumes of air.

5. E) The hypothalamus stimulates the thyroid gland in very cold environments to generate internal heat.

6. C) Applying a static stretch to the muscle inhibits the muscle spindle and stimulates the inverse myotatic reflex, which originates in the Golgi tendon organs and causes relaxation of the muscle.

7. C) A patient who is hypermobile/hyperflexible may be more susceptible to joint injuries, such as sprains and strains.

8. E) Interval training involves alternating intense, continuous periods of work with periods of active recovery. This type of training is very effective when conditioning patients who participate in sports that involve short bursts of activity and are followed by a period of recovery.

9. A) The off-season period should be a time when the patient is not training as frequently or as intensely as the in-season period, but he or she should participate in an activity that maintains a level of flexibility, strength, and endurance. The off-season can be broken down into the transition and preparatory periods, while the in-season may also be referred to as the competition period. In turn, these periods may be further divided into subphases.

10. C) The principles of overload, specificity of training, proper progression, and consistency must be adhered to in order to obtain optimal training effects.

11. B) Physiological adaptations to resistive exercise include increased ligament and tendon strength, increased mineral content of bone, and improved maximal oxygen intake.

12. A) When the muscle is in a position where there is maximum interaction of the cross-bridges between the actin and myosin myofilaments in a sarcomere, the tension within the muscle will be at its greatest point.

13. D) Heart rate and stroke volume determine the volume of blood that is pumped through the heart during a given period of time.

14. E) Target heart rate can be calculated with the following formula: 0.8 x (220 - age), or 0.8 x (220 - 20) = 160.

15. B) Contract-relax requires that the antagonist muscles contract isotonically just prior to the "relax" (stretch) phase of the exercise.

16. D) The triceps and pectoralis major must contract concentrically during the "lift" phase of a bench press.

17. C) Circuit training is one of the best means of improving muscle strength and flexibility because it includes weight training, flexibility, and calisthenics at various stages.

18. C) The hypothalamus is responsible for thermoregulation of the body.

19. B) Periodization includes the following phases: postseason, off-season, preseason, and in-season conditioning.

20. C) A proper cool down aids the return of blood to the heart and assists in decreasing lactic acid levels in the muscle.

21. E) Plyometric exercises emphasize a quick eccentric stretch prior to a forceful concentric contraction and are useful in building power.

22. E) The amount of testosterone present in the body has a significant impact on the amount of hypertrophy that will occur with weight training.

23. A) The greatest loss of heat from the body occurs at the head and neck. It is wise to keep these areas well covered in cold weather.

24. D) Those individuals with blonde or light hair and fair complexions are much more susceptible to severe sunburn as a result of prolonged exposure to ultraviolet light. This type of patient should use a sunscreen that has an SPF of 15 or greater.

25. C) The ozone levels are most diminished in the late afternoon because of the lower temperatures and decreased amount of traffic on the roads.

26. A) A patient with the sickle-cell trait who trains in high altitudes is susceptible to an enlarged or ruptured spleen.

27. A) Because sweat contains a lower concentration of salt than the blood, there is a much greater loss of water when the patient sweats. Therefore, fluids, especially water, should be unlimited.

28. C) Plyometric exercises include eccentric exercise, which is the most common cause of DOMS.

29. E) Hilton's law states that the joint capsule, the muscles that move that joint, and the skin that covers that joint are supplied by the same nerve source.

30. D) A protein level of "trace" or +1 by urinalysis is not considered an abnormal finding in an adolescent.

31. A) Women have a lower strength:body weight ratio (due to a higher percent of body fat) than men.

32. D) There is increased mitochondrial density in the skeletal muscle with endurance exercise.

33. C) During a 400-meter sprint, which lasts approximately 45 seconds to 1 minute, the anaerobic glycolysis system is the predominant source of energy.

34. C) The diastolic blood pressure should remain close to resting levels during endurance exercises.

35. A) Hemolysis is the destruction of red blood cells caused by the repeated impact of the foot on the ground.

Biomechanics

1. D) A contraction that occurs as the muscle is shortening is known as a concentric contraction. An eccentric contraction occurs as the muscle lengthens against resistance.

2. A) The foot becomes a rigid lever in preparation for push-off during gait when the foot is supinated in midstance.

3. E) The knee has 2 degrees of freedom, allowing for flexion and extension in the sagittal plane and rotation in the horizontal plane.

4. E) During shoulder abduction, the humerus and scapula move simultaneously. This is known as scapulohumeral rhythm. For every 30 degrees of shoulder abduction, 20 degrees of motion occurs at the glenohumeral joint and 10 degrees occurs with the scapula rotating on the thorax. During shoulder abduction, the scapula contributes 60 degrees of movement, while the remaining 120 degrees occurs at the glenohumeral joint.

5. B) The agonist muscle is the primary mover, while the antagonistic muscle is the muscle that causes the opposite action (ie, the quadriceps are the agonist muscle and the hamstrings are the antagonistic musculature during knee extension).

6. E) The most common lever system that exists in the body is the third lever system, where the point of attachment of the muscle causing the motion is closer to the joint axis than the resisting motion (ie, biceps flexing the forearm against gravity).

7. D) The movement arm of a force is always greatest when the angle of application is at 90 degrees to the lever being moved.

8. A) An anatomic pulley (such as the patella) can change the direction of the muscle force but not the magnitude of the force.

9. A) Muscular tension may be increased by increasing the frequency of the motor units firing or by increasing the number of motor units that are simulated.

10. C) Pronation of the foot is a complex movement. It is a combination of eversion, abduction, and dorsiflexion.

11. B) Plantar flexion of the ankle is an example of a second-class lever (ie, the resistance arm is shorter than the force arm).

12. C) Each lever has a force arm, which is the perpendicular distance from the line of force to the axis, and a resistance arm, which is the perpendicular distance from the resistance to the axis.

13. D) Running utilizes linear motion of the entire body and angular motion of the arms and legs.

14. B) Momentum = mass x velocity. Momentum is the force of motion that is acquired by a moving body as a result of its continued motion.

15. D) Potential energy is energy that is stored in a body when it is at rest. The amount of potential energy a body has depends on its position in space. Kinetic energy is the energy of a body in motion.

16. A) Cervical rotation occurs in the horizontal (transverse) plane around a vertical (longitudinal) axis of motion.

17. D) Applying an external force parallel to the tibia will result only in a distraction force.

18. E) An avulsion fracture of a bone is caused when tissue and bone are stretched and tension is produced beyond its yield point. This is known as a stretching injury.

19. A) This situation results in an isometric contraction.

20. E) The carpometacarpal joint is a saddle joint. A saddle joint has one articulating surface that is concave and one articulating surface that is convex.

21. E) The maximum degrees of freedom (number of axes of movement) a joint can have is 3 degrees.

22. E) The elbow joint is a hinge, or ginglymus, joint and has 1 degree of freedom.

23. D) The frontal plane divides the body into anterior and posterior parts.

24. B) When performing a push-up, the distal end of the upper extremity is in a fixed position.

25. A) The tibia externally rotates on the femur during knee extension. This action is known as the screw-home mechanism.

26. A) With compressive loading, the articular surfaces are brought closer together.

27. E) Loading of a joint that is unstable as a result of ligament rupture produces abnormally high stresses on the joint cartilage.

28. C) Shoulder abduction occurs in the frontal plane around an anterior-posterior axis.

29. D) In the anatomic position, hip rotation occurs in the horizontal plane around a vertical axis.

30. B) A spiral fracture occurs when the foot is planted on the ground and the body is violently rotated. The bone breaks in an S-shaped line. The mechanism of injury is a torsion force.

31. B) Blisters may form in the epidermal layer of the skin as a result of continuous friction to the area.

Psychology

1. B) Progressive muscle relaxation is a relaxation technique by which the patient learns to manage anxiety and control pain. This form of relaxation training incorporates systematically tensing and relaxing muscles in groups (such as the thighs and buttocks). This technique, when practiced routinely, allows the patient to tune into his or her body reactions and gain more control of these reactions.

2. B) A passive-aggressive personality procrastinates, makes excuses for delays, and tends to criticize individuals on which he or she is dependent, but cannot separate from their company. These individuals also lack assertiveness and are indirect with their needs.

3. D) Signs of anabolic steroid abuse include mania and depression, bouts of anxiety and insomnia, changes in libido, and aggressive behavior.

4. B) The general adaptation syndrome is a stress response theory developed by Dr. Hans Selye in which there are 3 stages an organism may pass through: the alarm stage, resistance stage, and exhaustion stage. The alarm stage consists of the flight-or-fight response, which prepares the body to take action; the resistance stage is when the body directs the stress to a particular body site (such as to the stomach); and the exhaustion stage is when the body may become dysfunctional because of chronic stress.

5. E) A patient who is "burned out" may display a variety of physical and emotional symptoms, including negative self-concept and attitudes regarding his or her sport and teammates, chronic fatigue, headaches, insomnia, and gastrointestinal problems.

6. D) The body passes through 3 distinct psychophysiological phases in response to an injury: alarm, resistance, and exhaustion. The adrenal glands secrete adrenaline, which stimulates the flight-or-fight response during the alarm stage.

7. C) It has been shown that an abrupt cessation of exercise can lead to "sudden exercise abstinence syndrome," which is characterized by depression, sleep disorders, arrhythmias, eating disorders, and emotional problems.

8. E) In order for the patient and athletic trainer to have a good relationship, it is crucial that the patient trusts the individual who is providing his or her health care.

9. B) Having the patient draw a mental picture of the healing process can have a positive impact on his or her recovery.

10. A) Two methods of cognitive restructuring are thought stopping and refuting irrational thoughts.

11. D) Obsessive-compulsiveness, mild feelings of denial, behavior that masks feelings of fear, providing self-worth, and taking extreme risks are factors that lead to overcompliant behavior.

12. A) Repeatedly rehearsing various plays in his mind while experiencing pain is a means of diverting his attention away from the pain.

13. E) Anger, loss of appetite, and chronic fatigue are signs of depression.

14. C) The patient must be cooperative and take responsibility if he or she is to completely rehabilitate an injury.

15. A) Purging by self-induced vomiting or self-administered laxatives is a symptom of bulimia.

16. D) If the patient is anxious, it is best to reassure him and not belittle his fear.

17. B) Staleness is characterized by an apathetic attitude, chronic fatigue, restlessness, and an increase in acute chronic injuries and infections.

18. C) Patients between the ages of 15 to 24 years, those sustaining a serious injury with a long rehabilitation process, and those with the prospect of losing their position to a teammate may become severely depressed.

19. A) Teaching the patient about his or her injury and the healing process can significantly reduce the patient's anxiety about rehabilitation.

20. E) This patient is demonstrating denial of his condition.

21. C) Arranging the rehabilitation sessions around the patient's daily routine will help the patient to be more compliant.

22. D) Patients who have little perceived control over their health care will tend to experience a greater amount of stress than those who feel they have some control over their environment.

23. A) A ritualistic cleaning of equipment is a sign of an obsessive-compulsive disorder.

24. B) Biofeedback is a technique that reflects the patient's efforts to control a specific physiological response, such as muscular tension.

25. B) Individuals diagnosed with anorexia nervosa tend to be perfectionists and overachievers.

26. D) It is best for the athletic trainer to remain empathetic and calm and help the patient to see the problem in proportion to the situation so she can deal effectively with the outcome.

27. B) A patient who threatens suicide must be taken very seriously. It is important to be empathetic and listen to the patient as he discusses what is troubling him. The team doctor should be immediately contacted so that a proper referral to a psychologist or psychiatrist may be made.

28. B) An inter-related set of pathologies affecting active women, including disordered eating, amenorrhea, and osteoporosis, is known as the female athlete triad.

29. D) Eliminating negative thoughts that are connected to the effects of anxiety by substituting a positive thought in its place is known as *thought stopping.*

30. E) According to the *Diagnostic and Statistical Manual of Mental Disorders* (DSM-IV-TR), substance abuse may be manifested by one or more of the following (occurring within a 12-month work period): recurrent substance abuse resulting in a failure to fulfill a major role obligation at work, school, or home; recurrent substance abuse in situations where it is physically hazardous (ie, driving a car while impaired); recurrent substance-related legal problems (ie, arrests for disorderly conduct); and continued substance abuse despite having persistent or recurrent social or interpersonal problems caused or exasterbated by the effects of the substance.

31. C) Desensitization is a cognitively based strategy to deal with stress. It is a commonly used treatment for anxiety and phobias.

32. C) A victim of sexual abuse may demonstrate a number of psychological and interpersonal issues. These symptoms may include negative self-concept, low self-esteem, shame about one's body and distorted body image, anxiety and guilt about sexuality, interpersonal distrust, depression, substance abuse, and a desire to perfect or purify one's body.

33. E) Signs and symptoms of addiction for the physically active individual may include attendance problems, deterioration of athletic performance, increasing infraction with school, job, or team and belligerent behavior.

34. A) A patient who uses mood-altering substances on a frequent basis in the belief that the substance helps him or her perform better in school, in sports relationships, sexually, or in any other key area of life may be developing a psychological dependence on that substance.

35. D) In order to be diagnosed with anorexia nervosa, a patient must be underweight by 85% or below what is considered normal weight for him or her.

36. A) Bulimia nervosa typically results in feelings of guilt after a binge.

37. E) An athletic trainer should make a psychological referral when he or she does not have the time or resources to meet the needs of the patient, when the patient becomes a danger to him or herself and others including the athletic trainer, when the athletic trainer does not have the support system or supervision to address the psychological needs of the patient and when the patient with psychological issues are affecting him or her in such a way that it is counterproductive to his or her daily functioning.

38. C) A stress management technique that involves systematic, purposeful tension followed by relaxation of predetermined muscle groups is known as *progressive relaxation.*

39. D) Achieving a deep state of relaxation by disciplining the mind against encroaching thoughts is known as *meditation.*

40. D) If an individual is demonstrating symptoms of depression for 2 or more weeks, he or she should be referred to a mental health professional.

41. E) Anxiety is often manifested by (but not limited to) tachycardia, nausea, intense worry, and paranoia. Other symptoms may include sweating, dizziness, poor concentration, crying, irritability, and avoidance.

42. A) Information regarding insurance coverage is unrelated to educating a patient about the rehabilitative process.

43. E) A normal emotional reaction to a recent injury may include trembling, nausea or vomiting, anxiety or fear, and tachycardia. Inappropriate overreaction may include inappropriate joke telling, excessive talking, hyperactivity, and being argumentative.

44. B) When providing "emotional first aid" to a newly injured patient, if the athletic trainer notices the patient is failing to answer questions, looks dazed or confused, and is lacking emotion, the athletic trainer should be empathetic and encourage the patient to express his or her feelings.

45. E) The outcome is linked to the process, not the effort.

46. A) Seasonal affective disorder (SAD) is most likely to occur during the winter months because of the decrease in sunlight.

47. D) An individual who has sustained a psychologically traumatic event may experience a numbing of general responsiveness, insomnia or increased aggression. This is known as *post traumatic stress disorder* (PTSD).

Nutrition

1. D) Vitamin A exists in 2 forms: provitamin A carotenoids, which are found in dark green and orange vegetables, and preformed vitamin A, which is found in liver, fish oils, fortified milk, and eggs.

2. C) Vitamin C is also known as ascorbic acid. Retinol is vitamin A, and thiamin and niacin are B vitamins.

3. B) Ultraviolet light in sunlight converts a form of cholesterol to vitamin D in the skin.

4. B) During glycolysis, glucose is broken down into pyruvate and adenosine triphosphate. Pyruvate is then

broken down into CO_2 and water aerobically or into lactic acid during anaerobic exercise.

5. A) The best time for a patient to consume carbohydrate-rich foods is within 2 hours after training, as glycogen synthesis is the greatest at this time.

6. C) Muscle cells primarily burn fat during low workloads (eg, a brisk walk) because the supply of adenosine triphosphate generated is able to handle that level of work. Intense exercise that may not last more than 30 seconds uses phosphocreatine and some anaerobic glycolysis to replenish adenosine triphosphate.

7. E) Phosphorus can be found in milk and cheese products, eggs, legumes, nuts, whole grain cereals, meat, fish, and poultry.

8. B) Proteins are long chains of organic compounds called amino acids. There are 22 amino acids, which are used by the body to produce hormones and enzymes. Because the body cannot store excessive protein, some protein is converted into energy or fat.

9. E) Sodium and chloride are electrolytes, which are lost in the greatest amounts while sweating.

10. D) Do not wait for the patient to complain of being thirsty before supplying fluids. Because the thirst mechanism does not function well when large amounts of fluids are lost by the body during activity, the patient may need to be reminded to consume fluids frequently.

11. D) The 6 classes of nutrients include carbohydrates, proteins, water, fats, vitamins, and minerals.

12. C) Water is the most abundant nutrient in the body and must be present in an adequate supply for the body to function normally.

13. C) The new nutrient food label format is known as reference daily intakes.

14. A) Hydrostatic weighing, electrical impedance, and skin-fold thickness measurements are all means of measuring body composition.

15. B) When more calories are expended than consumed, a negative caloric balance exists and the individual will lose weight.

16. E) Triglyceride, which is a form of fat, is stored in adipose cells and released as the intensity and duration of exercise increases.

17. B) Increasing muscular exercise and dietary intake in appropriate amounts are necessary to increase muscle mass.

18. C) A female patient who has been diagnosed with a combination of an eating disorder, amenorrhea, and osteoporosis has female triad syndrome.

19. E) Calcium supplements may be necessary to prevent osteoporosis in a patient who is at high risk for this disease.

20. B) Lactovegetarians eat a diet consisting of plant foods and milk products, but exclude meat products, eggs, and fish. Iron and zinc may be deficient in this diet.

21. A) The body will begin to utilize protein in the event that the patient's dietary carbohydrate supply is inadequate.

22. D) Patients who lack the enzyme lactase have a difficult time digesting dairy products, which causes the development of intestinal gas, diarrhea, and cramping.

23. D) If the body experiences significant electrolyte losses during exercise, the patient may experience muscular cramping and become susceptible to heat illnesses.

24. A) The kidneys and brain are responsible for regulating water excretion from the body.

25. C) A diet that is significantly lacking in vitamin A will cause poor night vision.

Pharmacology

1. B) Lomotil is an antidiarrheal medication.

2. E) Prozac is a medication used to treat depression, obsessive-compulsive disorder, and bulimia nervosa.

3. E) Pepcid is a medication used to treat heartburn and acid indigestion. It has no stimulant effects.

4. D) Ibuprofen (ie, Advil, Motrin) is available in 200-, 400-, 600-, and 800-mg tablets.

5. B) Diclofenac is known by the brand name Voltaren.

6. A) The recommended dosage for Naprosyn is 250 to 500 mg twice a day.

7. B) A patient who has overdosed on a stimulant will be agitated and excitable, demonstrate an increase in the respiratory and pulse rates with possible arrhythmias, exhibit tremors, and might become hyperthermic and have convulsions (cocaine affects central thermoregulation) if left untreated.

8. C) Because beta-blockers slow the heart rate, they are potentially performance enhancing during archery.

9. A) Caffeine consumed in moderate amounts will stimulate the cerebral cortex and the medulla, which will increase mental alertness.

10. E) Diarrhea is not a symptom of human growth hormone abuse.

11. D) When 2 drugs are combined and there is a response that is 2 times the response as when each drug is used alone, it is known as a *synergistic effect*.

12. E) Drugs may be classified according to chemical make up, mechanism of action (molecular basis) therapeutic effect (ie, pain relief, anti-hypertensive), or legal classification (OTC, controlled substance, etc).

13. A) The use of aspirin in treating children and teenagers with a viral infection has been linked to Reye's syndrome.

14. B) The primary mechanism of action of penicillin is inhibition of cell wall synthesis.

15. D) Opioid analgesics can cause drowsiness and constipation and is used to reduce anxiety and distress. Its primary use is to relieve moderate to severe pain.

16. E) Symptoms of caffeine withdrawal include fatigue, headache, irritability, yawning, restlessness, anxiety, and runny nose.

17. C) Klonopin and Tegretol are both anticonvulsant medications.

18. A) The abbreviation "GERD" stands for "gastroesophageal reflux disease." Proton-pump inhibitors are the most effective treatment for GERD.

19. D) The abbreviation "IBS" stands for "irritable bowel syndrome." Anti-diarrheal medications and laxatives are the primary choice of treatment for IBS.

20. B) Diuretics increase the excretion of sodium (Na+) and Chloride (Cl-) ions. With higher amounts of sodium chloride (NaCl) present in the body, there is an increased amount of extracellular fluid volume. This in turn can increase blood pressure. Diuretics are a common treatment for hypertension.

21. D) The routes of drug administration include oral, sublingual or buccal, rectal, parenteral, topical, or inhalation.

22. E) Hemorrhoids may be treated by the use of corticosteroids (reduces inflammation and itching), local anesthetics (blocks pain and burning), astringents (relieves irritation and inflammation), vasoconstrictors (decreases swelling), protectants (provides a skin barrier), counterirritants, (provides a feeling of cooling or tingling), and keratolytics (increases the rate of epidermal sloughing to allow medications to be more effective).

23. A) According to the hypertension guidelines set in 2014 by the Joint National Committee (JNC[8]) Panel, the blood pressure threshold for initiating drug therapy for an individual younger than 60 years old is a systolic BP ≥ 140 mm Hg and diastolic BP ≥ 90 mm Hg.

24. D) Benzodiazepines and antidepressants are used to treat panic disorders. Xanax is a commonly used benzodiazepine drug for anxiety.

25. D) Glucophage is an oral medication used in treating type 2 diabetes.

26. D) Acyclovir (Zovirax) is the drug of choice to treat the herpes simplex virus. Acyclovir interferes with DNA synthesis in cells.

27. A) To avoid gastric upset, NSAIDS should be taken with food or milk.

28. C) Adverse reactions related to skeletal muscle relaxants include drowsiness, dizziness, decreased liver and kidney function, hypersensitivity, physical dependence (in centrally acting skeletal muscle relaxants) and anticholinergic effects.

29. B) Crestor (Rosuvastatin) is a commonly used statin to treat hyperlipidemia.

30. E) Adverse effects of insulin use include hypoglycemia, weight gain, immune-based responses and lipohypertrophy.

Physics

1. C) The effective radiating area is the area of the applicator that emits ultrasound waves to the surface tissue.

2. A) The frequency range of therapeutic ultrasound is between 1.0 to 3.0 MHz.

3. A) Archimedes' principle states that an object immersed in water experiences an upward force that is equal to the weight of the water displaced by the object.

4. B) TENS is a modality for pain relief that is based on the gate control theory.

5. A) A pulsed current during electric stimulation may be monophasic or biphasic.

6. B) The most common frequency used with short-wave diathermy is 27.33 MHz.

7. C) Microwave diathermy produces electromagnetic radiation with a frequency of 2450 megacycles per second and has a wavelength of less than 1 meter.

8. E) There is no "surge" setting on a TENS unit.

9. E) With iontophoresis, ionized medication, such as dexamethasone, is driven through the skin by a direct electrical current.

10. C) Work = force x distance.

11. E) Medication delivered by iontophoresis must be ionized.

12. A) According to Joule's law, heat produced by high frequency electrical currents is directly proportional to the square of the current strength, resistance of the conductor, and the time during which the current flows.

13. E) Ohm's law states that the strength of an electric current is equal to the electromotive force divided by the resistance, or I = V/R.

14. A) Heat transfers to the skin from a moist heat pack via conduction, which is the transfer of heat by direct contact.

15. C) An alternating current is an electrical current that reverses direction at a regular interval. A TENS unit utilizes alternating current.

16. C) To change a temperature reading from Celsius to Fahrenheit, the following formula must be used: (temperature in Celsius x 9/5) + 32.

17. C) The impedance of a circuit is the resistance that exists within the circuit.

18. E) Moist heat applied during the acute phases of tendinitis will increase pain and enhance the inflammatory process.

19. C) Amperage is the strength of a current flow. It is expressed in amperes.

20. A) According to Poiseuille's law, the length and radius of a blood vessel are significant in determining resistance to blood flow.

21. A) Medium-intensity ultrasound is between 0.8 to 1.5 watts per square cm.

22. D) The transducer head should be kept between 0.5 to 1 inch from the skin surface during underwater treatment.

23. C) The anode is the positive pole of an electric source.

Evidence-Based Practice

1. B) When developing a specific clinical question that targets what the athletic trainer would like to focus on and will address the condition in a targeted approach, the PIO, PICO, PIOT, or PICOT Format can be used depending on the information that is being sought. PICOT is an acronym that stands for patient population, intervention of interest, comparison intervention or issue of interest, outcome(s) of interest, and time of interest.

2. E) A descriptive study examines something at a point in time and provides information concerning the findings. Descriptive studies are divided into 5 subcategories: Case Reports, Case Series, Time Series, Surveys and Questionnaires, and Cross-Sectional Studies.

3. E) All of the following are databases commonly used by health care professionals: Google Scholar, Cochrane Database, Cumulative Index to Nursing and Allied Health Literature (CINAHL), MEDLINE and PubMed, and Physiotherapy Evidence Database (PEDro).

4. A) A controlled vocabulary search utilizes medical subject headings (MeSH)

5. C) Data is classified as Nominal, Ordinal, Interval, or Ratio. Nominal data are the simplest level of measurement and are classified into predetermined categories (ie, blood type, gender, etc). Ordinal scales are used for data that have a rank order on hierarchy of meaning (ie, strongly agree to strongly disagree). Interval data involve a scale that incorporates an ordinal characteristic and equal distance between adjoining data. A Ratio scale is the highest level of measurement and is similar to an interval scale, but it includes an absolute 0 point (a 0 on this scale indicates a total absence of what is being measured).

6. B) A variable that is measured by an investigator is known as a *dependent variable.*

7. C) A statement made by an investigator indicating his or her expectations about the differences or relationships among variables being investigated is known as a *research hypothesis.*

8. D) Data that are continuous and primarily cluster around a central value, such as the mean, is known as *normal distribution.*

9. E) Researchers use a threshold value known as *significance level* to determine if the results of a study are significant.

10. A) A type I error is made when a researcher makes an incorrect decision to REJECT the Null Hypothesis when it is actually true.

11. C) When every person in the population of interest has an equal chance of being chosen, it is known as *random sampling.*

12. D) A blinding process is put into place by a researcher to eliminate bias.

13. B) Critical appraisal is the process of carefully and systematically examining research to judge its trustworthiness as well as its value and relevance in a particular context.

14. E) A Boolean operator is a logical word or symbol that is used to connect 2 or more words or phrases in the Internet database search.

15. A) An interval validity threat can include treatments, procedures, or participant experiences that threaten the researcher's ability to draw accurate conclusions from the research.

16. B) Confidence intervals commonly range from 85% to 99%.

17. E) Reliability is the consistency of a specific measurement.

18. C) The validity of a clinical diagnostic test is measured through mathematical equations that compare it to a reference or "gold standard" finding.

19. E) The most commonly utilized scales for examining evidence are the Oxford Centre for Evidence-Based Medicine (CEBM) scale and the Strength of Recommendation Taxonomy (SORT).

20. A) When there is a negative clinical diagnostic finding but a positive reference standard finding, the result is known as a *false negative finding.*

21. D) When there is a positive clinical diagnostic finding and a positive reference standard finding, the result is known as a *true positive finding.*

22. A) Percent accuracy of a clinical diagnostic test can be derived by the following formula:

$$\frac{\text{True positive finding} + \text{True negative finding}}{\text{Total number of patients}} \times 100$$

23. B) Prevalence is defined as the number of cases of a condition existing in a given population at any one time.

24. B) A feature in which a database will automatically attempt to match a keyword entered in the search box to a MeSH (Medical Subject Heading) term that already exists is known as *mapping.*

25. D) *Mutually exclusive* means that a subject or characteristic fits into only one category (such as gender).

26. C) The NAGI disablement model is a disablement model that describes the interaction between a health condition and the patient's environment.

27. A) A letter rating system assigned to a body of evidence by examination of a group of articles relating to the same topic is known as a *grade of recommendation.* This grade takes into consideration the validity of the study, cost and ease of implementation of the study, and reproducibility of the study.

28. E) Four response scales are commonly used for a patient-rated outcome (PRO) instrument: The Binary Response Scale, Visual Analog Scale (VAS), Adjectival Scale, and Likert Response Scale.

29. D) The short form 12, Disablement in the Physically Active Scale, Pediatric Quality of Life Inventory, and Patient-Reported Outcomes Measurement Information system are all patient-rated outcome (PRO) instruments. The Physiotherapy Evidence Database (PEDro) is a free database managed by the center for evidence-based physiotherapy at the George Institute for Global Health in Australia.

30. A) An incidence rate (or injury rate) can be defined by the following equation:
The number of New Injuries ÷ Total Exposure Time

31. E) The midpoint in which 50% of the values fall on either side of the value is known as the *median*.

32. B) The Alpha Value is assigned by an investigator to represent the threshold value at which the results of the statistical test will be declared significant or not is typically 0.05 or 5%.

33. C) The 3 main types of clinical prediction rules (CPR) used in health care are as follows: Interventional CPRs determine how likely a person would be to respond to a certain intervention or variety of interventions. A prognostic CPR is used to provide information about a likely outcome of patients with a specific condition. A diagnostic CPR determines the probability that a patient has a particular condition of interest.

34. D) A 1 to 2 page summary that focuses on appraising a single research study to help determine if the reported results are valid, reliable, and clinically applicable is called a *critically appraised paper* (CAP).

35. B) The Disabilities of the Arm, Shoulder, and Hand (DASH), Modified Oswestry, and the Lower Extremity Functional Scale are all patient-reported outcome instruments.

36. A) An electronic health record (EHR) combines the legal medical records from multiple entities, whereas an electronic medical record is a legal medical record that is restricted to one entity.

37. E) Clinical documentation, data storage, clinical messaging between providers and patients, and results reporting for clinical tests are all components of the EMR.

38. A) A level I validation of a clinical prediction rule means it can be used in a variety of settings with confidence that it improves outcomes. It is the highest level of validation.

39. D) An 11-item scale which was developed by physiotherapists to rate the methodological quality of randomized controlled trials is known as a *PEDro scale*.

40. E) Most critically appraised topics (CAT) include the following main sections: clinical scenario, focused clinical question, summary of search and key findings, clinical bottom line, strength of recommendation, search strategy, inclusion and exclusion criteria, results of search, summary of best evidence and implications for practice, education, and future research.

41. C) The first step in the use of evidence-based practice is developing an answerable clinical question.

42. B) The levels of the "5S" model of health care research evidence include Systems—computerized decision support systems that connect summarized evidence to the patient's clinical problem; Summaries—evidence-based textbooks and abstracts that integrate evidence from lower levels; Synopses—evidence-based journal abstracts that briefly describe systemic reviews and research studies; Syntheses—include systematic reviews and meta-analyses that are based on clinical question of interest and follow a specific process for identification, search, and selection of included investigations; and Studies—include original journal articles accessed through various databases.

43. B) A systematic review in which the data from the included studies are pooled for additional analyses and a summary estimate of effect is known as a *meta-analysis*.

44. E) Critical appraisal checklists include a Consort—consolidated standard of reporting trials; Strobe—strengthening the reporting of observational studies in epidemiology; Stard—standards for the reporting of diagnostic accuracy studies; Prisma—preferred reporting items for systematic reviews and meta-analyses; and Moose—meta-analysis or observational studies in epidemiology.

45. A) EBP ensures a scientific foundation for athletic training profession, improves critical thinking, may elevate the athletic training profession in the medical community, and can lead to the development of best practice guidelines.

46. E) Strength of recommendation (SOR) grades include A, B, C, D, or I, with the grade of "A" representing the evidence with greatest applicability and use in clinical practice. A grade of "D" or "I" indicates insufficient evidence available to make a clinical recommendation.

47. A) A collection of data on a single patient is known as a *case report*.

48. B) Clinical questions can be categorized into background and foreground questions. Background questions examine broader topics and obtain generic knowledge regarding the topic or issue at hand. A foreground question is specific to a specific patient or case and gives answers that directly lead to a clinical decision, which impacts your patient.

49. D) Foreground questions may be developed using the PICOT format (P = patient population, I = intervention, C = comparison intervention, O = outcome, T = time of interest).

50. E) A variable that is manipulated by a researcher is known as an *independent variable*.

TRUE/FALSE ANSWERS

EVIDENCE-BASED PRACTICE

1. *False.* Although evidence-based practice may improve third-party reimbursement for athletic trainers, other benefits include improved patient care, the development of the knowledge base specifically within the discipline of athletic training, and encouragement for an athletic training facility to evaluate its current practices.
2. *False.* All treatments should be reviewed and evaluated for scientific support and clinical relevance.
3. *True.* Evidence-based practice is best defined as the use of the consensus of scientific evidence to indicate the best clinical practices for managing specific conditions.
4. *True.* The number of quasi-experimental studies does not indicate that a treatment method or practice is acceptable. One randomized controlled trial is better than numerous quasi-experimental studies.
5. *True.* A clinical trial is any research project that prospectively assigns human subjects to intervention or comparison groups to study the cause-effect relationship between a medical intervention and a health-related outcome is a clinical trial.
6. *False.* An in vitro study is a study done outside the living body and in an artificial environment.
7. *False.* Each patient and each condition should be treated individually using sound judgment and clinical reasoning. Having a single approach to treatment further supports the need to utilize evidence-based practice within athletic training.
8. *True.* An experimental research design that allows for each subject to receive every condition in succession but provides a random treatment administration while at least 2 conditions are being evaluated simultaneously is a cross-over study.
9. *True.* A group of individuals who are involved with a common activity or event through its entire progression is a cohort.
10. *False.* All research articles and studies should be evaluated for content and validity as well as sound scientific practices and outcomes regardless of how many articles have been printed on the subject.

PREVENTION AND HEALTH PROMOTION

1. *False.* Fibroids, or leiomyomas, are the most common form of pelvic tumor and generally occur in approximately 1 out of every 4 or 5 women older than 35 years of age. They are benign neoplasms of smooth muscle origin. Most of the time they are asymptomatic, but they can cause menorrhagia, anemia, urinary frequency, rectal pressure/constipation, abdominal distention, and pain. Most leiomyomas regress with menopause.
2. *False.* Type 1 diabetes mellitus is also known as insulin-dependent diabetes mellitus. It is an autoimmune disease and destroys the insulin producing cells of the pancreas. The body cannot regulate blood glucose levels without insulin. A type 1 diabetic must control his or her disease with lifelong insulin injections and a strict dietary regimen to control carbohydrate metabolism.
3. *True.* Osteoporosis, a pathological disease in bone density, can be prevented in high-risk women by adhering to a daily regimen of weight-bearing exercises, calcium, and vitamin D consumption at the proper recommended daily allowance levels, and observing a balanced diet.
4. *False. Trichomonas vaginalis* is an anaerobic protozoa that can be transmitted sexually. *Trichinella spiralis* (Trichinosis) infection occurs after the ingestion of raw or undercooked pork. This disease is caused by parasites and/or their larvae in the intestinal tract, which causes abdominal pain, diarrhea, and myalgias.
5. *True.* Men who have an undescended or partially descended testicle are at a greater risk for developing testicular cancer and should perform a testicular self-examination on a monthly basis. This is the most common malignancy in males aged 15 to 35 years of age.
6. *True.* To reduce the risk of dehydration and heat stroke while exercising on hot, humid days, 24 ounces of fluid should be replaced for every pound of water lost.
7. *True.* Otitis externa ("swimmer's ear") can be prevented by protecting the ear from excessive moisture, reducing the chance of infection of the ear canal.
8. *True.* Conjunctivitis ("pink eye") can be prevented by good hand and eyelid hygiene, thereby reducing the chance of infection by direct inoculation of bacteria to the eye.
9. *True.* The cure rate of skin cancer is 95% with early detection and treatment. This includes basal cell, squamous cell, and malignant melanoma.
10. *False.* If an athletic trainer modifies a piece of equipment or does not follow the manufacturer's instructions for its proper use and maintenance, both the athletic trainer and his or her employer may be held liable for the injury.

CLINICAL EXAMINATION AND DIAGNOSIS

1. *True.* Huntington's chorea is an autosomal dominant disorder that is characterized by chronic progressive chorea, psychological changes, and dementia. The age of onset is most often in the fourth and fifth decades of life. Approximately 10% of cases involve children who rarely live into adulthood. There is no known cure.

2. *False.* Cerebral palsy is an anoxic, metabolic, or ischemic brain injury acquired during birth. The neurological deficits cannot be transmitted genetically and the disorder is not progressive in nature. Impairments vary depending on which area of the cerebrum is damaged. The most common symptom of cerebral palsy is hypertonicity of the limbs, although cognitive and behavior changes may occur.

3. *False.* Decorticate posturing may occur as a result of an elevated intercranial pressure secondary to brain injury. In decorticate posturing, the upper arms are held at the sides with the elbows, wrists, and fingers flexed. The legs are extended and internally rotated. The feet are plantar flexed.

4. *True.* Endometriosis is a condition in which functional endometrial tissue is found in ectopic sites outside the uterus. The classic symptoms of endometriosis are dysmenorrhea, dyspareunia, and infertility. The cause of endometriosis is unknown. An accurate diagnosis can only be made through laparoscopy.

5. *False.* Wernicke's aphasia is characterized by the inability to comprehend the speech of others or written material. It is a result of an insult to the posterior temporal or lower parietal lobe of the brain.

6. *False.* Emphysema is characterized by the loss of lung elasticity and abnormal enlargement of the air spaces distal to the terminal bronchioles with destruction of the alveolar walls and capillary beds. It is most commonly the result of smoking.

7. *False.* Acute compartment syndrome is considered a medical and surgical emergency because the neurovascular functions become compromised. Immediate intervention is necessary because irreversible damage can occur within 12 to 24 hours after injury.

8. *True.* Hyperthyroidism produces an increase in metabolic rate, oxygen consumption, increased use of metabolic fuels, and increased sympathetic nervous system responsiveness.

9. *True.* Graves' disease is one of the most common autoimmune diseases of the thyroid. An excessive amount of thyroid hormone is released, which causes weight loss, increased appetite, increased blood pressure and heart rate, tremors, anxiety, and increased peristalsis of the bowels. Systemic lupus erythematosus is an inflammatory condition of the connective tissues of the body. Symptoms of systemic lupus erythematosus include weight loss, fever, hair loss, fatigue, nose and mouth sores, joint pain, mental changes, and seizures. Up to 50% exhibit a "butterfly" rash on the nose and cheeks. Rheumatoid arthritis is a systemic disorder in which the immune cells attack and inflame the membranes that cover the joints. Symptoms include inflamed and deformed joints, edema, and loss of strength.

10. *True.* Cranial nerve V, or the trigeminal nerve, has been injured if the patient cannot masticate (chew).

THERAPEUTIC INTERVENTIONS

1. *False.* A C6 quadriplegic has full head and neck control, good shoulder and elbow flexion strength, and is able to flex and extend the wrist. At this level, the individual is able to independently transfer to and operate a manual wheelchair.

2. *False.* The primary goal when rehabilitating a patient with spondylolisthesis is abdominal strengthening. Dynamic core stabilization exercises help control the hypermobile vertebral segment.

3. *True.* Grade III joint mobilization is a large amplitude glide up to the pathological limit in the range of movement. It is used when pain and resistance are the result of muscle spasm, inert joint tissue stiffness, or tissue compression that limit end range joint motion. Adhesive capsulitis ("frozen shoulder syndrome"), which is characterized by a contracted and thickened joint capsule and contracted rotator cuff musculature, is a condition in which grade III joint mobilizations are an appropriate therapeutic technique in restoring movement.

4. *True.* The combined movements of 90 degrees of shoulder abduction and 90 degrees of shoulder external rotation are performed with caution in a patient with a history of anterior shoulder joint instability. The PNF D2 flexion pattern includes both shoulder abduction and external rotation motions.

5. *True.* A throwing program should progressively increase the throwing distances and speeds through a series of preset stages. The patient is allowed to progress from one stage to another as long as he or she does not experience any upper extremity pain or soreness. These stages should be designed to be sport-specific.

6. *False.* Kinesthesia is the ability to detect movement of a joint; proprioception is the ability to determine the position of a joint in space.

7. *True.* The functional progression program following an ankle injury should include a series of movements in which the sequence allows for an increased level of skill/agility that is sport-specific.

8. *True.* The conservative management of a mild case of thoracic outlet syndrome includes the strengthening of the posterior thoracic muscles and stretching of the anterior chest wall, which takes the pressure off the thoracic outlet and its structures.

9. *True.* Exercise may help to maintain muscular tone of a patient with multiple sclerosis, but care should be taken to exercise in the morning rather than late in the day when the individual may be fatigued. Excessive fatigue, emotional stress, and extreme environmental temperatures may exacerbate the symptoms of the disease.

10. *True.* Heparin is an anticoagulant drug used to prevent thromboembolic disorders, such as vein thrombosis and pulmonary embolism. Eating vegetables high in vitamin K may interfere with the action of heparin.

11. *True.* When an energy source such as ultrasound is applied to the body, the maximal effect occurs when energy raised strikes the body at a 90-degree angle. The level of absorption decreases as the angle deviates from 90 degrees (ie, tilting the transducer head).

12. *True.* A major disadvantage of using an instant (chemical) coldpack is the chemical inside the pack has an alkaline pH, which can cause burns if it comes in contact with the skin.

13. *False.* You should be concerned that the sympathetic actions may increase his blood pressure.

14. *True.* Narcan (naloxone hydrochloride) would be an example of an opiate antagonist drug.

15. *False.* Albuterol (beta 2 adrenergic agonist) would be a common drug for an acute asthma attack.

Psychosocial Strategies and Referral

1. *False.* The correct order for the Kübler-Ross reaction is denial, anger, bargaining, depression, and acceptance.

2. *True.* An individual suffering from burnout is usually experiencing both physical and emotional exhaustion. Some of the symptoms related to burnout are loss of interest, depressed mood, cynicism, irritability, and chronic fatigue.

3. *False.* Seasonal affective disorder occurs in adults during the winter months. Women are more common to suffer from this condition than their male counterparts.

4. *False.* Progressive relaxation is described as a mental training technique where the patient is either reclining or seated in a chair and progressively contracts and relaxes his or her muscles. The contracting of each muscle group should last from 5 to 10 seconds and then relax for 20 to 30 seconds.

5. *True.* Anxiety, denial, sleep disturbance, depression or grief, anger, and psychosocial isolation are all barriers to rehabilitation.

6. *True.* According to Hedgpeth and Gieck (2004), if the length of rehabilitation is categorized as "short" or less than 4 weeks the patient will react with shock and relief.

7. *True.* Sudden exercise abstinence syndrome symptoms include heart palpitations, chest pain, arrhythmias, sleep and digestive disorders, depression, and emotional instability.

8. *True.* Thought stopping is a strategy used to eliminate negative thoughts linked to anxiety by replacing the negative thought with positive ones.

9. *False.* An individual who is observed as having abnormally elevated, expansive, or irritable moods lasting a week or more would be characterized as having a manic episode.

10. *True.* When counseling a patient regarding his or her nutritional health, it is important that the athletic trainer take into consideration the patient's social influences and his or her attitudes in philosophy toward life.

Acute Care of Injury and Illness

1. *False.* A spontaneous anterior epistaxis (nosebleed) is caused by a direct blow to the nose/face, a sinus infection, allergies, high humidity, or a foreign body lodged in the nose. It is not considered a medical emergency and is usually self-limiting.

2. *True.* Guidelines for physician referral following a concussion include loss of consciousness on the field; amnesia lasting longer than 15 minutes; deterioration of neurologic function; increasing level of consciousness, respiration, or pulse rate; irregular respiration or pulse rates; increased blood pressure; unequal, dilated, or unreactive pupils; cranial nerve deficits; any signs of associated injury; spine or skull fracture or bleeding; mental status changes; vomiting or progressive motor deficits; sensory/balance deficits; worsening postconcussion symptoms; or symptoms that continue through the end of the game.

3. *True.* Scabies, which is a skin disease caused by the mite sarcoptes scabiei, produces severe nocturnal itching. The female mite burrows a tunnel that is approximately ¼- to ½-inch long in length into the skin and deposits its eggs. The irritation from the burrowing causes itching. Permethrin 5% cream (Elimite) should be applied from the neck down overnight. Anyone who is living with the patient or anyone who has come in contact with the patient should also be treated. All bedding and clothing should be thoroughly washed in hot, soapy water.

4. *False.* When a patient has a seizure, it is important for the athletic trainer to protect him or her from falling and move the patient to an open area away from objects that may cause further injury. Restrictive clothing should be loosened, and a soft cloth may be placed between the teeth to prevent biting. The patient should be allowed to awaken naturally on his or her own when the seizure subsides. The patient should not be restrained during the seizure as it may cause additional injury.

5. *True.* A paronychia is a purulent infection of the proximal and/or lateral skin-folds of the finger or toenail. The patient should soak the finger or toe in Epsom salts or boric acid 3 times a day and apply a topical antibiotic between soakings to control the infection.

6. *True.* When using lumbar traction, a force equal to half of the patient's body weight is appropriate for causing vertebral separation.

7. *True.* When covering an athletic event that is taking place in a pool, it is vital that the athletic trainer have access to a rescue tube and aquatic spine board in case an injured patient has to be removed from the pool.

8. *True.* The rapid form vacuum immobilizer is the best splint to use if the athletic trainer has to transport a patient who has sustained a fracture with a deformity. This type of splint is made of a pliable, airtight cloth sleeve that contains foam chips that can be molded to any angle/shape with Velcro straps. The air is then evacuated from the sleeve by use of a hand-held pump that gives the splint rigidity.

9. *False.* When there is a luxation of a tooth, the tooth is not fractured, but it is very loose. It is either forced forward (extruded) or backward (intruded) toward the mouth. When this occurs, the tooth should be moved back into its normal position if it moves freely, and the patient should be referred to a dentist as soon as possible.

10. *True.* A hordeolum, or sty, is an infection of an eyelash follicle or the sebaceous gland at the end of the eyelid. It is caused by a staphylococcal organism and is spread by rubbing the eye or by dust particles. Treatment includes the application of hot, moist compresses and the application of 1% yellow oxide or mercury to the affected area.

HEALTH CARE ADMINISTRATION

1. *False.* Not all insurance policies offer an out-of-network benefit.

2. *False.* An MCO is a managed care organization. Managed care organizations, which showed a rise in popularity during the presidency of Ronald Reagan, were originally designed to control Medicare payouts. There were a number of mechanisms put into effect to reduce "unnecessary" health care costs, which included incentives for physicians and patients to choose less costly forms of care, increasing beneficiary cost sharing, controlling inpatient hospital length of stay, reviewing medical necessity of treatment, contracting with health care providers, tight management of high cost cases, and cost sharing for outpatient surgeries. There are several forms of managed care plans, which range from most restrictive to less restrictive policies. These include health maintenance organizations, point-of-service plans, preferred provider organizations, and derivatives of traditional health care plans. These limitations in coverage vary on a plan-to-plan basis, but all cover short- and long-term illness/injuries to some degree.

3. *False.* Zero-based budget is an administrative process that requires budget unit heads to justify every expense without reference to previous spending patterns.

4. *True.* A certified athletic trainer is acting outside his or her scope of practice if he or she sutures a patient. Negligence is defined as an athletic trainer not acting in a reasonably prudent manner under the circumstances.

5. *False.* Preferred provider organizations, or PPOs, do not require a primary care physician in most situations. A PPO gives you the flexibility to use physicians that are a part of the PPO network.

6. *False.* Ground fault interrupters are required for all modalities. They act as a defense against power surges and any electrical malfunctions that may occur.

7. *True.* Current Procedural Terminology is utilized by the AMA and most insurance and billing companies. This is a standard coding language that is used in diagnosis, treatment, and billing of patients.

8. *True.* In the definition of "management," as it is used in administration of athletic training, the elements of leadership include decision making, planning, coordination of employees, and organization.

9. *True.* NCOSAE (National Operating Committee on Standards for Athletic Equipment) has been influential in producing research directed toward injury reduction. NOCSAE has developed test standards for football helmets, baseball/softball batting helmets, baseballs/softballs, lacrosse helmets/facemasks, and football facemasks.

10. *False.* Releasing medical records is not a function of human resources.

11. *False.* The laws of practicing athletic training vary in every state. In addition to BOC certification, most states require a separate licensure, registration, or certification process.

12. *False.* Principle 2 states, "Members shall comply with the laws and regulations governing the practice of athletic training." Principle 1 of the NATA *Code of Ethics* states, "Members shall respects the rights, welfare, and dignity of all."

13. *False.* Individuals who are unsupportive of both a program and a particular plan relative to the specific program are considered adversaries.

14. *True.* Omission is failure to act in an appropriate manner when the athletic trainer has a legal responsibility and duty to do so.

15. *False.* Prior to giving out personal information on any patient, the athletic trainer must have permission from the patient or guardian to do so. If permission is granted, the athletic trainer should have the patient sign a consent form during the annual preparticipation physical examination.

16. *False.* A health maintenance organization, or HMO, is a type of health insurance plan that requires the policyholder to use only those medical services and physicians contracted by the company. An HMO requires a primary care physician to coordinate the health care of its policyholders.

17. *True.* Point-of-service plans, or POS plans, are managed care plans that cover both in-network and out-of-network services. Policyholders are encouraged to use in-network providers. Patient out-of-pocket costs are higher when non-network providers are used. POS plans generally manage in-network services more tightly than preferred provider organizations. A POS plan uses a primary physician as a gatekeeper.

18. *True.* Secondary athletic coverage is utilized by an institution to cover the costs of medical bills not covered by a patient's personal insurance. In some cases, the secondary insurance will cover those patients who do not have primary coverage.

19. *True.* Primary insurance is the first insurance that medical bills will be filed on for those that received medical services and treatment. When a large number of patients do not have personal insurance, it is wise to have a large group primary policy to help reduce spending on medical bills.

20. *False.* Long-term permanent disabilities are usually excluded in an athletic accident insurance policy.

PROFESSIONAL DEVELOPMENT AND RESPONSIBILITY

1. *False.* The NATA has the *Code of Ethics* and the BOC has *Standards of Professional Practice.*

2. *False.* Specific patient outcomes are not ensured by following the standard of professional practice. An outcome is the result or consequence of a treatment, a drug, an event, or a disease. The standard of professional practice is an ethical guideline, rule of conduct, or standard of care that governs the profession of athletic training.

3. *False.* A certified athletic trainer must hold a CPR certification from a provider that certifies competencies for Emergency Cardiac Care. These include CPR/AED for the Professional Rescuer (through the American Red Cross) or BLS Healthcare Provider certification through the American Heart Association.

4. *False.* The BOC *Role Delineation Study/Practice Analysis* is intended to serve as a guideline for the practice of athletic training but is not the sole entity governing the practice of athletic training. The athletic trainer must also follow state laws.

5. *False.* Each state has its own regulatory guidelines and practice acts for athletic trainers.

6. *True.* You must accept all position statements put out by NATA. These include position statements on environmental cold injuries, emergency planning in athletics, exertional heat illnesses, fluid replacement for patients, head down contact and spearing in tackle football, lightning safety for athletics and recreation, management of asthma in patients, management of sport-related concussion, management of the patient with type 1 diabetes mellitus, and preventing, detecting, and managing disordered eating in patients.

7. *False.* States are getting stricter and enforcing the regulatory acts of athletic trainers more than has been done in the past. A large shift has been made for states to license athletic trainers.

8. *True.* This policy is stated within the preamble of the NATA *Code of Ethics.*

9. *True.* A few of such systems include the National Safety Council, the National Center for Catastrophic Sports Injury Research, and the NCAA Injury Surveillance System.

10. *True.* There are many actions an athletic trainer can take to avoid being sued. The athletic trainer must make sure he or she has done everything possible to provide a reasonable degree of care to the injured patient and closely follow athletic training procedures that conform to the legal guidelines governing liability for negligence.

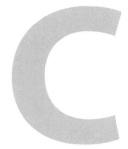

Answer Key

Applied Decision Making

PROBLEM I

Section A

The current situation: You know your patient has injured his right lower leg during a dismount off the rings.

Your immediate responsibility: To perform your initial evaluation to determine the type and severity of the injury.

1. (++) Since this injury was not witnessed, information should be obtained from the patient about what occurred as part of the "history" portion of the initial evaluation. (The patient tells you he was not balanced and landed on his right side.)

2. (++) Because the opening scene has implied there is a significant lower extremity injury, the athletic trainer should ask the patient if he heard/felt a "snap" or "pop," which may indicate a ligament injury or fracture. (The patient definitely felt a "snap.")

3. (++) This will give the athletic trainer an idea of the patient's willingness to move his leg. (The patient will not move his leg because of pain.)

4. (+) Observing for areas of swelling and/or bleeding is part of a secondary survey. (The distal lower extremity is swollen with deformity.)

5. (+) Palpation of the injured area is part of the secondary survey. (The patient has significant pain with palpation of the lower leg.)

6. (++) Because this appears to be a significant injury, it would be prudent for the athletic trainer to monitor the patient's vital signs. (Blood pressure is 128/88 and his pulse is 88.)

7. (++) The pulses of the lower leg should be assessed to make sure there is adequate circulation to the affected limb. (The right popliteal pulse is palpable and strong.)

8. (--) Heating the affected area is contraindicated during the acute phase of the injury. (The effusion becomes enormous.)

9. (-) The injured leg should not be moved until your initial evaluation is complete. (The patient screams in pain.)

10. (+) It has been determined this injury is serious enough to warrant calling for an ambulance.

11. (-) It has been determined that there is a significant injury to the right lower extremity. It is not necessary to spend a lot of time examining the patient's entire body for injuries. (A lot of time has been wasted.)

12. (+) If the area that is injured is not immediately accessible, it may be necessary to cut away the patient's uniform. (You can clearly see where the injury is located.)

13. (0) Until the severity of the injury is established, immobilization of the limb may be a premature action.

Van Ost L, Lew Feirman K, Manfré K. *Athletic Training Exam Review: A Student Guide to Success, Sixth Edition* (pp 221-254).
© 2017 SLACK Incorporated.

Section B

The current situation: The patient is complaining of severe right lower leg pain and the lower leg is swollen and obviously deformed. The patient's vital signs are stable.

Your immediate responsibility: Continue your evaluation, then stabilize the leg and make the patient comfortable.

14. (--) If a fracture is suspected, the athletic trainer should never manipulate the injured area, as this will cause further injury. (The deformity is worsened.)

15. (-) The patient should not be moved until the immobilizer or splint is in place and secured on the affected limb. (The patient screams in pain.)

16. (0) This action would only be necessary if a crowd is gathering and/or there is equipment that is in the way.

17. (+) This action is appropriate to decrease pain and minimize effusion. (The patient feels better with ice on his leg.)

18. (++) It is critical to check the pulses of the ankle and foot to determine if there is adequate circulation to the injured limb. (The right dorsalis pedis pulse is palpable, but weak.)

19. (++) If the leg appears hard and swollen, it may indicate the beginning of a Volkmann's contracture, which is a paralytic contracture that results from ischemia of muscles and nerves in an extremity. (The lower leg appears tight and swollen.)

20. (0) The competition should be stopped if the patient is in harm's way or an entrance/exit to the gym area is blocked because of crowding.

21. (--) Moving the patient may cause further injury; initial immobilization should take place with the patient in side-lying position. (The deformity is made worse by moving the leg.)

22. (-) It has been determined by this time that the patient has a significant lower leg injury. Evaluating the hip at this time is both unnecessary and inappropriate. (You wasted valuable time.)

23. (+) Assuming the leg is immobilized at this point, short-term elevation may help retard swelling.

24. (-) Checking for crepitus at this time is inappropriate. (The patient screams in pain.)

25. (++) If a fracture of the lower extremity is suspected, immobilization is a priority in preventing further injury. (The leg is immobilized while the patient is in side-lying.)

26. (--) Massaging the area of injury is inappropriate and will cause increased pain and swelling. (The patient screams in pain.)

Section C

The current situation: You have determined the patient has sustained a lower leg fracture. The patient's leg is immobilized.

Your immediate responsibility: Prepare to transport the patient to the hospital and monitor the patient until the rescue squad arrives. Document the event and your actions.

27. (+) This is an appropriate action to assess circulation and neurological function. (The patient complains his foot feels numb.)

28. (--) This action would be inappropriate. The patient should be transported by a gurney to minimize movement of the lower body. (The patient trips with the crutches.)

29. (--) Issuing any medications to this patient would not be an appropriate action at this point in time because it is unknown what other medications he will be given at the hospital. (The team physician finds out and is furious.)

30. (-) It is not necessary for the coach to accompany this patient to the hospital. It is the duty of the athletic trainer to follow up with this patient after the meet is finished. (A parent substitutes for the coach and the team loses.)

31. (--) It is unknown what the patient will be given at the hospital (eg, medications, etc) or if he may need anesthesia. It is dangerous to allow the patient to eat or drink until he is told it is okay by the medical staff at the hospital. (The patient aspirates in the operating room and dies.)

32. (-) It is unknown what this patient's status is at this time, and the decision to return to play will be up to the team physician. (The coach wants to know if you spoke with the team physician.)

33. (0) If the athletic trainer has a personal rapport with the emergency room staff, this is a nice touch, but not necessary. The rescue squad will alert the hospital of their arrival. (The emergency room nurse politely thanks you for your call.)

34. (++) Monitoring the patient for symptoms of shock is always appropriate with a traumatic injury, and your findings should be passed along to the EMS team. (The patient appears pale, and his blood pressure has dropped to 90/60 with a pulse rate of 90.)

35. (++) It is important that the athletic trainer emotionally support the patient. Realize he is in pain and scared and will need reassurance that he is in good hands. (The patient is calm with your presence.)

36. (0) Fitting the patient for a pair of crutches is unnecessary. (The hospital will handle it.)

37. (+) If this patient is a minor, his parents should be contacted and given information on what occurred, what actions were taken to care for the patient, and to which hospital he was sent. (The parents leave for the hospital and are grateful you called.)

38. (+) An injury report should be filled out to ensure the circumstances surrounding the injury and what steps were taken during his care are documented. (You avoid a potential malpractice lawsuit.)

PROBLEM II

Section A

The current situation: You know your patient has sustained a traumatic injury to her eyes and/or face as a result of a blow by a hockey ball.

Your immediate responsibility: To perform your initial evaluation to determine the nature and severity of the injury.

1. (0) With the exception of the goalie, there is no head/face protective equipment in field hockey.

2. (-) From the information provided by the opening scenario, you know the patient has an eye and/or facial injury. Testing the patient's fine motor skills is inappropriate. (There is no problem with the patient's fine motor skills.)

3. (-) It has been determined that this is an injury to the eye and/or face. Attempting to test this patient's balance is inappropriate. (The patient wonders why you want her to balance on one leg.)

4. (--) The use of an ammonia capsule would be unnecessary and inappropriate. The patient may jerk her head, possibly causing further injury. (The patient sustains a retinal detachment.)

5. (--) This patient may have a potentially serious eye injury. The patient should remain in a recumbent position until the initial injury assessment is complete. (The patient complains of "throbbing" pain.)

6. (+) This is an appropriate action but does not directly relate to your evaluation. (The patient is more comfortable.)

7. (0) Asking the patient who made the shot is an inappropriate question. (Who cares?)

8. (+) This is an appropriate question during an injury assessment as part of the "subjective" information portion of the evaluation. (The patient complains of pain above the right eye.)

9. (0) Although examining the shoulders will not harm the patient, it has been determined the injury is to the eye. (The patient has no shoulder pain.)

10. (++) It is important the athletic trainer perform a primary survey and thoroughly examine the head, face, or neck as indicated once the mechanism of injury has been determined. (It is determined this is not a life-threatening situation.)

11. (++) Gently palpating the orbital rim and nose for point tenderness, crepitus, or deformity is part of the initial assessment of an eye injury. (There is tenderness over the left eyebrow with a large hematoma. No crepitus is noted.)

12. (++) Because this was a traumatic injury involving a small high-velocity projectile, it is highly likely blood will be present. (Donning gloves is part of universal precautions.)

13. (-) Battle's sign is present when there is a basilar skull fracture. It is known from the opening scene that the patient has suffered an eye/facial injury.

14. (0) Asking the patient if she is a scholarship patient is unnecessary and inappropriate. (The patient asks why that matters.)

15. (++) Checking the area for bleeding is a fundamental component of your initial examination of this patient. (There is a profuse amount of blood present.)

16. (+) This is an appropriate question when assessing the severity of injury to the eye itself. (The patient's vision is blurred.)

Section B

The current situation: You know the patient has a deep laceration above the left eyebrow. It does not appear that the patient has sustained any facial fractures.

Your immediate responsibility: To clean and dress the wound and treat the patient for pain and swelling.

17. (++) It is important to check pupillary response for possible cerebral injury. (The pupillary response is normal.)

18. (--) This would be contradicted in an acute injury to the eye. (The bleeding and swelling increase dramatically.)

19. (+) Rinsing the wound with saline solution will help to remove any dirt or debris that may cause an infection.

20. (0) Because this is a deep laceration, the patient will have to be referred to a physician for treatment. Application of an antiseptic or antibiotic to the area after a thorough cleansing will be done by the physician.

21. (+) Both eyes should be covered during the patient's transport to the hospital to minimize eye movement. (The patient feels better with her eyes closed.)

22. (0) The mechanism of injury was determined by the opening scenario. (This is obvious.)

23. (+) Because there is no apparent injury to the eye itself, an ice pack applied lightly to the surrounding area of the eye will help minimize swelling. (The pain and swelling are controlled.)

24. (+) The application of butterfly strips will help to minimize bleeding and approximate the wound until the physician sutures it. (You are able to close the wound.)

25. (-) It is inappropriate to ignore the patient. It is the job of the athletic trainer to answer her questions honestly and be reassuring to minimize her anxieties. (The patient appears fearful.)

26. (--) Only a physician can suture a wound; an athletic trainer is not qualified or licensed to do so. (You are sued for malpractice.)

27. (+) If there is a suspected serious eye injury, the patient should be transported to a hospital while lying in a recumbent position. (You act cautiously.)

28. (--) The patient should be kept calm and comfortable while waiting for the ambulance and should not be left alone. (The patient passes out in the parking lot.)

29. (-) In case of a serious eye injury, no direct pressure should be applied to the eye. (You find out later you might have made the injury worse.)

30. (++) A secondary evaluation is a detailed assessment that focuses on the nature and extent of the injury. (You know the patient has a bad laceration and suspect a potentially serious eye injury.)

Section C

The current situation: The patient has sustained a deep laceration over the left eyebrow with a potential eye injury.

Your immediate responsibility: Keep the patient calm while waiting for the rescue squad and document the course of events.

31. (+) The athletic trainer should be a source of reassurance. This is an appropriate action. (The patient is grateful you are staying with her.)

32. (-) The patient's condition and playing status have not been determined. Announcing the patient's condition is inappropriate. (You anger the coach and parents with this announcement.)

33. (-) The student's insurance coverage should not be a deterrent for an emergency room visit. (You delay treatment.)

34. (-) It is not the duty of the school nurse to accompany the patient to the emergency room. (She reminds you that this is part of your job.)

35. (--) Once the initial dressing is applied and the bleeding is controlled, it is inappropriate to change the bandage multiple times. (The butterfly strips come off, and the cut bleeds again.)

36. (+) The patient may need reassurance from her coach that her position is not in jeopardy. (The coach tells the patient there is no need to worry.)

37. (-) Speaking with the press about the patient's condition is not appropriate. (You are reprimanded by your athletic director.)

38. (++) Washing your hands thoroughly after handling a "blood spill" is a fundamental universal precaution.

39. (++) Documenting the incident and treatment given is appropriate.

40. (0) Dispensing vitamins to the patient is unnecessary and inappropriate.

41. (+) Once the patient is stable and not in any immediate danger, it is wise to inform the patient's coach of the nature and severity of the injury and what is being done for her. (The coach thanks you for doing a thorough job.)

PROBLEM III

Section A

The current situation: You know your patient has been injured after incorrectly landing on a crash mat. He is not moving.

Your immediate responsibility: To evaluate the injury to determine the type and nature of the injury.

1. (-) This would be a premature action as you have not completed your initial evaluation of the injury.

2. (+) This question should be asked as part of the history portion of the initial assessment. (The patient complains of dull neck pain.)

3. (++) A primary survey is necessary to determine if there is a life-threatening injury. (The patient is conscious and is breathing without difficulty. Blood pressure is 130/90 and pulse is 82.)

4. (+) Noting the position of the patient is important when deciding how the patient is to be treated and transported. (The patient is lying on his right side with his knees flexed.)

5. (-) The patient should not be moved unless the airway is blocked and there is additional help available. (The patient is breathing without difficulty.)

6. (+) This is a quick screen to assess motor function of the upper and lower extremities. (The patient states he cannot move his fingers or toes.)

7. (+) If the patient is conscious and can answer questions, it is appropriate to ask this as part of the history portion of the evaluation. It helps in determining the mechanism of injury. (He reports he did not tuck his chin in and landed on his head, snapping his head forward.)

8. (0) Applying an ice pack to the patient's neck is unnecessary and inappropriate.

9. (0) It is known from the opening scenario that the area of injury is not the lower extremity.

10. (+) It is an appropriate action as part of the primary survey to assess the patient for areas of significant bleeding. (The patient's face is uninjured.)

11. (0) Until the initial evaluation of the injury is completed, this would be a premature and inappropriate action. (You waste valuable time.)

12. (++) Checking the patient's level of consciousness is a necessary step during the primary survey. (The patient is coherent and responds appropriately to questions.)

Section B

The current situation: The patient is conscious and coherent and is breathing without difficulty. His vital signs are stable, but he is unable to move his extremities.

Your immediate responsibility: To continue your evaluation to determine the patient's neuromuscular function, protect the patient from further injury, and prepare him for transport to the hospital.

13. (--) Moving the patient at this time without securing him to a spine board may cause further injury. (The patient sustains a complete spinal cord injury and is quadriplegic.)

14. (--) Having the patient move his head may be a potentially fatal or debilitating action. (The patient sustains a vertebral fracture/dislocation and dies.)

15. (++) Determining sensation to the extremities is important in assessing the severity of the injury. (The patient complains he cannot feel anything from his armpits down to his feet.)

16. (++) This is a fundamental action in preventing further injury to the patient.

17. (0) This is an unnecessary action, as you have ruled out a head injury. (The patient is conscious and alert.)

18. (-) The findings of the primary survey do not indicate there is a head injury. (You waste time.)

19. (++) Log-rolling the patient with assistance onto his back is necessary for stabilization and transport of the patient. (You successfully position the patient into supine.)

20. (0) Unless the patient is in an area where he may be subjected to further injury, it is not necessary to stop the meet at this time. (You keep the area clear of spectators.)

21. (++) Securing the patient to a spine board is an appropriate action. (You successfully secure the patient onto a spine board with help.)

22. (++) While you stay with the patient, an ambulance should be summoned to the field. (The ambulance is close by and arrives in 5 minutes.)

23. (+) This is an appropriate action with a suspected neck injury. (You successfully apply a cervical collar.)

24. (++) Monitoring the patient's vital signs is a fundamental aspect of your care. (The patient's vital signs remain stable.)

Section C

The current situation: You have evaluated the injury and suspect the patient has sustained a serious cervical spinal injury. The patient is transported to the hospital via ambulance.

Your immediate responsibility: To contact the team physician, parents, and other appropriate individuals with information regarding the accident. Document what occurred and who was involved.

25. (+) Communicating with the team physician would be appropriate at this time. (Your athletic training student contacts the team doctor's office.)

26. (+) It is important to document the incident. (You protect yourself against a malpractice lawsuit.)

27. (0) If another certified athletic trainer is available to cover the rest of the meet, it would be appropriate to go to the hospital. Otherwise, you should follow up with the patient at the hospital after the meet.

28. (0) The patient is coherent and able to provide this information to the EMS and hospital personnel.

29. (0) Whether or not the patient is on a scholarship is not pertinent to the treatment of this patient.

30. (+) Contacting the parents of the injured patient would be an appropriate step. (The parents go directly to the hospital.)

31. (-) Leaving an athletic training student in charge of covering a state track meet without direct supervision of a certified athletic trainer is inappropriate. (You are reprimanded by your athletic director and are lucky no one else is hurt while you are gone.)

32. (-) This is an inappropriate comment. (The athletic director suggests that you stick to your duties as an athletic trainer.)

PROBLEM IV

Section A

The current situation: A patient comes to your office complaining of chronic left anterior knee pain. No specific mechanism of injury has been identified.

Your immediate responsibility: To perform your initial evaluation to determine the nature and severity of the condition.

1. (0) Applying an ice pack will not cause further injury, but may not help the patient either because the problem has not been thoroughly evaluated at this time.

2. (+) A postural assessment is part of the evaluation of anterior knee pain. (Both knees are in genu valgum.)

3. (+) Palpation of the knee joint is a basic element of a knee evaluation. (The patient complains of patellar tendon and medial knee pain.)

4. (+) With subjective complaints of anterior knee pain, it is highly likely the patient's iliotibial band will be tight. Both sides must be tested for comparison. (Ober's test is positive on the left lower extremity.)

5. (+) This question should be asked while taking the patient's history, as a "popping" sensation is often associated with patellofemoral pain syndrome. (The patient reports it "pops" intermittently while running.)

6. (-) It is known from the patient's subjective complaints that this is a knee injury. (The patient tells you her feet are fine.)

7.   (0) Patrick's test is a special test of the hip that when positive is indicative of degenerative joint disease.

8.   (+) This is an appropriate question to ask when gathering information regarding the mechanism of injury. (The patient has pain going down stairs and running downhill.)

9.   (++) Because activity appears to increase the pain, it would be wise to advise the patient to stop running when it hurts. (The patient feels much better when she is not landing on it.)

10.   (-) Temporary orthotics may not be necessary or appropriate; the initial evaluation is not complete. (You waste time making them and the patient reports no change in her pain.)

11.   (+) Observing the knee for swelling or deformity is a fundamental component of the initial evaluation. (No swelling is noted.)

12.   (+) Palpating the knee joint and surrounding soft tissue structures is a fundamental component of the initial evaluation. (The patient complains of pain with palpation of the medial facet.)

13.   (-) A KT-1000 arthrometer is used to test for anterior cruciate laxity and would not be appropriate in this situation. (It is known from the opening scenario that this is not an acute injury, and injury to the anterior cruciate ligament is unlikely.)

Section B

The current situation: The patient has pain running downhill, especially over the patellar tendon and medial aspect of the knee. She has pain over the same areas with palpation, although there is no swelling present. She also experiences a "popping" sensation with running. She stands in genu valgum and presents a tight iliotibial band on the left leg.

Your immediate responsibility: Make recommendations to the patient to decrease her pain with activities and teach the patient lower limb stretching and strengthening exercises to realign the patella.

14.   (+) A soft knee brace designed to help stabilize the patella may help decrease the patient's pain during activity. (The patient reports a decrease in pain and feeling of "popping" while wearing the knee sleeve.)

15.   (0) Strengthening the hamstrings does not have a direct effect in stabilizing the patella.

16.   (+) Strengthening the vastus medialis obliquus will help to improve the tracking of the patella in the femoral groove. (The patient has fewer episodes of "popping.")

17.   (--) Repetitive deep squatting exercises cause high compressive loading on the patellofemoral joint and will aggravate the patient's knee. (The patient complains of significant anterior knee pain.)

18.   (+) Patella taping is a useful tool in evaluating and treating patellar misalignment problems. (There is reduction of pain with taping.)

19.   (++) A tight iliotibial band will cause mistracking of the patella. (There are fewer episodes of "popping.")

20.   (++) Tight hamstrings may cause mistracking of the patella in the femoral groove. (The patient has bilateral hamstring tightness.)

21.   (-) Recommending an oral NSAID might be appropriate, but a certified athletic trainer is not qualified or licensed to dispense a prescription drug such as Voltaren. (The patient has an adverse reaction to the medication and you are sued for malpractice.)

22.   (-) The patient should avoid hard or hilly surfaces. (The patient continues to complain of "popping" and knee pain with running.)

Section C

The current situation: You have determined from your evaluation that this patient has a subluxing patella secondary to weak anteromedial thigh musculature and a tight iliotibial band and hamstrings.

Your immediate responsibility: Continue to work with the patient to develop a structured rehabilitation program to encourage proper alignment of the patella, which will in turn eliminate the pain.

23.   (0) A TENS unit is a modality that can be used temporarily for pain. A TENS unit will not contribute directly to the elimination of the origin of the problem. (The patient has no pain when she is not running.)

24.   (-) The patella subluxes as a result of weak anterior and medial thigh musculature; PNF exercises that emphasize motions that encourage hip abduction with internal rotation facilitate strengthening of the lateral thigh musculature. (The patient experiences an increase in episodes of patella subluxation.)

25.   (0) Ultrasound treatments will not have a direct impact on the cause of the problem.

26.   (--) Because plyometric exercises employ ballistic movements, which generate high forces, the initiation of this type of exercise would not be appropriate. (The patient now complains of anterior knee pain at rest.)

27.   (++) Strengthening the quadriceps musculature in both open- and closed-chain positions is appropriate as long as the exercise is pain-free.

28.   (+) It may be beneficial to evaluate the patient's running gait to assess what is occurring at the knee. (The patient's feet severely pronate during midstance.)

29.   (++) Strengthening the hip adductors will augment the strength of the vastus medialis obliquus.

30.   (+) The continual application of ice to the knee will help minimize any pain or inflammation from exercises. (The patient is able to control postactivity soreness.)

PROBLEM V

Section A

The current situation: A patient comes to you complaining of right shoulder pain that occurs after throwing. He is able to voluntarily sublux both his shoulders.

Your immediate responsibility: To perform an initial evaluation to determine the nature and severity of the problem.

1. (++) Asking the patient how long the problem has existed is a fundamental question to ask during the history portion of the evaluation. This will give the athletic trainer an idea if this is an acute or chronic problem. (The patient states it has hurt over the past 3 weeks.)

2. (+) A more appropriate question might be to ask the patient if the right shoulder had ever been injured in the past and when the injury occurred. (The patient states he has not had a shoulder injury prior to this recent episode.)

3. (+) This is an appropriate question to ask during the history portion of the evaluation. (The patient states that he cannot specifically tell you what position[s] make the pain worse.)

4. (0) This would be an inappropriate question. Whether or not the patient is consuming an adequate amount of protein has nothing to do with this problem.

5. (++) This would be an appropriate question given the information that has been provided in the opening scenario. (The fact that the patient is able to voluntarily sublux his shoulder.)

6. (0) This question is unnecessary and inappropriate. The patient has already provided you with information in the opening scenario relating to his joint laxity.

7. (0) This question is unnecessary and inappropriate. Whether or not the patient is taking supplemental vitamins has no direct correlation to the present problem.

8. (+) Asking the patient about the intensity of his pain will provide the athletic trainer information regarding the severity of the condition. (The patient reports his pain level is moderate, 5/10 after pitching.)

9. (-) This is an inappropriate question. Whether or not his father played baseball is irrelevant and whether or not his father had injured his shoulder has no direct correlation to the present problem. (The patient has no idea if his father ever had a shoulder problem.)

10. (+) Asking the patient about any medications he may be taking is appropriate during the history portion of the initial evaluation. (The patient reports he has been taking aspirin for the pain with temporary relief.)

Section B

The current situation: The patient has subacute right shoulder pain with joint laxity. He is able to voluntarily sublux both his shoulders. Aspirin provides minimal pain relief.

Your immediate responsibility: Perform special tests to identify the etiology of the patient's pain.

11. (-) This is an inappropriate test for this problem. Phalen's test is performed when carpal tunnel syndrome is suspected.

12. (+) A clunk test is an appropriate test to perform if a glenoid labral tear is suspected. (The patient has a negative clunk test.)

13. (-) The pivot shift test is performed to evaluate the knee for anterolateral instability secondary to tearing the anterior cruciate ligament. This is an inappropriate test for this problem.

14. (-) Patrick's test is performed to evaluate the hip for iliopsoas, sacroiliac, or joint pathology. This is an inappropriate test for this problem.

15. (-) Thompson's test is performed when the possibility of an Achilles tendon rupture exists. This is an inappropriate test for this problem.

16. (+) The apprehension test (anterior and posterior) is an appropriate test to perform for this problem. A positive test may be indicative of either anterior or posterior glenohumeral instability. (The patient has a positive apprehension sign.)

17. (+) The Hawkins-Kennedy impingement test is used to test for pain and apprehension relating to shoulder impingement. This would be an appropriate test to perform for this problem. (The patient has a positive test.)

18. (+) Neer's sign is used to test for pain and apprehension relating to shoulder impingement, primarily of the biceps long head and supraspinatus tendons. (The patient has a negative Neer's sign.)

19. (+) The posterior drawer test of the shoulder is used when there is suspicion of posterior instability of the glenohumeral joint. This would be an appropriate test for this problem. (The patient has a negative posterior drawer sign.)

20. (-) Ober's test is used to determine iliotibial band/tensor fasciae latae tightness of the lower extremity. This is an inappropriate test for this problem.

21. (-) Trendelenburg's test is used to determine if there is weakness of the gluteus medius muscle. This is not an appropriate test for this problem.

22. (+) Testing for a sulcus sign is appropriate when assessing the patient for multidirectional instability of the shoulder. This is an appropriate test for this problem. (The patient has a positive sulcus sign.)

Section C

The current situation: The patient has a positive impingement test, a positive sulcus sign, and a positive apprehension test.

Your immediate responsibility: Instruct and supervise an upper extremity strengthening program.

23. (+) Shoulder shrugs strengthen the upper trapezius muscle, which helps to stabilize the scapula superiorly.

24. (-) Although biceps curls are not inappropriate for general upper extremity strengthening, they will not contribute to strengthening the rotator cuff or scapula musculature.

25. (+) Shoulder abduction strengthening exercises are appropriate, as they stabilize the scapula laterally and posteriorly.

26. (-) Cervical isometric exercises are unnecessary and inappropriate for this particular problem, as they will not have a direct effect on stabilizing the scapula or strengthening the rotator cuff.

27. (++) Resistive exercises involving internal and external rotation of the shoulder directly strengthen the rotator cuff musculature.

28. (+) Resistive exercises performed in the D2 extension pattern work the shoulder extensors, adductors, and internal rotators. This type of exercise would be appropriate for this problem.

29. (-) Because the long head of the triceps brachii muscle arises from the infraglenoid tuberosity of the scapula, shoulder extension exercises would assist in scapular stabilization, but triceps curls (ie, elbow extension) would not have a direct effect on either the scapula or the rotator cuff.

30. (+) Rowing exercises strengthen the rhomboids, triceps (long head), and latissimus dorsi, stabilizing the scapula medially and posteriorly.

31. (+) Exercises involving resisted scapular protraction strengthen the serratus anterior muscle, stabilizing the scapula laterally.

32. (-) Partial sit-ups strengthen the upper abdominals, which is unnecessary and inappropriate for this problem.

33. (-) Prone trunk extensions strengthen the erector spinae musculature of the back, which is unnecessary and inappropriate for this problem.

34. (-) Calf raises strengthen the triceps surae complex of the lower leg, which is unnecessary and inappropriate for this problem.

PROBLEM VI

Section A

The current situation: You know your patient has sustained a left lower leg injury and the mechanism of injury was an indirect trauma.

Your immediate responsibility: To perform your initial evaluation of the injury to determine the type and extent of the injury.

1. (-) It is obvious from the opening scenario that the patient is breathing fine. (The patient is howling in pain.)

2. (-) It is obvious from the opening scenario that the patient has a significant lower extremity injury; it is inappropriate to have the patient attempt to walk until your initial evaluation is complete. (The patient asks if you are an athletic training student.)

3. (+) Asking the patient what happened is an appropriate question that should be asked during the history portion of the initial evaluation. (He states he stopped suddenly and the left lower leg "gave out.")

4. (-) It is obvious from the opening scenario that the patient has not sustained a head injury. This would be an inappropriate action. (The patient is very alert and in severe pain.)

5. (+) Examining the patient's leg for areas of external or internal bleeding (ecchymosis) is an appropriate action. (There are no obvious signs of bleeding at this time.)

6. (++) Asking the patient where the pain is located is fundamental in determining what structures of the lower leg are involved. (The patient points to the musculotendinous junction of the gastrocnemius and Achilles tendon.)

7. (++) Observing the area of injury is an appropriate and necessary action as part of the initial assessment of an injury. (There is mild edema of the posterior lower extremity at the musculotendinous junction.)

8. (++) Asking the patient whether or not he felt or heard a "pop" or "snap" provides the athletic trainer information regarding the nature and severity of the injury. (The patient states he felt a "pop" with severe pain in the calf.)

9. (0) Applying ice at this point of your evaluation will not hurt the patient but is premature, as your evaluation is not yet complete.

10. (-) Asking the patient if he has ever injured his uninvolved leg would be inappropriate at this time, as it is not a priority. (The patient states his left lower extremity has never been hurt.)

11. (--) It is obvious from the opening scenario that the left lower extremity has been significantly injured. Asking the patient to stand and hop would be inappropriate and could cause further injury if attempted. (The patient completely ruptures his gastrocnemius muscle.)

Section B

The current situation: You know from your evaluation that the patient felt a "pop" accompanied by severe pain at the musculotendinous junction of the gastrocnemius and Achilles tendon. There is mild edema present in the area.

Your immediate responsibility: To continue your evaluation to determine the severity of the injury.

12. (++) Palpating the injured extremity for swelling and deformity would be an appropriate action at this time. (There is now a moderate effusion of the lower extremity and a palpable defect at the musculotendinous junction.)

13. (-) Performing a Lachman's test bilaterally would be an unnecessary and inappropriate action. The injury is to the left lower extremity, not the knee. (The patient wonders why you are checking his knee.)

14. (-) Performing a Thomas test bilaterally would be an unnecessary and inappropriate action. The Thomas test is performed to assess for tight hip flexors. (You have now wasted time examining the patient's hip flexibility.)

15. (+) Checking the active range of motion of both ankles is appropriate to assess the patient's functional ability and willingness to move. (The patient is unable to actively plantar flex his foot and has pain with the attempt.)

16. (-) Checking the patient's Q-angle is unnecessary and inappropriate. It is also known from the opening scenario that it is the left lower extremity, not the right, that is injured. (Be sure to carefully read through all the information provided.)

17. (0) Whether or not the patient has bunions has nothing to do with this injury.

18. (++) Performing Thompson's test bilaterally would be an appropriate action to take during your assessment of this injury. (The test is positive on the left leg.)

19. (-) Performing a Hawkin's test bilaterally would be unnecessary and inappropriate. The patient's left lower extremity has been injured, not his shoulder. (The patient wonders why you are examining his shoulder.)

20. (-) Performing an anterior drawer test bilaterally on both ankles is unnecessary and inappropriate. The patient's left lower leg has been injured, not his left ankle. (The patient wonders why you are examining his ankles.)

21. (0) Palpating the femoral pulse is unnecessary and inappropriate for this problem. (The patient's femoral pulses are fine.)

22. (0) Testing the patellar tendon reflexes bilaterally is an unnecessary and inappropriate action. (The patient's patellar tendon reflexes are fine.)

23. (+) Testing the strength of the ankle plantar flexors would be an appropriate action to take when initially assessing the severity of the injury. (The strength of the ankle plantar flexors is -2/5 and painful.)

Section C

The current situation: You suspect a torn left gastrocnemius muscle.

Your immediate responsibility: To begin treatment to control the pain and swelling and protect the patient from further injury.

24. (--) If the lower limb still has a significant amount of swelling, warm whirlpool treatments would be inappropriate. (The patient's leg swells significantly during this treatment.)

25. (++) Applying ice to the injured area is an appropriate action to ease the pain and control the effusion. (The patient is much more comfortable with the ice.)

26. (++) Applying a compression wrap to the injured area is an appropriate action to ease the pain and control the effusion. (The patient is much more comfortable with the compression wrap.)

27. (+) High-volt galvanic stimulation can be used to modulate pain and assist with edema reduction. (The patient is much more comfortable after the treatment.)

28. (++) The application of a posterior leg splint is an appropriate action. This puts the lower extremity at rest and protects the area from further injury. (The patient is much more comfortable with the lower leg immobilized.)

29. (-) Attempting to use the BAPS board too early in the treatment may increase pain and swelling. This is an inappropriate action at this time. (The patient complains of increased calf pain and is frustrated he is unable to move the board.)

30. (--) Based on your initial assessment, this patient has sustained a torn gastrocnemius muscle. This would be an inappropriate action if your assessment is correct. (The patient howls in pain during the attempt to come up on his toes.)

31. (+) This is an appropriate action, especially if the lower extremity is immobilized.

32. (-) This is an inappropriate action. The defect is a result of a torn muscle, not an infection. (The patient questions why you are smearing gel on him.)

33. (0) The patient may or may not be able to perform hamstring curls early in the rehabilitation. (The patient is able to lift light weights.)

34. (--) Because this is an acute muscle tear, ultrasound treatments are contraindicated at this time. (The calf swells and becomes ecchymotic.)

35. (-) While gentle range of motion exercises are appropriate, the injured limb is the left lower extremity, not the right. (The patient reminds you that his right leg is fine.)

Section D

The current situation: Your patient sustained a torn gastrocnemius muscle, which is now subacute in nature. The motion of his ankle and knee is normal, but he still has some strength deficits in plantar flexion.

Your immediate responsibility: Develop a strength and conditioning program designed to improve the patient's left lower extremity strength and maintain his level of fitness.

36. (++) Stationary bicycling would be appropriate at this point of this patient's rehabilitation. (The patient is grateful to be aerobically active.)

37. (--) Uphill jogging would be inappropriate. Based on the information provided, the patient's strength in plantar flexion is still weak. This exercise is premature and may cause further injury. (The patient retears the muscle.)

38. (0) Although push-ups will not harm the patient, it is not a necessary exercise for this patient's rehabilitation.

39. (++) Having the patient performing progressive-resistive ankle exercises in all directions would be appropriate at this point of the patient's rehabilitation. (The patient has no pain or significant difficulty with resistive exercises.)

40. (--) Knowing from the information given thus far that the patient is weak in plantar flexion concentrically, plyometric exercises would be inappropriate and may cause further injury if initiated too soon. (The patient retears the gastrocnemius.)

41. (0) Using the upper body ergometer during the patient's rehabilitation would be appropriate to maintain aerobic fitness but is not directly related to rehabilitating a lower extremity injury.

42. (+) Initiating exercises that enhance proprioception is a necessary and appropriate action to take in preparing the patient to return to his sport. (The patient demonstrates some difficulty in maintaining his balance on the injured leg.)

43. (++) Having the patient perform exercises that directly work in strengthening the plantar flexors of the ankle is appropriate. (The patient has no pain performing this exercise but still has difficulty performing unilateral calf raises.)

44. (+) Partial squats with and without additional resistance is appropriate for lower extremity strengthening. (The patient is able to do this without pain or difficulty.)

45. (++) Having the patient perform resisted hamstring curls would be appropriate, as the gastrocnemius not only functions to plantar flex the ankle but is also a flexor of the knee.

46. (+) It is important to make sure the rest of the leg is strengthened in addition to the specific area of injury, because the entire lower extremity loses strength during the initial phases of treatment when the limb is immobilized. (The patient has normal quadricep strength bilaterally.)

47. (+) Making sure the patient maintains his lower extremity flexibility is appropriate in preparing the patient to return to his sport. (The patient's flexibility is normal bilaterally.)

48. (-) Focusing attention on upper extremity strengthening would not be necessary or appropriate during the rehabilitation of this injury.

49. (-) Focusing attention on upper extremity strengthening would not be necessary or appropriate during the rehabilitation of this injury.

50. (-) Until the strength of the patient's plantar flexors on the injured limb is equal to the strength of the uninjured limb, initiating agility exercises would be inappropriate.

Section E

The current situation: This patient has been performing a general lower extremity flexibility and strengthening exercise program as instructed without complaints of pain or difficulty. He is anxious to return to playing competitive tennis.

Your immediate responsibility: Reassess the patient and have the patient perform a series of functional exercises to determine if the patient is ready to play.

51. (+) Making sure the patient can walk without a limp would be appropriate. (The patient has no difficulty with this task.)

52. (++) The patient should be completely pain-free at rest and during activity prior to returning to full-time competition. (The patient is completely pain-free.)

53. (++) There should be no visible edema or ecchymosis at the site of injury. (There is no visible swelling or ecchymosis.)

54. (+) The patient should have no complaints of pain with deep palpation of the injured area. (The patient reports he has no pain with palpation of the injured area.)

55. (+) The patient should have no complaints of pain with a resisted hamstring curl. (The patient is pain-free with this motion.)

56. (++) The patient should have full range of motion of both the ankle and knee before returning to full activity. (The range of motion of the injured ankle and knee is equal to the uninjured side.)

57. (--) The athletic trainer should only return the patient to competition when the athletic trainer and team physician determine the patient is fully recovered. (The patient returns too soon and is reinjured.)

58. (+) The patient should be able to hop on the injured lower extremity without pain before returning to full activity. (The patient has no pain or difficulty pushing off or landing on the injured leg.)

59. (+) The patient should be able to jog a reasonable amount of time in a straight line before returning to full activity. (The patient has no difficulty doing this.)

60. (--) Although the patient may not be as interested in his rehabilitation program as he is in his sport, the patient's level of interest is not a credible parameter by which to determine whether or not he can return to full activity.

61. (++) The strength of the patient's involved ankle should be equal to the strength of the uninvolved ankle before returning the patient to full activity. (Both ankles are now graded as 5/5 during manual muscle testing.)

62. (++) It is prudent to have the team physician clear the patient for return to full activity before the patient participates in his sport. (The patient is cleared for competition.)

63. (0) Whether or not the patient can bench press 50 pounds or more has nothing to do with whether or not this patient can compete in tennis. (The patient can bench press 90 pounds.)

PROBLEM VII

Section A

The current situation: You know your patient has sustained an indirect traumatic injury to his right knee. He is able to bear weight without assistance.

Your immediate responsibility: To perform your initial evaluation to determine the nature and severity of the injury.

1. (++) Having the patient locate the area of pain is appropriate during the initial assessment of the injury. It is important in determining the nature of the injury. (The patient reports he has pain along the medial side of the right knee.)

2. (+) Observing for areas of swelling is appropriate during the initial assessment of the injury. (There is minimal edema noted along the medial side of the right knee.)

3. (0) Applying ice to the area prior to completing the initial exam is a premature action.

4. (0) Applying a knee immobilizer prior to completing the initial examination is a premature action.

5. (0) Issuing a cane to the patient prior to completing the initial examination is a premature action. A cane may or may not be an appropriate assistive device for this injury.

6. (++) Palpation of the knee joint and the surrounding structures is a fundamental task of the initial evaluation. (The patient reports he has a small amount of pain with palpation of the anteromedial joint line.)

7. (-) Palpating the gluteus medius muscle is an inappropriate and unnecessary action. It is obvious from the opening scenario that this is a knee injury, not a hip injury. (The patient asks why you are palpating his hip.)

8. (-) Having the patient perform multiple calf raises is not an appropriate action. It is known from the opening scenario that the patient has pain in full weight-bearing. (The patient is unable to perform a calf raise because of knee pain and instability.)

9. (++) Evaluating the range of motion of both knees is appropriate during your initial evaluation of the injury. It assists the athletic trainer in determining the severity of the injury and the patient's willingness to move. (The patient has significant difficulty bending and completely straightening his knee because of pain.)

10. (++) Asking the patient if he has injured his right knee before is an appropriate question during the history portion of the initial evaluation. (The patient reports he had a minor knee injury 3 years ago but has been fine since that time.)

11. (+) It is appropriate during the initial evaluation to assess the strength of the hip musculature bilaterally. (The strength of the hip flexors on the injured limb is +4/5.)

12. (+) It is appropriate during the initial evaluation to assess the strength of the quadriceps musculature bilaterally. (The strength of the quadriceps musculature on the injured limb is -3/5.)

13. (+) It is appropriate during the initial evaluation to assess the strength of the hamstring musculature bilaterally. (The strength of the hamstring musculature on the injured limb is -3/5.)

14. (0) Checking the patient's pupillary reaction is an unnecessary and inappropriate action. (The patient tells you to get the light out of his eyes.)

Section B

The current situation: You have determined from your evaluation that the patient has pain along the medial aspect of the knee with palpation, there is minimal edema present, and the patient has pain with movement into knee flexion and extension.

Your immediate responsibility: To continue your evaluation by performing special tests on the right knee.

15. (++) Performing a Lachman's test bilaterally would be appropriate to assess the integrity of the anterior cruciate ligament. (The Lachman's test is negative.)

16. (--) The vertebral artery test is performed to test the patency of the vertebral arteries. This would be inappropriate. (The patient does not trust you at this point in the exam.)

17. (--) Tinel's test is performed when carpal tunnel syndrome is suspected. This would not be an appropriate test for this problem. (The patient reminds you that it is his knee that is injured, not his wrist or hand.)

18. (++) The valgus stress test is performed to test the integrity of the medial collateral ligament. Performing this test bilaterally would be appropriate. (The patient complains of medial knee joint pain and there is increased valgus movement on the injured side.)

19. (++) The varus stress test is performed to test the integrity of the lateral collateral ligament. Performing this test bilaterally would be an appropriate action. (There is no complaint of pain with this test and minimal/no varus movement on the injured knee joint.)

20. (+) Performing a posterior drawer test bilaterally would be appropriate to test the integrity of the posterior cruciate ligament. (The posterior drawer test is negative.)

21. (--) The empty can test is performed to assess for supraspinatus weakness and is an inappropriate test for this problem. This patient has a knee injury, not a shoulder injury. (The patient's shoulders are fine.)

22. (--) Finkelstein's test is performed to assess for tenosynovitis of the abductor pollicis longus and extensor pollicis brevis tendons and is an inappropriate test for this problem. (The patient asks you what this test has to do with his knees.)

23. (-) Yergason's test is performed bilaterally when bicipital tendinitis is suspected. (The patient asks you what this test has to do with his knees.)

24. (++) Performing a McMurray's test bilaterally would be appropriate to test the knee for a meniscal tear. (McMurray's test is inconclusive because of the limitation in range of motion.)

25. (+) Performing an anterior drawer test bilaterally would be appropriate to test the knee for an anterior cruciate tear. (The anterior drawer test is negative.)

26. (+) Performing a pivot shift test would be appropriate to test the knee for anterolateral rotary instability secondary to a torn anterior cruciate ligament and posterolateral capsule. (The pivot shift test is inconclusive because the patient is guarding.)

27. (+) Performing a patellar apprehension test bilaterally would be appropriate to test the knee for patellar subluxation or dislocation. (The patellar apprehension test is negative.)

Section C

The current situation: You suspect from the results of your evaluation that this patient has a medial collateral ligament sprain with a possible meniscus tear of the right knee.

Your immediate responsibility: Begin a treatment program with emphasis on pain control and early motion.

28. (--) The application of heat early in the rehabilitation when the knee is swollen would be inappropriate. (The knee swells severely after the heat is applied.)

29. (-) Massaging the knee joint is unnecessary and inappropriate. (This causes great pain to the patient, and he avoids you the following week.)

30. (--) Having the patient attempt to use a rowing machine would be inappropriate during the initial stages of rehabilitation. (The patient has significant knee pain and is unable to move the knee enough to operate it.)

31. (++) Placing the patient on crutches to protect the joint is an appropriate action during the initial phases of treatment. (The patient is much more comfortable and mobile with crutches.)

32. (+) Assessing the strength of the quadriceps is important in determining the starting point for a rehabilitation program. (The patient is unable to fully extend his knee against gravity.)

33. (-) Starting isotonic hamstring strengthening exercises would be an inappropriate action if the goal is to treat the patient for pain and swelling. (The patient is unable to fully flex his knee against gravity.)

34. (++) Applying ice to the injured joint is appropriate for pain management and reducing edema. (The patient reports pain relief with the ice packs in place.)

35. (++) It is important to have the patient move his knee as soon as possible to his tolerance to maintain joint mobility. (The patient is able to actively flex and extend his leg to a limited degree while lying in a supine position.)

36. (0) This would not be an appropriate suggestion. It is the right knee that has sustained the injury, not the left knee. (Make sure you read through the scenario carefully.)

37. (--) It is not within an athletic trainer's scope of practice to issue medication with codeine as an active ingredient. (You are sued for trying to practice medicine.)

38. (++) The use of high-volt galvanic stimulation is indicated for reducing pain and swelling. (The patient has good results with this treatment.)

Section D

The current situation: The patient's pain is controlled well with modalities, and he is moving his knee with greater ease.

Your immediate responsibility: To begin the patient on a rehabilitation program with an emphasis on maintaining the patient's aerobic conditioning and beginning functional exercises.

39. (+) Functional activities should be introduced into the rehabilitation program as soon as possible; swimming is an appropriate activity to increase aerobic conditioning. (The patient is able to swim with minimal discomfort.)

40. (+) Having the patient perform calf raises is an inappropriate activity as an early functional exercise.

41. (-) Having the patient attempt to run on a treadmill 1 week after sustaining a second-degree medial collateral tear of the knee would be inappropriate and may subject the patient to further injury. (The patient reinjures his knee while trying to run.)

42. (+) Introducing closed-chain exercises, such as stair-climbing (eg, Stairmaster), into the rehabilitation program as early as possible is an appropriate action. (The patient is able to perform stair-climbing activities.)

43. (++) Having the patient use the upper body ergometer to maintain aerobic fitness is appropriate. (The patient is able to get a vigorous workout on this machine.)

44. (0) Wall pulley exercises for the upper extremity will not harm the patient but are unnecessary and inappropriate if the goal is to maintain the patient's aerobic capability.

45. (++) Introducing closed-chain exercises, such as stationary bicycling, into the rehabilitation program as early as possible is appropriate. (The patient has minimal/no difficulty using the stationary bike.)

46. (--) Fartlek training involves a type of cross-country running, which is varied in speed and terrain. This would be an inappropriate activity for the patient to attempt early in the rehabilitation. (The patient is unable to run, much less perform long-distance running through varied terrain.)

47. (--) Plyometric exercises would be inappropriate in the early stages of rehabilitation. (The patient attempts to jump up onto a stool from the floor and reinjures his knee.)

48. (--) Resisted rowing early in the rehabilitation would be inappropriate. The ballistic motion may cause further pain or injury. (The patient complains of significant pain during this activity.)

PROBLEM VIII

Section A

The current situation: You know this patient has sustained a significant abdominal injury after being kicked by an opponent.

Your immediate responsibility: To perform an initial evaluation to determine the nature and extent of the injury and assess if it is a life-threatening situation.

1. (++) Performing a primary survey would be an appropriate action. (The patient is conscious, coherent, and in obvious pain.)

2. (0) Giving the patient oxygen is unnecessary and inappropriate. (The patient angrily pushes the oxygen mask away from his face.)

3. (-) Auscultating the patient's heart is an inappropriate and unnecessary action. (The patient's heart is fine.)

4. (++) It is appropriate to gently palpate the patient's abdomen to assess for areas of pain and firmness. (The patient has significant pain with palpation of the lower right quadrant and a moderately sized hematoma over the injury site.)

5. (++) It is appropriate during the history portion of the initial assessment to ask the patient where the pain is located. This will give the athletic trainer an idea regarding the nature of the injury. (The patient reports his pain is located in the lower right quadrant of his abdominal area.)

6. (--) Having the patient attempt to stand and jog is a premature action. You have not yet completed your evaluation and may cause further injury by excessively moving the patient. (This patient cannot stand, much less jog, because of the pain.)

7. (0) Having the patient count backward from 100 would be inappropriate and unnecessary. It is known from the opening scenario that a head injury has not been sustained.

8. (0) Having a stretcher brought out to the field is a premature action, as the initial evaluation has not been completed.

9. (0) Unless there is any evidence of bleeding, donning latex gloves is not necessary.

10. (++) Observing the abdominal area for signs of edema or ecchymosis is fundamental during the initial assessment of the injury. (There is a contusion over the lower right quadrant.)

11. (++) Asking the patient whether the pain radiates anywhere is essential in determining if there are any possible internal injuries and assessing the severity of the injury. (The pain is local to the area of injury.)

Section B

The current situation: Your evaluation reveals a localized injury to the patient's lower right abdominal area. The injury is not life threatening.

Your immediate responsibility: Monitor the patient's vital signs as a precaution. Begin treatment to control pain and minimize effusion.

12. (++) Applying an ice pack to the injured area would be appropriate to minimize pain and local effusion. (The patient is much more comfortable with the ice treatment.)

13. (+) Applying a compression wrap as soon as possible after the injury is appropriate to minimize pain and local effusion. (The patient reports he feels a little better with the compression wrap in place.)

14. (-) Massaging the patient's lumbar area would be unnecessary and inappropriate. (The patient questions what "rubbing his back" will do for him.)

15. (--) Massaging the contused area will be irritating and encourage further bleeding into the area. (The patient winces in pain.)

16. (+) It would be appropriate to assist the patient off the field so he can be monitored. (The patient is able to walk off the field unassisted.)

17. (0) The application of a rib belt would be inappropriate for this injury.

18. (+) It is appropriate to place the patient in a position in which he is most comfortable, preferably a position in which he is not placing pressure on the abdominals.

19. (++) It is important to monitor the patient for any changes in pain location or intensity. This will alert the athletic trainer to any deterioration in the patient's condition. (The patient has no increase in pain 30 minutes after the injury.)

20. (++) Because of the possibility of internal injury, it is prudent to monitor the patient's vital signs including his pulse and blood pressure. (The patient's vital signs remain stable 1 hour after the incident.)

Section C

The current situation: You have determined the patient has sustained a moderate contusion to his lower right abdominal area. The pain and effusion have been well controlled with your initial treatment.

Your immediate responsibility: Continue to use modalities to control the pain, monitor any changes in the patient's condition, and protect the patient from further injury.

21. (++) As long as the patient has any pain, swelling, or ecchymosis present, it is appropriate to continue to apply ice to the injured area. (The patient reports his pain is much less with the ice pack applied.)

22. (-) Because the patient is still complaining of pain, the application of moist heat packs would not be appropriate. (The patient has some increased pain and swelling over the area of injury after treatment.)

23. (--) A contusion to the abdominals is very painful and disabling to the patient. Manually muscle testing the abdominals during the early phases of treatment is inappropriate. (The patient has a difficult time rising from a supine position secondary to abdominal pain.)

24. (+) It would be appropriate to re-evaluate the injury in greater depth the next day when the patient is not in acute pain and there is more time to do so. (Your findings generally remain the same.)

25. (0) Although it is always important to keep a patient well hydrated, drinking a glass of Gatorade (PepsiCo, Chicago, IL) will not have any significant impact on the recovery of this patient. (The patient states he is not thirsty, but thanks you for your offer.)

26. (++) Protecting the injured area from further harm is appropriate and will give the patient a sense of security. (The patient is less apprehensive with the pad in place.)

27. (+) Because this can be an incapacitating injury, maintaining the patient's aerobic conditioning is critical during his recovery. Utilizing an upper body ergometer would be appropriate as long as the activity does not cause any discomfort. (The patient has no difficulty with this activity.)

PROBLEM IX

Section A

The current situation: You know that your patient has been injured as a result of a collision with another soccer player.

Your immediate responsibility: To perform your initial evaluation to determine the type and severity of the injury.

1. (+) If the patient is coherent, it is important for him to identify where there is pain. This gives the athletic trainer an idea of the severity and nature of the injury. (The patient is awake and complains of neck pain.)

2. (--) The patient should not be moved until a neck or back injury has been ruled out. (The patient is now a quadriplegic.)

3. (++) This is a quick screen to assess for possible spinal injury. (The patient can move his fingers and toes.)

4. (+) Gathering as much information as possible from those who witnessed the injury is important in understanding how the injury occurred and what the nature of the injury may be. (Another player states he saw the patient's head "snap" back.)

5. (+) As part of a primary survey, it is important to note if there is any bleeding (from a cut or from an orifice). (There is no evidence of bleeding.)

6. (0) Calling an ambulance prior to evaluating this patient's status would be premature. (The ambulance crew wastes a trip.)

7. (++) It is necessary to assess the patient's level of consciousness during the primary survey to determine if there is a life-threatening problem. (The patient is awake and alert.)

8. (++) The primary survey is an assessment of any life-threatening problems involving the patient's airway/breathing, circulation, or severe bleeding. (The patient's airway is fine and his pulse is 80.)

9. (+) If the patient is conscious and oriented, it is important to have basic knowledge concerning the patient's prior injuries, especially of the head/neck or back, to prevent potential problems even though there may not be any immediate threat to life. (The patient states he has never had a head injury.)

10. (+) The athletic trainer should make a mental note of the patient's body position in case the patient must be moved to be treated or transported. (The patient is lying in supine.)

11. (--) Asking the patient to get up and walk during an initial evaluation is not appropriate until the injury is completely assessed. (The patient stands and collapses.)

12. (+) Checking the pupillary reactions will give the athletic trainer information concerning a possible head injury. (Both pupils react normally.)

13. (0) This action would not be appropriate while performing your initial evaluation on the field. (The patient wonders why you are placing ice on his shoulder.)

14. (--) Unless the patient is in harm's way while lying on the field, he should not be moved until a complete assessment of his injuries is conducted. (The patient complains of dizziness and passes out.)

15. (+) If the patient can communicate what occurred, it is important to elicit this information to determine the mechanism and nature of his injury. (The patient remembers colliding with the other player and felt his head "hit something hard.")

16. (+) As part of your primary survey, it is imperative to monitor the patient's vital signs to detect changes in status. (All vital signs remain stable.)

17. (0) Asking a member of your support team to get a spine board at this time may be a premature action. (The patient feels okay, is moving, and asks if he is allowed to stand up.)

18. (--) The patient should not be moved until a head, neck, or back injury has been ruled out. (The patient becomes dizzy.)

Section B

The current situation: You know that the patient is conscious and coherent, his vital signs are stable, but he may have sustained a concussion and/or a neck injury.

Your immediate responsibility: Continue with a more in-depth evaluation of his neuromuscular function.

19. (++) Once the patient is on the sidelines, an assessment of his injuries may be conducted in greater detail. (He is able to move his arms but is complaining of left arm "tingling" and a slight headache. There is a small hematoma on his forehead.)

20. (++) It is appropriate to assess the patient's cognition if there is any evidence of a head injury. (The patient knows who you are, the date, place, and event.)

21. (--) Unless a significant head injury has been completely ruled out, the patient should be kept awake in order to monitor any changes in level of consciousness. (The patient becomes lethargic and difficult to arouse.)

22. (--) Aspirin has anticoagulant properties; administration of aspirin is contraindicated with a possible head injury. (The patient has an epidural hematoma and dies.)

23. (+) It would be necessary to palpate the cervical area while evaluating the patient for a possible neck or shoulder injury. (The patient complains of left upper trapezius soreness.)

24. (+) Palpating the trapezius and shoulder girdle musculature may elicit information regarding a musculoskeletal injury to the neck and shoulders. (The patient is complaining of left-sided neck soreness.)

25. (+) This action is a quick screen for the function of C7,T1. (The patient's left grip strength is weak.)

26. (+) The patient should not return to the game until a secondary survey is complete and the team physician feels confident there are no significant injuries and clears the patient to play. (A doctor has not examined the patient yet.)

27. (+) Observing the patient's "body language" will give the athletic trainer an idea of where the injury may be located. (The patient is holding his left arm.)

28. (0) Assessing the patient's skin color is not a priority at this time unless the patient is bleeding severely or the athletic trainer suspects the patient's circulation may be compromised. (The patient's skin color is normal.)

29. (-) This is not an appropriate action because it does not apply to this situation at this time. (The parents are insulted.)

30. (-) The team physician would not need to be notified of the injury at this time unless there was a life-threatening/potentially disabling injury. (The team physician is surprised you do not have the ability to assess the patient's condition.)

31. (-) Calling the patient's parents would be a premature action. (The parents panic.)

32. (0) This is not an appropriate action because it does not apply to this situation. (The patient shows no sign of shock.)

33. (-) If the patient can ambulate under his own power without difficulty, he will not need crutches. (There is no evidence of a lower extremity injury.)

Section C

The current situation: The patient's vital signs remain stable, and he appears alert and oriented. You suspect the patient may have sustained a concussion and an upper quarter injury.

Your immediate responsibility: Continue with a detailed examination of the patient to determine the severity of the injury.

34. (0) Unless there is evidence of a significant problem at this time, monitoring vital signs as frequently as every 10 minutes may or may not be necessary. (The patient's blood pressure is 120/80 and pulse is 74 and stable.)

35. (+) Manually muscle testing the upper trapezius muscle would be appropriate during your evaluation of this injury. (The patient can shrug but complains that the left side hurts.)

36. (-) Adson's test is performed when thoracic outlet syndrome is suspected; this patient has an acute injury. (Review this test and its indications.)

37. (+) Manually muscle testing the deltoids would be appropriate during your evaluation of this injury. (The patient has some difficulty abducting his left arm. Grade = 3/5.)

38. (+) Manually muscle testing the rotator cuff musculature would be appropriate during your evaluation of this injury. (The patient has some difficulty with external rotation of his left arm. Grade = +3/5.)

39. (-) If the patient has potentially injured his neck or back, this may make the injury worse. If the patient was feeling light-headed, it would be better to position him in supine with both legs elevated. (The patient now has a headache.)

40. (-) You have already determined from your sideline evaluation that there is no significant lower extremity injury. A functional movement test is not appropriate at this time. (The patient is steady while standing and walking.)

41. (0) You have already determined from your sideline evaluation that the patient is oriented. (The patient counts backward by increments of 7 without difficulty.)

42. (+) As part of an upper quarter screen, it may be necessary to check upper extremity deep tendon reflexes. (The left triceps deep tendon reflex is a little sluggish.)

43. (-) The patient is not in any respiratory distress. (The patient refuses the mask.)

44. (++) If the physician is available at this time, it would be important for him or her to evaluate the patient and determine his status for play. (The team physician will arrive in 10 minutes.)

45. (--) With a suspected head injury, it would be poor judgment on the athletic trainer's part to allow the patient to drive. (The patient gets dizzy and hits a parked car in the parking lot.)

46. (+) Checking the sensation of the upper extremities should be included in a detailed evaluation of the patient in the athletic training facility. (There is hypersensitivity in the C7,8 dermatomes.)

47. (+) Checking the range of motion of the patient's neck should be included in a detailed examination of the patient. (The patient has full cervical active range of motion.)

48. (-) A positive Tinel's sign is indicative of carpal tunnel syndrome and would be inappropriate, as this was a known traumatic event. (No information is gained from this test.)

49. (0) Palpation of the lateral epicondyle would not provide any helpful information in the evaluation of this patient. (The patient states his elbow feels fine.)

50. (+) Manually muscle testing the biceps would be appropriate during your evaluation of this injury. (The patient has some difficulty with resisted elbow flexion. Grade = +3/5.)

51. (+) Manually muscle testing the triceps would be appropriate. (The patient has significant difficulty extending his elbow against resistance. Grade = 3/5.)

Section D

The current situation: You know that your patient has sustained a concussion and a left-sided "burner."

Your immediate responsibility: Monitor the patient for any changes in his condition and protect the patient from further harm until he is cleared by the team physician to play.

52. (0) A "burner" is an injury to the nerves of the brachial plexus. An ice pack applied to the upper arm would be ineffective.

53. (++) Persistent sensory changes of the upper extremity would be significant in determining the extent of nerve involvement. (The patient states his sensation is returning to normal.)

54. (-) The patient has to be cleared by the team doctor in order to return to play. (The patient returns the next day and is reinjured.)

55. (0) This action would be at the discretion of the physician, not the athletic trainer. (You are reprimanded by your athletic director and team physician.)

56. (--) Shoulder strengthening exercises are not indicated with an acute nerve injury. (This action causes further injury to the left upper extremity.)

57. (--) This exercise would be contraindicated for an acute upper extremity nerve injury. (The patient complains of increased pain.)

58. (++) It is prudent to monitor the patient for a few days after a concussion to be sure there is no change in his status. (The patient's condition returns to normal the next day.)

59. (++) It is imperative that the physician clear the patient before he returns to full-time activity. (The patient is cleared to play the second day after the injury.)

60. (0) Giving the patient a soft neck collar will not cause further injury, but it may not help the patient either. (The patient receives a lot of attention from his teammates.)

PROBLEM X

Section A

The current situation: You know the patient has sustained a direct blow to the nose causing recurrent nose bleeds.

Your immediate responsibility: Evaluate the patient for a possible nasal/facial fracture. Stop the bleeding.

1. (+) This question is important to ask as part of the history and in understanding the severity of the problem. (The patient states he saw "stars.")

2. (+) Asking whether or not there has been a similar problem in the past is a question that should always be asked when taking a history. (He has had one episode of recurrent nosebleeds 2 years ago from a blow to the nose.)

3. (0) Whether or not the patient's parents are aware of his nosebleed is irrelevant at this time.

4. (0) Whether or not the patient has any allergies is insignificant information. (He tells you he is allergic to cats.)

5. (-) This action may increase the flow of bleeding. (The bleeding becomes copious.)

6. (+) The patient should be seated in case he becomes faint from the bleeding or pain. (The patient has no complaints of dizziness.)

7. (0) This action is not necessary in this situation.

8. (0) A noseguard should not be necessary. (This should not be a chronic problem.)

9. (--) This action is inappropriate, as heating the area will cause further bleeding. (You have difficulty stopping the bleeding.)

10. (0) It is known from the opening scenario that the origin of this nosebleed was from a blow to the nose, not from chronic high blood pressure.

11. (-) Pressure should be applied to the affected nostril, not to the cheek. (This action does nothing to slow the bleeding.)

12. (++) The athletic trainer should palpate the patient's nose and surrounding areas to be sure no other areas were injured as a result of the earlier trauma (eg, nasal fracture). (The patient reports tenderness over the bridge of his nose, but there is no crepitus with palpation or deformity.)

13. (++) Swelling with or without deformity may be indicative of a possible nasal fracture. (A small hematoma is noted over the bridge of the nose.)

14. (0) An ice pack placed behind the patient's neck will be ineffective—it should be placed over the nasal area.

15. (--) Under no circumstances should the patient blow his nose, as this will increase the bleeding. (The bleeding becomes heavy.)

16. (++) Placing a cotton plug under the patient's top lip will assist in stopping the bleeding. (The bleeding slows down considerably.)

Section B

The current situation: The patient has a nosebleed. There is no evidence of a nasal or facial fracture.

Your immediate responsibility: Stop the bleeding.

17. (-) This is an unnecessary step at this time. (It is obvious that this is not a life-threatening problem.)

18. (-) This is an inappropriate step at this time. (The patient shows no signs of shock.)

19. (++) Having the patient maintain pressure on the affected nostril will help completely stop the bleeding. (The bleeding stops.)

20. (+) It is a prudent step to take, since you will not be following this patient on a long-term basis. (The coach appreciates your assistance.)

21. (-) Most nosebleeds are a minor problem and relatively easy to control. Unless the bleeding cannot be stopped within a 5-minute period, the patient should be able to return to the competition. (The patient is furious with you for not allowing him to compete.)

22. (0) This is only necessary if it is determined that this patient has fractured his nose. (So far there is no indication of a fracture.)

23. (-) The patient should sit upright with his head in a neutral position. (The patient becomes nauseated from the taste of blood.)

24. (-) Calling the visiting team's athletic trainer during your initial treatment is not an appropriate action. (The other athletic trainer wonders why you are calling him during your treatment.)

25. (++) A cotton nose plug soaked with epinephrine hydrochloride will enhance clotting. (The bleeding stops.)

26. (--) Aspirin should never be given during active bleeding, as it is an anticoagulant. (The bleeding increases again.)

27. (++) Checking to see that no blood is present on the patient, his clothing, the mat, and floor are appropriate steps in following universal precautions. (You do a thorough job making sure the blood is cleaned up.)

Section C

The current situation: The patient has sustained a nosebleed secondary to a traumatic blow to the nose, which is beginning to resolve.

Your immediate responsibility: Stop the bleeding and return the patient to competition.

28. (-) As long as the nosebleed has been brought under control, it is not necessary to call your team doctor. (The doctor is upset you wasted time calling him.)

29. (--) It is not your place to call the visiting team's doctor regarding a minor nosebleed. (The physician thinks you are incompetent.)

30. (0) This action may only serve to unnecessarily alarm the patient and his parents and should only be initiated if the nose needs to be cauterized by a doctor. (You panic the parents.)

31. (-) There is no reason to restrict this patient's fluid intake. (The patient becomes dehydrated.)

32. (++) As long as the bleeding has completely stopped, the patient can return to competition. (He wins his match.)

33. (-) This is an unnecessary action if no swelling or deformity of the nose is evident, as the bleeding has stopped. (The team physician is upset that you suggested this.)

34. (++) It would be a responsible step to contact the patient's home athletic trainer to report the incident and what treatment was administered. (The athletic trainer appreciates your information.)

35. (--) Sit-ups temporarily increase blood pressure and capillary pressure, which may produce another spontaneous nosebleed. (The patient's nose begins bleeding again.)

36. (++) Biohazard bags should be used as a universal precaution. (The athletic director appreciates you following protocol.)

37. (+) The patient should be monitored during the competition for any further problems. (The patient has no further episodes of bleeding.)

38. (+) The patient should keep an ice pack on his nose while he is not competing to minimize pain and encourage clotting. (He reports the pain and swelling have decreased.)

Problem XI

Section A

The current situation: You know your patient has injured his left ankle.

Your immediate responsibility: To perform your initial evaluation to determine the nature and severity of the injury.

1. (-) You witnessed the injury. It is obvious that his left ankle is involved, not his back. Evaluating this patient's low back is unnecessary. (The patient thinks you are incompetent.)

2. (-) It is obvious from the information given in the opening scenario that the patient is able to bear weight on the ankle without assistance. Getting a wheelchair is inappropriate. (The patient wonders for whom you are getting a wheelchair.)

3. (0) This is an unnecessary action. It has been determined that the patient has injured his left ankle. (Now the patient definitely does not trust you.)

4. (+) It is important to make a bilateral comparison of both ankles when observing for swelling, ecchymosis, or deformity during the initial evaluation. (The left ankle is swollen on the lateral side.)

5. (--) This is an inappropriate action and may cause further injury. (The patient reinjures his ankle.)

6. (--) This is an unnecessary and inappropriate action that may cause further injury. (The pain and swelling increase.)

7. (-) Lachman's test is not a special test for the ankle. (The patient's knees are fine.)

8. (+) An anterior drawer test should be performed bilaterally to determine if there is any ankle joint instability. (There is a positive result on the left ankle.)

9. (++) Palpation is an integral portion of the initial evaluation. (There is tenderness over the anterior talofibular and calcaneofibular ligaments.)

10. (++) Checking the patient's willingness to move is an integral segment of the initial evaluation. Comparing the active range of motion of the involved joint to the uninvolved side is a necessary step in an orthopedic assessment. (The patient complains of pain with active movement into dorsiflexion and eversion.)

Section B

The current situation: The patient has a grade II inversion sprain of the left ankle with injury to the anterior talofibular and calcaneofibular ligaments.

Your immediate responsibility: To begin treating the injury to reduce the pain and swelling.

11. (++) During the acute stages of treatment, the patient should be kept in nonweightbearing or partial weightbearing to minimize pain and swelling. (There is less pain in nonweightbearing.)

12. (-) Although aspirin is an anti-inflammatory with analgesic properties, it would be contraindicated at this time because it may cause further bleeding into the joint. (The swelling increases.)

13. (++) Rest, ice, compression, and elevation are primary components of the initial treatment of an acute musculoskeletal injury. (The pain and swelling decrease.)

14. (0) Calling the team doctor at this time is unnecessary and inappropriate. (The doctor wonders why you do not know how to treat an acute ankle sprain.)

15. (--) Ultrasound is a deep-heating modality. This is a definite "no-no" during the acute stage of treatment. (The pain and swelling increase significantly.)

16. (--) As with ultrasound, a warm or hot whirlpool will only make the pain and swelling worse. (The ankle is very swollen.)

17. (+) Keeping the patient in nonweightbearing at this time is proper protocol in the immediate care of an acute injury. (The patient is able to ambulate comfortably with crutches.)

18. (0) Unless you suspect a more significant injury at this point, this action is inappropriate. (The patient has not seen a doctor.)

19. (0) The immediate care of an acute ankle sprain does not include upper body reconditioning.

20.   (+) It is the athletic trainer's duty to keep the patient's coach well informed about the patient's injury and treatment. (He appreciates your report.)

21.   (-) Resistive ankle strengthening exercises would be inappropriate at this time. (The ankle is too weak and the pain is increased with resistance.)

Section C

The current situation: You have determined the patient has sustained a grade II inversion sprain with injury to the anterior talofibular and calcaneofibular ligaments. Treatment has been initiated to reduce the pain and swelling.

Your immediate responsibility: To ensure the patient knows how to care for his injury at home.

22.   (-) Although going to the emergency room would not hurt the patient, it may not be necessary either. (The patient spends 3 hours in the emergency room to be diagnosed with a sprain.)

23.   (0) It is courteous to contact the parents if the patient is a minor, but this may be an unnecessary step. (The patient is able to follow your instructions overnight.)

24.   (--) Closed-chain exercises would be contraindicated with such an acute ankle injury. (The ankle pain increases.)

25.   (++) This is a fundamental component of treatment of an acute musculoskeletal injury. (The pain and swelling are controlled.)

26.   (+) This is a fundamental component of treatment of an acute musculoskeletal injury. (The swelling is controlled.)

27.   (0) Wearing high-top sneakers will not change the patient's condition. (Although they look "cool.")

28.   (--) Attempting to hop on an acutely injured ankle is inappropriate and will cause further injury to an already traumatized joint. (The patient falls and sprains his ankle again.)

Problem XII

Section A

The current situation: You have been made aware of a patient who may have a serious eating disorder.

Your immediate responsibility: Educate and advise the coach not to encourage her current behavior, but to emphasize the importance of proper nutritional habits and to keep the athletic training staff informed of her behavior.

1.   (--) Because anorexia nervosa is an eating disorder that is characterized by a distorted body image and is caused by a deep-seated and complex interaction of psychological and sociocultural factors, the patient must be gently confronted and not attacked. Unless the patient is in immediate danger, threatening the patient is inappropriate. (The patient is so upset she quits the team.)

2.   (+) Continual fixation on the patient's weight changes in relation to her athletic performance may encourage destructive behavior.

3.   (0) Keeping a diary of the time or place the patient eats is unnecessary. Treatment should be implemented by those qualified to do so, such as a psychologist or physician. (The coach wastes a lot of paper.)

4.   (+) Emphasizing the importance of good nutritional habits in optimizing athletic performance is an appropriate action. (The patient seems to respond in a positive manner and begins eating a small but regular breakfast.)

5.   (++) Any behaviors associated with eating disorders that become prominent must be relayed to the athletic training staff so the patient can be immediately referred for professional help. (You are able to provide the team physician with valuable information.)

Section B

The current situation: You have identified a patient who has an eating disorder and you have advised the coach how to properly handle the situation.

Your immediate responsibility: Continue to monitor the patient's behavior and educate and support the patient.

6.   (+) Providing constructive advice is an appropriate action. (The patient agrees to try to reach the set goals.)

7.   (-) Using an approach that threatens the patient in any fashion is not appropriate. (The patient feels challenged and continues to abuse laxatives anyway.)

8.   (+) Encouraging the patient to express her feelings is an important and necessary step in her recovery. (She states she feels her parents will not love her if she is not the best gymnast on the team.)

9.   (0) Addressing the issue with the athletic director is not necessary. (He tells you to discuss the matter with the team doctor.)

10.   (-) To make the assumption that the patient will be removed from the team is premature and is ultimately a decision that will be made by the coach. (The patient panics.)

11.   (--) It is not wise to make promises that you may not be able to keep. If this patient is seriously ill, the coach may cut her from the team. (The coach is debating what to do.)

12.   (-) This patient will need the support of the coaching and athletic training staff to actively seek professional counseling. (The patient does not have the self-esteem to initiate counseling on her own.)

13.   (++) The patient needs to be gently confronted with specific behaviors that the coach and athletic trainer have observed to move the patient toward recovery. (The patient admits she has a problem.)

Section C

The current situation: You have identified a patient with a significant eating disorder. The patient acknowledges she has a problem.

Your immediate responsibility: Make sure the patient is referred to a psychologist for treatment.

14. (++) The team physician needs to be aware of the problem to arrange for psychological or psychiatric treatment. (The team doctor tells you he will make a referral to a psychiatrist.)

15. (0) This is an appropriate action but should occur in conjunction with the team physician.

16. (-) Anorexia nervosa and bulimia are primarily psychological disorders. Placing the patient on a diet intended to encourage weight gain will not be enough to solve this problem. (She follows the diet for 2 days.)

17. (0) Weighing the patient will not have an impact on changing her behavior at this time.

18. (--) The athletic trainer is not qualified to arrange for this type of intervention. (The team doctor is very upset with your actions.)

19. (-) This would be an inappropriate referral for this patient. (The sports nutritionist reminds you she does not have a degree in psychology.)

20. (0) Although having the patient eat these foods would not hurt her, she is not likely to comply. She needs professional psychological treatment, so this action would not be appropriate. (This patient is a vegetarian and hates bananas.)

PROBLEM XIII

Section A

The current situation: Your patient presents to you with abdominal cramping and diarrhea of unknown origin, which has lasted 2 days.

Your immediate responsibility: To try to identify the etiology of the problem and perform an initial evaluation to determine the extent of the problem.

1. (++) It is important to evaluate what types of food and drink the patient has consumed because certain foods (such as spicy foods) may lead to dyspepsia or diarrhea. (The patient states he has not eaten any spicy foods.)

2. (+) Anxiety can contribute to gastrointestinal upset. This is an appropriate question to ask the patient during the history portion of your initial assessment. (The patient admits he is nervous.)

3. (++) This is an appropriate question to ask during the history portion of the initial evaluation because it will help to identify if the patient has an underlying gastrointestinal problem. (The patient states this frequently happens at the beginning of the season.)

4. (0) This action would be appropriate if you suspect the patient is dehydrated. (The patient complains his lips feel dry, but he is not excessively thirsty. Blood pressure is 115/70.)

5. (+) This is an appropriate action because the patient might have a fever secondary to an infection. (The patient's oral temperature is within normal limits.)

6. (0) This is an inappropriate action. It does not directly relate to the patient's condition.

7. (0) This is an unnecessary and inappropriate action. (The patient complains of "gas pain" with palpation of his abdomen.)

8. (--) Running or increased activity will only contribute to gastrointestinal upset and is an inappropriate action at this point. It will not provide any information regarding the cause of the problem. (The patient has a severe episode of diarrhea after running).

Section B

The current situation: You have determined that the patient has developed gastrointestinal upset because of precompetition anxiety.

Your immediate responsibility: Treat for abdominal cramping, diarrhea, and prevent dehydration.

9. (+) If the patient is very uncomfortable and is feeling "weak," this would be an appropriate action to take. (The patient feels better at rest.)

10. (++) This would be an appropriate action to monitor the patient for degree of dehydration. (The patient loses 3 pounds after a strenuous workout.)

11. (++) An over-the-counter antimotility medication, such as Imodium or Pepto-Bismol, may reduce the cramping and diarrhea. (The patient responds well to this and the diarrhea stops.)

12. (-) Certain vegetables may cause intestinal gas formation and would be inappropriate to add to the patient's diet at this time.

13. (--) It would be best to give the patient clear fluids. Milk may cause nausea and increased flatulence; soda and tea contain caffeine, which has a diuretic effect. (The patient becomes significantly dehydrated.)

14. (0) This would be an inappropriate action. Only one of your patients is complaining of gastrointestinal distress. (The hotel management finds out what you are doing and is outraged.)

15. (0) Although this is not necessary, drinking bottled water will not be harmful to the patient.

PROBLEM XIV

Section A

The current situation: You know your patient has injured his right knee while playing soccer, and he is only able to partially bear weight on the involved limb.

Your immediate responsibility: To perform your initial evaluation to determine the type and severity of the injury.

1. (+) Palpating the joint and the surrounding soft tissue structures is an appropriate action during the initial evaluation of the injury. (The patient is significantly tender over the anteromedial joint line and the medial retinaculum.)

2. (--) Performing a functional movement such as a deep squat is inappropriate during the initial assessment. (The patient refuses to do this.)

3. (++) Since you were not present during the actual injury, you must rely on the patient's account of what occurred to determine the mechanism of injury. (The patient reports feeling a "pop" and sharp knee pain after planting his right leg to kick the ball with his left leg.)

4. (+) It is an appropriate action to check the circulation of the injured limb distal to the injury site. (The circulation is fine.)

5. (+) This is an appropriate question to ask during the history portion of the evaluation. (The patient has told you he felt a "pop.")

6. (-) This is an inappropriate test for a knee injury. Speed's test is used to assess for the presence of bicipital tendinitis.

7. (++) Based on information given in the opening scenario and the mechanism of injury, this would be an appropriate special test to perform. (Lachman's test is positive on the right knee.)

8. (0) Although this was a traumatic incident, there was no direct insult. Crepitus would be present with a possible fracture or a chronic problem, such as patellofemoral joint disease.

9. (++) Asking the patient if he ever sustained a prior knee injury is an appropriate question during the history portion of the initial evaluation. (The patient states he had a partial anterior cruciate ligament tear of the right knee a year ago.)

10. (+) Assessing the range of motion of the knee joint would be appropriate at this time. This demonstrates the patient's willingness to move and assists in determining the level of disability. (The patient has difficulty fully flexing and extending the knee.)

11. (0) Testing the strength of the patient's hip abductors will not provide any information that will lead to determining the nature and extent of the knee injury.

12. (0) It is obvious from the opening scenario that this is a knee injury; having the patient attempt toe raises would be unnecessary and inappropriate. (The patient has difficulty doing this.)

13. (++) From the information given at the opening scenario and the mechanism of injury, performing a pivot shift test would be appropriate and should be performed bilaterally for comparison to the uninvolved extremity. (The test is inconclusive because the patient is so guarded.)

Section B

The current situation: The patient is complaining of pain along the anteromedial joint line and medial retinaculum. The patient felt a "pop" and has significant edema of the right knee. He has difficulty flexing and extending the knee and has a positive Lachman's test on the right knee.

Your immediate responsibility: Protect the knee from further injury and control the pain and swelling.

14. (+) Issuing crutches with a toe-touch weightbearing status would be an appropriate action. (The patient is more comfortable ambulating with crutches.)

15. (++) Applying ice and elevating the injured extremity are appropriate actions during the initial phases of treatment. (The pain and swelling are controlled.)

16. (++) The team physician should be contacted to evaluate the patient. (The team physician has athletic training facility hours that afternoon.)

17. (0) At this point, you realize this is not a patellofemoral joint problem. McConnell taping would be unnecessary and inappropriate. (The patient questions why you are taping his kneecap.)

18. (--) Applying heat to a swollen joint is contraindicated in the initial treatment of this injury. (The pain and swelling increase significantly.)

19. (0) Ordering a functional knee brace at this phase of treatment would be premature.

20. (-) The application of pulsed ultrasound would be an inappropriate action. (The pain and swelling increase.)

Section C

The current situation: The team physician has examined the patient and agrees with your suspicions. The MRI results are pending.

Your immediate responsibility: Instruct the patient in a home program emphasizing pain and edema reduction, early joint mobilization/range of motion, and isometric strengthening.

21. (+) It is important to restore normal joint range of motion as soon as possible. This would be an appropriate action. (The patient's range of motion improves 50% over the following week.)

22. (++) Applying ice on a routine basis during the initial stages of recovery is critical. (The pain and swelling decrease significantly.)

23. (-) The patient should remain on the crutches to protect the injured limb until the diagnosis is confirmed. (The patient's knee buckles while walking with a cane and he falls.)

24. (0) Working on the proprioception of the unaffected limb is unnecessary. (The patient's balance is fine.)

25. (++) Instructing the patient to perform early isometric exercises is an appropriate step in preventing atrophy of the musculature around the knee joint. (The patient is compliant.)

26. (0) The pain is controlled well with ice; a TENS unit is not contraindicated but is not necessary.

27. (--) The patient should be restricted from activities that may cause further injury until the diagnosis is confirmed and the patient is cleared by the doctor. (The patient reinjures his knee.)

PROBLEM XV

Section A

The current situation: A patient has requested assistance in developing a lower body strength and general conditioning program. He is currently in preseason.

Your immediate responsibility: Educate the patient about the goals of preseason training and in proper methods to develop good habits to develop lower extremity flexibility strength. Assist the patient in progressing his program and in preparing for his sport.

1. (--) An athletic trainer is not qualified to administer steroids. This is an inappropriate action. (The athletic director finds out and you lose your job.)

2. (+) A good flexibility program is a fundamental aspect of a general conditioning program. (The patient's flexibility improves.)

3. (--) Having the patient participate in such a vigorous activity is inappropriate. (The patient develops heat exhaustion.)

4. (0) There is nothing in the opening scene to indicate the patient has a respiratory problem. This is an unnecessary action.

5. (+) Adequate warm-up and cool-down periods are fundamental elements of a comprehensive fitness program. (The patient had spent little time warming up prior to your recommendations.)

6. (++) Optimal results occur from training when the patient mimics movement patterns and speeds that are similar to the activities in which he participates (eg, training a soccer player by performing short, high-intensity sprints).

7. (-) Having the patient participate in another sport during the preseason may not be wise because of the increased risk of injury just before the season begins. (The patient sprains his ankle and cannot participate for the first 2 weeks of the season.)

8. (++) Having the patient work on the strength of his lower extremities would be appropriate.

9. (-) The patient should be assisted in maintaining a well-balanced nutritional diet. Limiting the patient to 1 or 2 food groups is not appropriate. (The patient complains of feeling lethargic.)

10. (--) A regular training schedule should be maintained during the preseason period to allow for a progressive program. (Because of the many changes in the schedule during the preseason, the patient is not in an acceptable state of fitness by the beginning of the season.)

11. (--) Keeping the training schedule intense is acceptable, but often coaches prolong the workout, increasing the quantity rather than the quality of the session. (The patient becomes overly fatigued and pulls a hamstring.)

12. (++) Progressing the conditioning program gradually is an appropriate action. (The patient is at his physical peak going into the season.)

13. (+) Making sure the patient has acclimated to the heat prior to the season is appropriate. (The patient avoids episodes of heat cramps or heat exhaustion.)

Section B

The current situation: The patient has started a preseason conditioning program as per your instructions to improve his lower body strength and general conditioning. He is now in-season.

Your immediate responsibility: Continue to supervise his program to maintain a proper level of fitness that is tailored for his sport and position, and add variety to prevent staleness.

14. (+) Establishing a regular aerobic exercise routine while in-season is an appropriate action. (The patient maintains a good aerobic conditioning level.)

15. (++) Maintaining a regular strength training program throughout the season is appropriate. (The patient maintains a good strength level for his lower extremities.)

16. (--) Rest is important, but too much time off while in-season is counterproductive. (The patient starts to show signs of deconditioning.)

17. (0) This action is unnecessary unless the patient has a known or suspected cardiovascular problem.

18. (+) This is an appropriate action depending on the patient's position. (The patient is a running back.)

19. (++) Establishing a maintenance program for training while in season is necessary and appropriate. (The patient maintains a good level of aerobic and strength conditioning.)

20. (-) Putting the patient on a clear diet is inappropriate. (The patient begins to show signs of fatigue and malnutrition.)

21. (+) Cross-training during the season may serve to maintain a good fitness level and prevent staleness during training. (The patient swims 1 to 2 times per week.)

22. (0) Although this action is not harmful, it is not sport-specific and is not a necessary activity.

23. (--) This action is not necessary and is inappropriate. (The patient is thrown during a competition and is injured.)

Section C

The current situation: It is now postseason. The patient has done well thus far with the conditioning program you have designed.

Your immediate responsibility: Continue to educate the patient regarding proper flexibility and strengthening techniques. Adjust the workload so that the patient will avoid boredom and maintain a good level of fitness at a lower intensity.

24. (++) Maintaining a good flexibility program year-round is appropriate. (The patient remains injury-free during the off-season.)

25. (++) Cross-training is appropriate during the entire year but is especially effective during the off-season period to maintain proper fitness levels and prevent boredom with training. (The patient uses a rowing machine during the off-season.)

26. (--) The off-season is a period of detraining in which there is a gradual decrease of the workload. Jogging 4 to 5 days a week would be inappropriate. (The patient shows signs of overtraining and quits the team.)

27. (--) Along with a decrease in activity intensity during the off-season, there should be a decrease in the calorie intake by the patient. Having the patient consume a high-calorie diet during the off-season is inappropriate. (The patient reports to preseason practice 10 pounds overweight.)

28. (0) Having the patient learn the skill of visual imagery may enhance performance techniques but is not a necessary activity in maintaining fitness during the off-season.

29. (--) Having the patient become completely sedentary during the off-season period is inappropriate. (The patient gains 20 pounds during this time and becomes aerobically unfit).

30. (+) Allowing the patient time off from training will prevent burnout. (The patient appreciates the much-needed break.)

31. (+) Participating in another sport during the off-season will help the patient maintain a proper level of fitness. (The patient plays basketball during the off-season.)

Problem XVI

Section A

The current situation: You know your patient has suffered a serious traumatic injury after colliding with the boards.

Your immediate responsibility: To perform your initial evaluation to determine the nature and severity of the injury and assess if it is a life-threatening situation.

1. (-) Performing a secondary survey prior to doing a primary survey would be premature and inappropriate. (The patient is in respiratory distress and you have wasted valuable time.)

2. (++) If the patient is lying prone and it has been determined he is not breathing, this would be an appropriate action. (The patient is unconscious and not breathing.)

3. (--) This is an inappropriate action. The helmet should not be removed until a neck or spinal injury has been ruled out. (The patient has sustained a spinal cord injury and is now a quadriplegic.)

4. (++) Determining responsiveness and the ABCs is the immediate priority. This is an appropriate action. (The patient is unconscious and not breathing.)

5. (++) This is an appropriate action. Determining level of consciousness is part of the primary survey.

6. (--) Chest compressions should not be started unless it has been established that the patient has no pulse. (The patient has a weak carotid pulse.)

7. (0) This would be an inappropriate action. It is apparent from the opening scenario that the primary site of injury is not an extremity.

8. (-) This is an unnecessary action. It is known from the opening scenario that the patient hit the boards with his head. (You spend too much time asking questions instead of evaluating the patient.)

9. (--) This is an inappropriate action. The patient should not be moved until a neck or back injury has been ruled out.

Section B

The current situation: The patient has been carefully placed into supine and is unconscious and not breathing. He has a weak pulse.

Your immediate responsibility: Establish an airway and ventilate the patient. Activate the EMS system.

10. (-) The immediate priority is establishing an airway. Performing a secondary survey is inappropriate at this time. (The patient has now been without oxygen for 1.5 minutes.)

11. (+) This would be an appropriate action, as a true emergency has been determined. (The ambulance arrives within 5 minutes of the call.)

12. (--) This is an inappropriate action and may cause further injury to the patient.

13. (0) Although this action is appropriate, it is not a priority at this time.

14. (++) Cutting the facemask off the helmet is a necessary step to allow for CPR and artificial respiration. (You are now able to ventilate the patient.)

15. (-) This is an unnecessary and inappropriate action.

16. (-) This is an unnecessary and inappropriate action. (Romberg's sign is a test used to assess balance.)

17. (--) This is an inappropriate action. (The patient vomits, aspirates, and dies.)

18. (++) This is an appropriate action; opening the airway and ventilating the patient is a priority. (You are able to open the airway and administer mouth-to-mouth respiration.)

19. (0) This action is unnecessary as it has already been determined the patient has a pulse.

20. (+) Removing the mouthguard is necessary to clear the airway. This is an appropriate action.

21. (+) Using a jaw-thrust to open the airway is an appropriate action. (You suspect a possible spinal cord injury.)

Section C

The current situation: The patient responds to your resuscitation efforts, becomes conscious, and is able to respond to questions. He reports feelings of gross anesthesia.

Your immediate responsibility: Assess and monitor the patient's vital signs, assess the extent of loss of sensation and motor control, and document what occurred and who was involved. Prepare to transport the patient to the hospital via ambulance.

22. (++) Once the patient is conscious and breathing independently, it is a priority to perform a secondary survey. (Respiratory rate is 14 breaths per minute, blood pressure is 110/70, and pulse is 88. Gross sensation is absent from the armpits caudally, and no significant bleeding or deformities are noted.)

23. (+) Monitoring the patient's vital signs is appropriate. (You are able to give the EMS team vital information.)

24. (-) This is an inappropriate action. (You do not have enough information regarding the patient's permanent outcome.)

25. (+) This is an appropriate action. (The patient is ready to be transferred to the hospital.)

26. (0) This would be an inappropriate action at this time. (This would not be helpful at this time.)

27. (+) Checking the pupillary response is an appropriate action to determine if the patient has sustained a head injury. (Both pupils respond normally.)

28. (-) This is an inappropriate action. (The policy on helmet removal should be established before a catastrophic injury occurs.)

29. (-) This is an inappropriate action. Once the patient is transferred into the care of the emergency medical team, you are still responsible for the remaining patients. (You leave the practice area and a second patient gets injured.)

30. (+) This would be an appropriate action. (You avoid a malpractice suit.)

Section D

The current situation: Your patient has suffered a serious spinal cord injury and has been transported by the rescue squad to the hospital.

Your immediate responsibility: Provide emotional support to the patient and his teammates. Provide accurate information of what occurred to the team physician and provide support for the patient's parents.

31. (++) This would be an appropriate action. (The patient is very scared and is grateful you came.)

32. (+) This is an appropriate action. (The team doctor documents what occurred.)

33. (+) This is an appropriate action. (The parents meet you at the emergency room.)

34. (--) This is an inappropriate action. An athletic trainer is not qualified to determine the patient's prognosis. (You have given the patient false hope, and he becomes severely depressed.)

35. (0) This is an unnecessary action. (It is too late to change this now.)

36. (--) This is an inappropriate action. (You are reprimanded by the school administration.)

37. (+) This is an appropriate action. (The coach appreciates the information.)

38. (+) This is an appropriate action. (The rest of the hockey team expresses how they are feeling.)

39. (-) This is an inappropriate action. (The physician never makes the phone call and the athletic director finds out about the accident the following day from a coach.)

PROBLEM XVII

Section A

The current situation: You know from this patient's complaints that his low back pain is chronic in nature and localized to the lumbar area.

Your immediate responsibility: To perform an initial evaluation to determine the etiology of his pain.

1. (++) When assessing a low back injury, it is appropriate to observe the patient's posture in standing and sitting. (The patient stands with a forward head and rounded shoulder posture and slouches when he sits. The patient also has a slight scoliotic curve.)

2. (+) Having the patient describe his pain is appropriate, as it gives the athletic trainer information about the nature of the injury. (The patient reports the pain is a "dull ache.")

3. (0) Checking the range of motion of the patient's knees would not contribute any helpful information. This patient has a low back problem, not a knee injury.

4. (-) A Scour test of the hip is performed when the possibility of hip arthritis exists. This test would be unnecessary and inappropriate. The patient is not complaining of any hip pain.

5. (++) Palpating the lumbar erector spinae is an appropriate action and is a fundamental component of the initial assessment. (The patient reports mild muscle discomfort.)

6. (+) Although it is not likely that muscular wasting will be observed, it is appropriate to visualize the area of injury for any unusual changes, such as atrophy, swelling, or deformity. (There is no evidence of muscular atrophy.)

7. (+) Palpation of the entire lumbar and sacral regions is appropriate during the initial evaluation to check for any areas of point tenderness. (The patient is pain-free with palpation of both posterior superior iliac spine and sacroiliac joints.)

8. (0) Genu varum is a "bow-legged" deformity of the lower extremities and has no correlation to the patient's low back pain.

9. (++) Assessing the patient for a leg-length discrepancy is appropriate. Even a subtle leg-length discrepancy can cause chronic low back pain. (The patient's legs are of equal length.)

10. (0) Having the patient perform a partial squat is unnecessary and inappropriate during the initial evaluation. (Whether or not the patient can perform this action will not provide the athletic trainer with significant information concerning the nature of the problem.)

11. (++) Evaluating the range of motion of the lumbar spine will help the athletic trainer assess the patient's willingness to move and provide information concerning the nature and severity of the problem. (The patient complains of pain with lumbar flexion, right side-bending, and right rotation.)

12. (-) Evaluating the patient's hip abduction with a goniometer is not appropriate. (This patient does not have a hip injury.)

13. (+) It would be appropriate to check the flexibility of the muscles around the hip because tight hip flexors or hamstrings can contribute to chronic low back pain. (The patient has tight hamstrings bilaterally.)

Section B

The current situation: You have determined from your initial evaluation that the patient's pain is muscular in origin and he has tight bilateral hamstrings.

Your immediate responsibility: To provide immediate pain relief during rest and activity.

14. (-) Friction massage is a deep, local massage technique that is most commonly performed around joints and over thin tissue areas that are hypomobile because of scarring or local spasms. This type of massage is inappropriate for this problem. (The patient complains of significant pain during treatment.)

15. (++) The application of ice in the form of ice packs can break the pain-muscle spasm-pain cycle, allowing the patient to move more comfortably, and is an appropriate modality to use. (The patient reports pain relief during treatment.)

16. (+) Because the injury is chronic in nature and the patient is not in severe pain, moist heat in the form of a whirlpool may be useful in helping the patient relax and will reduce discomfort. (The patient reports pain relief with the heat treatments.)

17. (++) Because this is a chronic problem, ultrasound would be an appropriate modality choice. Deep heat improves circulation, which enhances healing.

18. (-) Iontophoresis is a technique in which ions of a chemical substance are delivered through the skin through use of an electrical current. The most common application is the delivery of a steroid to reduce a local inflammatory response (eg, tendinitis). Iontophoresis would not be an appropriate modality choice for this problem. (The patient complains of irritation under the active electrode.)

19. (0) Although an ice massage would not harm the patient, it would not be the optimal choice for decreasing chronic, diffuse low back pain. The application of ice massage would be more appropriate for decreasing pain in areas of point tenderness. (The patient is not pleased with you rubbing ice all over his lower back.)

20. (-) Sending the patient for chiropractic treatments would not be appropriate. It is within the athletic trainer's scope of practice to be able to comprehensively manage this patient's problem. (The chiropractor sends you a thank you note.)

21. (+) TENS therapy would be an appropriate choice of modality in managing the patient's pain. (The patient reports pain relief when the unit is used.)

22. (++) The application of moist heat packs (especially prior to exercise) would be appropriate to enhance relaxation and reduce pain. (The patient reports pain relief with moist heat treatments.)

23. (+) Short-wave diathermy would be an appropriate modality choice for treatment of chronic low back pain. Short-wave diathermy is a deep heater, which improves local circulation and enhances healing. (The patient reports feeling better after treatment.)

24. (0) Although stationary bicycling would be appropriate for aerobic conditioning, it has no direct effect regarding pain reduction of the low back or improving lumbar movement.

25. (--) Functional electric stimulation is not an appropriate modality choice in the treatment of chronic low back pain. It is primarily used for neuromuscular re-education. (The patient has more pain because of the muscular stimulation.)

26. (--) Cervical traction would not be an appropriate modality for this problem. This patient has a low back problem, not a neck injury. (Please read the opening scenario.)

27. (--) Paraffin bath would not be an appropriate modality choice for this problem. Paraffin treatments are most commonly used for hand and foot conditions. (The patient is very upset that you are pouring a very warm, waxy substance on his back.)

28. (++) Effleurage would be an appropriate action to take. This massage technique can be very effective in relaxing the patient and in encouraging improved venous and lymphatic drainage. (The patient reports significant relief of his muscular discomfort after your treatment.)

29. (+) A neoprene lumbar support would be an appropriate item to recommend to the patient to use during activity. It provides warmth and a sense of support that is effective in reducing pain with movement. (The patient reports he is able to move easier during practice.)

Section C

The current situation: The patient's low back pain is beginning to reduce with the treatment he has been receiving.

Your immediate responsibility: To instruct the patient in a series of exercises to improve his lumbar mobility and strength.

30. (-) Active trunk extensions against gravity would be inappropriate in the initial stages of rehabilitation, especially while the patient is still complaining of lumbar pain with active movement. This may aggravate his lumbar pain. (The patient is fine extending his back while standing but reports increased pain attempting this in prone.)

31. (+) Gentle active-assisted low back flexibility exercises, such as knee-to-chest exercises, are useful in the initial phases of rehabilitation to restore lumbar movement. (The patient has minimal discomfort with these exercises.)

32. (0) Resisted knee extensions will not cause further injury to the patient but are not necessary in the initial treatment of chronic low back pain. (The patient has strong hip flexors and quadriceps.)

33. (++) Stretching the hamstrings would be an appropriate action to take. Tight hamstrings can contribute to chronic low back pain. (The patient has bilateral tight hamstrings.)

34. (++) Having the patient perform active posterior pelvic tilts would be an appropriate exercise to initiate during the early phases of rehabilitation. (The patient has no difficulty or pain with this exercise.)

35. (+) Stretching the hip flexors would be appropriate if it is found during the initial evaluation that the muscles were tight. If the hip flexors are too tight, it can place a strain on the low back area. (The patient's hip flexors flexibility is within normal limits bilaterally.)

36. (+) Strengthening the muscles around the hip is important because these muscles also serve to support the pelvis and lumbar areas. This would be an appropriate exercise only if it does not cause the patient further discomfort.

37. (+) Lower trunk rotations in supine are useful in the initial phases of rehabilitation to restore lumbar movement. (The patient has no discomfort with these exercises.)

Section D

The current situation: The patient now has no complaints of low back pain during rest or activity.

Your immediate responsibility: Progress the patient's program with an emphasis on lumbar stabilization to prevent a reoccurrence of low back pain.

38. (++) PNF exercises for the trunk would be appropriate as long as the chosen exercises cause the patient no discomfort. (The patient fatigues easily.)

39. (++) Resistive abdominal strengthening would be appropriate exercises to initiate during the later stages of rehabilitation as long as the exercises cause the patient no discomfort. (The patient fatigues easily.)

40. (0) Resistive cervical strengthening would be unnecessary and inappropriate for this problem.

41. (+) Resisted prone hip extension requires activation of the lumbar musculature. This would be an appropriate exercise to perform for lumbar stabilization. (The patient has no discomfort with this but fatigues easily.)

42. (-) Achilles stretching exercises are unnecessary and not appropriate for this problem. (The patient questions why stretching his calves is important.)

43. (-) Groin stretching exercises are unnecessary and not appropriate for this problem. (The patient's groin musculature is not tight.)

44. (--) Shoulder press exercises are unnecessary and inappropriate during the rehabilitation of this problem. Loading the spine with overhead exercises could cause further harm. (The patient complains this exercise bothers his back.)

45. (0) Jogging would be appropriate to maintain aerobic conditioning but would not be the optimal choice of exercise for a patient with a low back injury. Swimming would be a safer choice if a pool is available. (The patient complains of mild lumbar discomfort with this activity but is able to jog short distances.)

46. (++) Swimming would be the optimal exercise for aerobic conditioning. (The patient has no lumbar discomfort while swimming.)

47. (++) Resisted bridging exercises are an effective exercise for lumbar stabilization and an appropriate exercise choice. (The patient has no pain with this exercise.)

48. (++) In the late stages of rehabilitation, trunk extensions against gravity are appropriate to strengthening the erector spinae. (The patient now has no complaints of lumbar discomfort but continues to fatigue easily with this exercise.)

Problem XVIII

Section A

The current situation: This patient is complaining of ear pain and itching. You suspect the patient has an ear infection.

Your immediate responsibility: Protect the patient's ear to prevent the infection from getting worse and refer the patient to a physician for treatment.

1. (--) Dispensing antibiotics is a medical task, not an athletic training task. It is illegal for an athletic trainer to dispense antibiotics. (You are brought up on charges for practicing medicine.)

2. (-) Cleaning the patient's ear with epinephrine is an inappropriate action. Inserting any foreign object into the ear canal should be avoided. Epinephrine is a vasoconstrictor and is an inappropriate chemical for the treatment of external otitis. (The patient hollers in pain during your attempt to "clean" his ear.)

3. (+) It is important that the patient is referred to the team physician as soon as possible so the patient can begin treatment. (The patient is placed on antibiotics by the team doctor.)

4. (-) Protecting the ear that has an ear infection is best accomplished by plugging it with lamb's wool that is soaked with lanolin. (The patient complains that the gauze pad is "not doing anything" and he removes it.)

5. (+) It is best to avoid having the infected ear exposed to cold wind. Wearing a hood or hat that covers the ears will help protect the ear and reduce pain. (The patient is much more comfortable when wearing a hood outside.)

6. (--) The use of a TENS unit would not be appropriate in this situation. (Even the patient knows this is wrong!)

7. (-) Because swimmer's ear is caused by an infection as a result of fluid trapped in the ear canal, the application of a moist heat pack would not be an appropriate action. (The infection gets worse.)

8. (+) It is appropriate to allow the patient to continue swimming as long as he habitually dries the affected ear with a soft towel and uses ear drops containing a 3% boric acid and alcohol solution before and after swimming.

Section B

The current situation: The patient has begun treatment by a physician.

Your immediate responsibility: Instruct the patient in methods to prevent the infection from getting worse.

9. (++) Using ear plugs while swimming to protect the infected ear is appropriate to reduce the amount of water entering the ear canal.

10. (0) Having the patient utilize a bathing cap may help decrease the amount of water entering the ear while swimming but may not be totally effective in doing so if ear plugs are not used.

11. (-) If properly managed, the patient should be able to return to swimming on a regular basis.

12. (0) Wearing goggles is unnecessary and inappropriate regarding treatment of this problem.

13. (++) Having the patient refrain from inserting any foreign objects into the ears is appropriate in protecting the patient from further injury or additional infection.

Problem XIX

Section A

The current situation: You know this patient has suffered a traumatic mouth/facial injury resulting from a blow by a hockey stick.

Your immediate responsibility: To perform an initial evaluation to determine the type and extent of the injury.

1. (++) Having the patient clear the mouth with water and cleansing the face with water will allow the athletic trainer better visualization of the injured area.

2. (-) Cleaning the patient's mouth out with a paper towel is inappropriate. (The patient is not pleased with pieces of paper sticking to her teeth and the roof of her mouth.)

3. (++) Anytime there is blood present during an injury, universal precautions must be observed.

4. (-) The patient has just received a significant blow to the mouth; wouldn't you be crying? (The patient is upset with your insensitivity.)

5. (+) It would be appropriate to check to see if the patient was wearing a mouthguard. If she was wearing it, the fit must be checked. (She states she forgot it today and was not wearing it.)

6. (-) Reviewing the school's liability insurance policy would be inappropriate. (It does not matter at this time.)

7. (+) It would be an appropriate action to observe the mouth and surrounding areas for lacerations or abrasions. (There is an abrasion on the inside of the upper lip.)

8. (+) Palpating the mouth and surrounding structures for deformity would be appropriate to check the patient for a possible facial or jaw fracture. (Although edema is present, no gross deformity is palpable.)

9. (-) Placing the patient in a cervical collar would be unnecessary and inappropriate.

10. (+) Having the patient open and close her mouth will provide the athletic trainer some information concerning the extent of the injury. (The patient is able to open and close her mouth, although it is painful.)

Section B

The current situation: Your findings indicate that the patient's inner upper lip has been abrased and there is some swelling present with a moderate amount of bleeding. There is no gross deformity of the face/jaw, and the patient is able to open and close her mouth. One of the patient's front teeth is missing.

Your immediate responsibility: Recover the tooth, if possible, and try to reposition it, if possible. Refer the patient to a dentist as soon as possible.

11. (-) Asking the officials to stop the game would be unnecessary and inappropriate. (The officials deny your request.)

12. (0) Having a athletic training student bring the patient to the school nurse would be unnecessary and inappropriate. (There is nothing the school nurse could do that you could not do.)

13. (+) Speaking with the patient's parents would be appropriate, especially since the patient is a minor. (The parents are grateful you filled them in on the situation.)

14. (-) Calling the team physician would not be appropriate. (He wonders why you need his assistance.)

15. (+) Applying ice to the injured area would be appropriate to control the patient's pain and reduce the bleeding. (Although the patient still has pain, she is more comfortable.)

16. (+) Applying a cotton plug between the lip and injured gum will help control the bleeding and decrease the swelling. (The bleeding begins to stop.)

17. (++) Placing the displaced tooth in a container of sterile saline solution would be appropriate and is an important step toward saving the tooth if it is not possible to reposition the tooth in its socket.

18. (+) The displaced tooth should be rinsed off with water to clean it of any dirt or debris.

19. (++) Sending the patient and the tooth to a dentist within 30 minutes is critical if the tooth is to be saved. (The parents immediately leave with the patient.)

20. (--) Discarding the tooth is inappropriate unless it is a known fact that the tooth is no longer alive. (The parents threaten to sue you when they find out the tooth could have been saved.)

21. (0) Having the patient lie down in a side-lying position has no bearing on this situation.

Problem XX

Section A

The current situation: You have been asked by a patient to assist him in losing weight during his off-season period.

Your immediate responsibility: Assist the patient in developing a nutritionally balanced diet and proper eating habits. Assess the patient's current condition.

1. (--) Having the patient consume a protein drink daily with one of his regular meals will not encourage weight loss and should not be used in lieu of a regular meal. (The patient gains another 7 pounds in 2 weeks.)

2. (+) Using calipers to measure the patient's percent body fat would be appropriate to obtain a baseline measurement. (The patient's body fat is 12%.)

3. (--) It is unrealistic to give the patient a cookbook and expect him to lose weight as a result of that one action. This would be an inappropriate action. (The patient admits he never even opened the book.)

4. (--) Sending the patient to an acupuncturist for this problem is not appropriate. (The patient refuses to go.)

5. (++) Having the patient record his food and drink intake in a personal log will assist the athletic trainer in adjusting the patient's diet to ensure he is eating a nutritionally sound diet. (The patient's current diet is high in fatty food and fluids high in sugar.)

6. (++) Monitoring the patient's weight once a week will help the athletic trainer modify the patient's diet accordingly and ensure the patient is losing weight at a safe pace. (The patient begins to lose weight after 3 days from initiating the new diet.)

7. (--) Having the patient fast is an inappropriate and potentially dangerous action. Fluids in particular should not be restricted. (The patient becomes significantly dehydrated and ends up at the hospital.)

8. (+) It is important that the patient consume plenty of water while losing weight to avoid dehydration. (The patient is compliant with this recommendation.)

9. (++) Weighing the patient prior to beginning his program will provide the athletic trainer with a baseline weight so weight reduction can be tracked. (The patient is overweight by 10 pounds.)

10. (--) Having the patient sit in a sauna is an inappropriate and potentially dangerous suggestion. (The patient sits in a sauna for an extended period of time and becomes significantly dehydrated.)

11. (++) Monitoring the patient's exercise program is essential in providing a comprehensive weight loss program.

12. (++) Sitting down with the patient to put together a balanced diet that he will adhere to is appropriate. Having the patient be an active participant in his own care will help to maintain compliance. (The patient is satisfied with the diet that is developed.)

13. (--) Wearing a rubber suit during activity to encourage rapid dehydration is an inappropriate and very dangerous practice. (The patient becomes severely dehydrated during a workout and collapses.)

14. (0) Although having the patient perform progressive-resistive exercises for his lower extremities certainly will cause no harm to the patient, it will serve no specific purpose in decreasing this patient's weight. (In fact, the patient's weight might increase with the increased muscle bulk.)

Section B

The current situation: You have concluded from your assessment of this patient that he is somewhat overweight and is eating a diet that is high in fat and sugar. He is compliant with your program and is beginning to show signs of success.

Your immediate responsibility: Continue to encourage the patient in maintaining good eating habits and monitor the patient on a regular basis to track his progression.

15. (+) It would be appropriate to have the patient keep a diet log so he can continue to keep track of what he eats and drinks. This will make it easier to make adjustments in his diet as necessary. (The patient thinks this is a good idea.)

16. (-) Having the coach monitor the patient's food intake is inappropriate and not practical. (The coach has enough to do just coaching the team.)

17. (++) Having the patient maintain a good level of hydration is always important. (This poses no problem.)

18. (-) Increasing the level of physical activity does not necessarily require the patient to exercise twice as long as his current exercise program requires. How the intensity and duration of the exercise program is modified will depend on the patient's current level of activity. (The patient becomes chronically fatigued.)

19. (--) The use of laxatives to lose weight is inappropriate and potentially dangerous because of their dehydrating effects. (The patient overdoses and collapses from dehydration and an electrolyte imbalance.)

20. (0) Involving a sports nutritionist is not necessary unless complicating conditions exist, such as medical problems (eg, diabetes, ulcerative colitis, etc) or the patient desires to seek help from a professional nutritionist.

21. (++) To discourage binge eating, encouraging the patient to eat numerous small meals throughout the day would be an appropriate suggestion. (The patient nibbles on fruit, crackers, and small amounts of cheese during the day.)

22. (0) Although having the patient perform progressive-resistive exercises for his upper extremities will cause him no harm, it serves no specific purpose in decreasing this patient's weight. (The patient sees no change in his weight since beginning an upper extremity strength program.)

PROBLEM XXI

Section A

The current situation: You know this patient has sustained a traumatic lower extremity injury from a hard landing.

Your immediate responsibility: To perform an initial evaluation to determine the type and extent of the injury.

1. (--) Manipulation of the limb is premature until the severity of the injury is established.

2. (++) Blood pressure is 110/78, and the pulse is 90.

3. (0) This is unnecessary at this point.

4. (-) You can see the primary deformity has occurred at the hip. Performing a Lachman's test is a premature action.

5. (0) The patient is breathing without difficulty.

6. (++) The patient tells you his right hip is "killing him."

7. (-) You have caused disruption of the blood supply to the head of the femur and injury to the sciatic nerve.

8. (+) Both extremities are grossly intact to light touch.

9. (-) Moving the patient at this time is inappropriate; you have not established the nature/severity of the injury or stabilized the patient for transport.

10. (--) The patient screams in pain.

11. (+) This would be an appropriate action.

12. (+) You rule out injuries to the neck, upper body, and left lower extremity.

13. (+) The patient states, "I don't know; I got whacked on my right side."

14. (++) You prevent additional injury to the right lower extremity.

15. (+) You do not find any areas of deformity or pain with palpation of the right knee or ankle.

Section B

The current situation: You realize from your initial findings that the patient's right hip is grossly malaligned and that there is no injury to the right knee or ankle.

Your immediate responsibility: Monitor (and treat as necessary) the patient for shock, minimize pain, and prevent further injury.

16. (0) This is not a priority at this time.
17. (++) The patient's respiratory rate is 16 breaths per second; blood pressure is 100/70, pulse rate is 94 and thready.
18. (-) Competition was stopped at the time of the injury, and the patient has not yet been removed from the field.
19. (+) You have the room you need to work without obstruction, and the patient feels less anxious without his teammates watching him.
20. (-) You have just caused a sciatic nerve injury as a result of moving the patient.
21. (-) The patient screams in pain as you try to straighten his knee.
22. (+) The pain is minimized with the application of an ice pack.
23. (-) The aspirin causes increased internal bleeding at the site of the injury.
24. (-) The patient screams in pain.
25. (-) The patient tells you that he cannot move his right leg.
26. (++) The popliteal and dorsalis pedis pulses are palpable but weak.
27. (+) This helps to prevent additional injury.

Section C

The current situation: You have stabilized the patient in anticipation of the EMS team's arrival.

Your immediate responsibility: Assist the EMS team with the transfer of the patient onto a spine board, ensure the patient's family and your athletic director are informed of the patient's status, and properly document the incident.

28. (0) The EMTs have taken care of this.
29. (-) The patient should not eat or drink anything prior to arriving at the hospital.
30. (0) The coach is needed at the venue to keep his team together. You go to the hospital after the game.
31. (+) The patient tells you he is scared and thanks you for staying with him.
32. (0) The patient has already done this.
33. (++) You assist the EMTs with the transfer and stabilization of the patient onto a spine board successfully.
34. (+) You protect yourself from a possible malpractice suit.
35. (+) The parents thank you for your care and proceed to the hospital.
36. (+) Your athletic director appreciates being kept informed.

Problem XXII

Section A

The current situation: The referee presents with a quick onset of nausea and chest discomfort with associated diaphoresis. His past medical history is unknown.

Your immediate responsibility: To perform an initial evaluation to determine the type and origin of his condition.

1.   (++) He states he was jogging up the court and suddenly has "pressure in his chest" and "just felt bad."
2.   (-) There is no such thing as an ACE.
3.   (--) You ignore obvious signs of physiologic distress and are eventually sued for negligence.
4.   (0) This is an inappropriate action at this time.
5.   (+) It would not be wise to continue the game while you are attending to an ill referee.
6.   (++) The referee's blood pressure is 130/80, and his pulse is 100 and regular.
7.   (+) The referee tells you he takes nitroglycerin for angina pectoris, Claritin for allergies, and naprosyn for knee arthritis.
8.   (--) You lose your certification, state license, and are sued for practicing medicine without a license.
9.   (-) The referee states he is dizzy and unable to stand at this time.
10. (++) The referee tells you he had a "mild heart attack" 10 years ago.
11. (+) The referee states, "I've been trying to quit…."
12. (+) The referee tells you he definitely has pain in his right shoulder area.

Section B

The current situation: You determine from your initial evaluation that the referee has a past medical history of cardiac issues and he is a smoker. Although his vital signs are stable, he is exhibiting signs/symptoms of a myocardial infarction.

Your immediate responsibility: Monitor vital signs and escalating symptoms, keep the referee calm, and activate EMS.

13. (0) The team doctor is not immediately available for assistance.
14. (++) This is an appropriate action based on your assessment of the situation.
15. (-) The referee tells you lying on his back "makes it hard to breathe."
16. (--) The referee panics and his symptoms exacerbate.
17. (--) This is an inappropriate action.
18. (0) Placing ice on the back of the referee's neck is an inappropriate action.
19. (0) Why? Having the referee cough has no purpose.

20. (+) The referee tells you that he is having a hard time "catching his breath."

21. (0) Poor capillary refill of the digits is a sign of peripheral vascular problems and is not a symptom of a myocardial infarction.

22. (+) The referee may experience anxiety and a feeling of "impending doom," so it is important to keep him calm and be supportive.

23. (++) This should be obvious; you are informed that an ambulance has been dispatched.

Section C

The current situation: The referee suddenly collapses.

Your immediate responsibility: To confirm that he is unresponsive and begin the sequence for CPR and the application of the AED.

24. (++) This is the first step in CPR.

25. (--) The referee dies as you waste time in the stands looking for assistance.

26. (++) The referee is breathing and you palpate a carotid pulse.

27. ( ) This is an inappropriate action.

28. (-) You do not need a spine board right now. CPR can be performed on the court.

29. (0) A facial droop is a sign of a stroke, not of a myocardial infarction.

30. (++) This action could save the referee's life.

31. (-) This action is inappropriate for this situation.

32. (++) This action could save the referee's life.

33. (0) This will not make the referee's condition better or worse, but it will impede your ability to perform CPR.

Section D

The current situation: The paramedics have stabilized and transported the referee to the hospital.

Your immediate responsibility: Document the incident and give a verbal report to your athletic director.

34. (--) You are severely reprimanded by your athletic director and the superintendent for giving confidential information to the media.

35. (++) It is important to document how the incident occurred and what actions you took to ensure the victim's care.

36. (+) The athletic director appreciates you keeping him updated and commends you on a job well done.

37. (-) Play resumes without you present and one of your patients gets injured. You are reprimanded by the athletic director for leaving the game unattended.

38. (+) The rest of the game is uneventful and you check on the referee's condition the next day.

PROBLEM XXIII

Section A

The current situation: Your patient presents to you with dyspnea and chest discomfort.

Your immediate responsibility: To perform an initial evaluation to determine the etiology of his condition.

1. (-) Shortness of breath is not a symptom of diabetes. The patient denies that he is a diabetic.

2. (+) The patient tells you he is asthmatic.

3. (0) Imodium is a drug used to slow peristalsis. The patient denies having any symptoms of diarrhea.

4. (-) The patient experiences increased difficulty in breathing.

5. (++) The patient acknowledges he owns an inhaler.

6. (+) You are able to keep the patient's respiratory rate at 14 breaths per second.

7. (--) This is a premature action. You have not determined the nature/severity of the problem.

Section B

The current situation: The patient reveals he is an asthmatic and owns an inhaler.

Your immediate responsibility: Make the process of breathing easier by instructing the patient to breathe through his nose and slow down his pace of activity. Monitor the patient for further symptoms at least 4 hours after his episode of EIB.

8. (++) Breathing through the nose warms and humidifies the air.

9. (0) The patient's pulse rate is 74 and regular.

10. (-) The patient is not hyperventilating.

11. (-) A short-acting inhaler works best as a pretreatment after a warm-up routine to prevent an attack for 2 to 6 hours.

12. (++) A 10- to 30-minute cool-down after vigorous activity will help to avoid thermal changes in the airways.

13. (0) The patient thanks you for the offer, but hot tea or chocolate will not help him breathe.

14. (0) The patient states he feels better if he "just walks around".

15. (+) Taking the patient out of the game is an appropriate action.

16. (++) It is important to monitor the patient after the symptoms decrease or subside because the patient may develop another bout of bronchospasm 4 to 12 hours after exercise. He has no symptoms after 5 hours of observation.

PROBLEM XXIV

Section A

The current situation: Your patient presents to you with low back pain and radiating symptoms down his right leg after a weight-lifting session.

Your immediate responsibility: To perform an initial evaluation to determine the type and severity of the injury.

1. (-) There is no reason to use iontophoresis when the nature/severity of the injury has yet to be determined.
2. (-) The initial evaluation should be completed before any modality is used.
3. (++) Palpation of the injured area is a vital step in the evaluative process. The patient tells you the right side of his lower back and right sacroiliac joint are sore.
4. (++) A right lateral shift is observed.
5. (0) The patient tells you his knees feel fine.
6. (++) The patient has a positive Slump test.
7. (+) The patient states that he has pain down the back of his right leg to just below the knee joint.
8. (+) The patient states he had similar pain 2 years ago after helping a friend move into his apartment.
9. (0) The patient reports the massage feels great but it has not changed his leg pain.
10. (-) The patient replies he now feels sharp pain in his right calf.

Section B

The current situation: The pain is significantly increased with forward flexion and his pain is radiating to the L5-S1 dermatome.

Your immediate responsibility: Decrease the radicular pain with prone press-ups and pain modalities.

11. (++) The patient reports his pain is now out of his calf and thigh and is concentrated in his right buttock.
12. (-) The patient reports his pain has intensified to the back of his right knee.
13. (0) The patient reports the tape has not changed his pain level.
14. (--) Administration of a medication without the direction of a physician is beyond the scope of practice for an athletic trainer.
15. (--) It is the physician's decision whether or not an MRI is ordered.
16. (-) The patient loses confidence in your skills to evaluate his condition.
17. (++) The patient reports the pain has moved from his leg to his right buttock.

18. (+) The patient reports good relief of low back pain with the ice.

Section C

The current situation: The patient is responding favorably to the prone press-ups and pain modalities.

Your immediate responsibility: Instruct the patient in proper body mechanics while lifting and make sure the patient continues to perform lumbar extension exercises to counteract any forward flexion he performs during the day (ie, sitting or lifting).

19. (0) The patient is able to side bend with greater ease, but it does not affect his pain intensity or location.
20. (+) The patient agrees not to lift any heavy objects at this time.
21. (++) You observe the patient bending at the knees as he picks up his sweatshirt off the floor.
22. (+) The patient has decreased spasm of the lumbar area as he moves.
23. (-) NSAIDs may ease the immediate discomfort but do not eliminate the underlying problem involving the intervertebral disc.
24. (--) The patient bends over to tie his sneakers and winces in pain.
25. (-) The patient experiences peripheralization of his pain.
26. (+) The patient's low back pain is reduced.

PROBLEM XXV

Section A

The current situation: A patient presents to you with changes in cognition, skin temperature, texture, and color after running for a prolonged period of time.

Your immediate responsibility: To perform your initial evaluation to determine the etiology of his condition.

1. (--) You are sued for practicing medicine without a license.
2. (+) The patient replies "nothing."
3. (++) The patient's core temperature is 102°F.
4. (++) The patient's blood pressure is 90/60, and his pulse rate is 122.
5. (0) The patient has no cranial nerve dysfunction.
6. (0) The patient does not have a deep vein thrombosis.
7. (0) The patient's capillary refill is fine.
8. (+) The patient is oriented to self, time, and place.

Section B

The current situation: You determine from your evaluation that the patient is suffering from symptoms of heat exhaustion.

Your immediate responsibility: Monitor and treat for shock, reduce the patient's core temperature as soon as possible, rehydrate him, and instruct him on the signs and prevention of heat illness.

9. (-) The patient has no symptoms of hyperventilation.
10. (++) It is imperative to get the patient's core body temperature reduced as soon as possible.
11. (++) You are able to prevent symptoms of shock.
12. (0) The patient is indifferent to your attempt to relax him.
13. (--) The patient becomes completely disoriented, his temperature rises, and his blood pressure falls.
14. (+) The patient's vital signs begin to stabilize as his core temperature returns to normal and he is rehydrated.
15. (--) There is no decrease in the patient's core temperature.
16. (++) The patient's core temperature returns to normal.
17. (+) The patient thanks you and follows your recommendations.

PROBLEM XXVI

Section A

The current situation: You know this patient has sustained a blunt trauma injury to the right side of her chest.

Your immediate responsibility: To perform an initial evaluation to determine the severity of the injury.

1. (+) The patient's skin color/lips appear normal.
2. (--) The patient loses consciousness.
3. (0) The patient is obviously able to move her extremities.
4. (--) The patient experiences respiratory distress.
5. (++) The patient is breathing, and the pulse rate is 90 BPS.
6. (--) The patient screams in pain as she tries to elevate her right arm.
7. (-) You have determined there is no neck injury.
8. (+) You notice the patient coughing up small amounts of frank blood.
9. (++) The patient winces from pain as you palpate the right lower ribs, and you feel some crepitus.

Section B

The current situation: You find the patient's vital signs are stable, but you suspect a rib injury with a possible lung injury as a result of blunt chest trauma.

Your immediate responsibility: Monitor vital signs, splint the chest area to make inspiration easier, keep the patient calm, and activate EMS. Follow-up with the team physician and document the incident.

10. (++) The patient's respiratory rate is 18 breaths per minute and is shallow.
11. (++) The patient's vital signs remain stable.
12. (--) The bandage is too constrictive and limits the patient's ability to breathe freely.
13. (0) The patient asks you what that "cold stuff" is.
14. (++) The patient reports she feels much more comfortable.
15. (+) You notice an indentation over the eighth rib.
16. (--) The patient screams in pain.
17. (0) The patient does not have thoracic outlet syndrome.
18. (0) The patient does not have carpal tunnel syndrome.
19. (+) An ambulance has been dispatched.
20. (++) The patient is able to breathe easier.
21. (++) You contact the team physician as soon as the game is over.

PROBLEM XXVII

Section A

The current situation: Your patient presents with a change in level of cognition and you are aware that he is diabetic.

Your immediate responsibility: Perform an initial evaluation to determine the extent of his condition.

1. (0) The patient is breathing with difficulty.
2. (+) The patient is profusely diaphoretic.
3. (+) The patient's pulse rate is 74 BPS.
4. (++) The patient tells you he injected himself with regular insulin at 7:00 AM this morning right after breakfast.
5. (0) The patient's face appears to be fine.
6. (0) There are no signs of cranial nerve involvement.
7. (0) The Romberg's test is not indicated for this problem.
8. (--) The patient is highly insulted by your suggestion of drug abuse, and you miss signs of the patient's problem.
9. (+) The patient does not have fruity smelling breath.

Section B

The current situation: Based on your initial findings, you determine the patient has become hypoglycemic secondary to increased activity.

Your immediate responsibility: Monitor vital signs and administer a mixture of sugar and juice to increase the blood glucose levels.

10. (--) The patient goes into a coma and dies.
11. (0) Lack of protein is not this patient's problem.
12. (0) There is no change in the patient's condition.
13. (+) The patient's vital signs are stable.
14. (++) The patient responds quickly and feels much better. He is alert and asks, "What happened?"
15. (0) There is no change in the patient's status.
16. (0) The patient recovers minimally.

Section C

The current situation: The patient has fully recovered from the hypoglycemic event.

Your immediate responsibility: Instruct the patient in the prevention of hypoglycemia during exercise.

17. (++) The patient reports he "forgot" to eat some fruit and crackers before coming to the athletic training facility.
18. (--) The patient goes into insulin shock as a result of injecting himself prior to his rehabilitation session.
19. (+) The patient has no problem during his events.
20. (+) The patient tells you he has hard candy in his duffle bag.
21. (0) Do they have diabetic support groups?

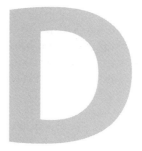

Answer Key
Critical Thinking

NEUROLOGY
(DIFFERENTIAL DIAGNOSIS)

1. Answer: I, A

    The most likely diagnosis for this scenario is Parkinson's disease. Parkinson's disease is a degenerative disorder of the basal ganglia. The cardinal manifestations of this disease are intentional tremors, rigidity, and bradykinesia. Advanced stage Parkinson's signs include fluctuations in motor function, falls, neuropsychic disorders, and sleep disturbances.

    This disease must be differentiated from multiple sclerosis, which is a neurodegenerative, chronic disease primarily affecting young adults. Myelin cells in the brain are destroyed and replaced by hard sclerotic tissue, causing gradual accumulation of focal plaques of demyelination in the brain. It is manifested by vague, insidious signs and symptoms including generalized fatigue, optic neuritis, numbness and tingling of the extremities, coordination/balance deficits, and changes in mental status (eg, memory loss or difficulty concentrating).

2. Answer: H, K

    The most likely diagnosis for this scenario is hemorrhagic stroke. The manifestations of acute stroke will vary depending on the specific cerebral artery that is affected, by the area of the brain tissue that is supplied by that particular artery, and by the amount of collateral circulation that is available. The symptoms of a

stroke or transient ischemic attack are always sudden, focal, and are usually one sided.

A brain tumor or neoplasm is an overgrowth of cells that serve no purpose. If they are malignant, they often metastasize from the breast, lung, or colon but can also arise directly from the meninges, glial tissue of the brain, cranial nerves, or cells living in the ventricles. The symptoms of a brain tumor depend on the size and location of the lesion. As a result, the neurological disturbances can vary greatly. Headache is a common initial manifestation because of the increased volume within the cranial cavity.

3. Answer: D, A, L

    The most likely diagnosis for this scenario is Guillain-Barré syndrome. Guillain-Barré syndrome is an acquired demyelinating polyneuropathy. This disorder is characterized by progressive, ascending muscle weakness of the limbs producing a symmetric flaccid paralysis. Paresthesias and numbness of the extremities may accompany the motor loss ("glove and stocking" paresthesias). Cognitive function is maintained, but the individual may experience difficulty speaking. Paralysis may rapidly progress to the respiratory muscles and therefore this condition is considered a medical emergency. Thirty percent of those afflicted with Guillain-Barré need the assistance of a ventilator at some point of their care. Eighty to 90% of those with Guillain-Barré experience a spontaneous recovery.

    See Answer #1 regarding the signs and symptoms of multiple sclerosis.

Van Ost L, Lew Feirman K, Manfré K. *Athletic Training Exam Review: A Student Guide to Success, Sixth Edition* (pp 255-261). © 2017 SLACK Incorporated.

Amyotrophic lateral sclerosis affects both the cortical and cranial/spinal motor neurons, which leads to weakness and eventual flaccid paralysis of the muscles of the body. Death usually results from respiratory failure, often complicated by a secondary pulmonary infection. ALS is also known as *Lou Gehrig disease.*

4.   Answer: C, A

The most likely diagnosis for this scenario is myasthenia gravis. Myasthenia gravis is an autoimmune disorder of the neuromuscular junction and is characterized by ptosis, diplopia, muscle fatigue, dysarthria, dyspnea, and dysphagia. There is no known cure for this disease. See Answer #1 regarding the signs and symptoms of multiple sclerosis.

RESPIRATORY
(DIFFERENTIAL DIAGNOSIS)

1.   Answer: C, B

The most likely diagnosis for this scenario is asthma. Asthma is an abnormal autonomic regulation of the bronchial muscles. It causes bronchospasm, partial airway obstruction, chronic brachial inflammation, and edema. Manifestations of this disease are wheezing upon inspiration, panting speech, coughing, hyperpnea, and cyanosis. Bronchospasm can be triggered by allergens, cold or dry air, drugs, and emotional stress. See Answer #2 for the signs and symptoms of chronic bronchitis.

2.   Answer: B, A

The most likely diagnosis for this scenario is chronic bronchitis. Chronic obstructive bronchitis is characterized by excessive bronchial secretions and airway obstruction, which causes an imbalance of ventilation and profusion. As a result, these patients are unable to maintain normal blood gas levels by increasing their ventilation rate and become hypoxic and cyanotic. They are commonly referred to as "blue bloaters." Over a period of time, they may develop pulmonary hypertension and cor pulmonale.

This must be differentiated from emphysema, which is a disease characterized by the destruction of the alveolar structures of the lungs resulting in large, cystic air spaces with diminished capillary beds and narrowed bronchioles. The destructive process usually begins in the upper lobes and progresses throughout all the lobes of both lungs. It is often accompanied by chronic bronchitis and results in severe dyspnea and generalized cyanosis secondary to poor gaseous perfusion. Cigarette smoking and air pollution are thought to be the primary causes of this disease.

3.   Answer: I, D

The most likely diagnosis for this scenario is upper respiratory tract infection. An upper respiratory tract infection, otherwise known as the common cold, is viral in nature and runs a self-limiting course. The hallmark signs of an upper respiratory tract infection include rhinorrhea, nasal congestion, and a sore throat. Other symptoms may include a nonproductive cough, headache, coughing, and sneezing. Fever is uncommon in the adult.

Rhinosinusitis is an inflammatory condition of the paranasal sinuses and the associated nasal passages. It stems from the impairment of mucociliary flow within the paranasal sinuses secondary to obstruction related to inflammation or anatomic narrowing. It is usually preceded by a viral upper respiratory tract infection, acute allergic reaction, or dental/facial trauma. Signs and symptoms not only include purulent rhinorrhea, fever, and nasal congestion, but facial discomfort and an impaired sense of smell.

4.   Answer: E, I, D

The most likely diagnosis for this scenario is viral influenza pneumonia. Influenza A is the primary type that affects the adult population; influenza B causes mild influenza in both children and adults. Influenza usually occurs in the winter and is spread by droplet infection. Mild influenza usually resolves in a couple of days without complication, but severe influenza A in adults can be fatal.

See Answer #3 regarding the signs and symptoms of upper respiratory tract infection and rhinosinusitis.

CARDIOVASCULAR
(EVALUATIVE TESTS)

1.   Answer: B, A, H

The most likely diagnosis for this scenario is angina pectoris. Angina is usually described as heavy chest pressure with a squeezing or burning characteristic and is associated with heavy breathing. The pain can radiate to the jaw, left shoulder, arm, or neck. Stable angina builds over several minutes of physical exercise or psychological stress and it subsides with a few minutes of rest. Angina is the result of a mismatch of myocardial oxygen supply and demand secondary to atherosclerotic coronary artery disease. The 3 most appropriate diagnostic tests for angina pectoris are electrocardiography, echocardiography, and cardiac stress testing.

2. Answer: A, B

The most likely diagnosis for this scenario is mitral valve prolapse. Mitral valve prolapse is a very common valve disorder. It is caused by deformed mitral valve flaps that flip back into the aorta during ventricular systole causing a backflow of blood. Diagnostic testing for this condition includes echocardiography and electrocardiography to image the defect and detect any arrhythmias.

3. Answer: I, C

The most likely diagnosis for this scenario is deep vein thrombosis (DVT). DVT results from blood pooling in large veins resulting in a thrombus. This may occur as a consequence of immobilization or prolonged bed rest. The most appropriate diagnostic tests for DVT include venography and ultrasonography.

4. Answer: J, H, C, F

The most likely diagnosis for this scenario is peripheral arterial disease (PAD). PAD is atherosclerosis of the peripheral artery tree. Although it can manifest itself in any artery or arteriole of the body (with the exception of those found in the heart, lungs, and brain), it is most commonly diagnosed in the lower extremities. The prevalence of PAD increases after the age of 50 and is a common finding in diabetic individuals. The most appropriate diagnostic testing for PAD includes arterial Doppler studies, stress testing, ultrasound testing, and CT scans.

ORTHOPEDIC (DIFFERENTIAL DIAGNOSIS)

1. Answer: C, A

The most likely diagnosis for this scenario is lumbar herniated nucleus propulsus. Hallmark signs and symptoms of a herniated nucleus propulsus of the lumbar vertebral disc include radicular pain of the lower extremity, localized lumbar muscle spasms, a positive Valsalva's maneuver, a positive straight leg raise, and Slump test. Deep tendon reflexes may be diminished on the affected limb with concurrent muscular weakness.

See Answer #3 regarding the signs and symptoms of lumbar degenerative joint disease.

2. Answer: L, J

The most likely diagnosis for this scenario is Legg-Calvé-Perthes disease. Legg-Calvé-Perthes disease is an osteonecrotic disease of the proximal femoral epiphysis. It is also known as *coxa plana*. It usually occurs in children between the ages of 4 and 9 and is more commonly found in White males. Although it can be associated with an acute traumatic event, it usually has an insidious onset and occurs in otherwise healthy children. There is no known cause for the disease, but malnutrition is a possible factor. In the majority of cases, only one limb is affected, but it can occur in both lower extremities. Treatment includes the use of abduction braces to decrease the weightbearing load and maintain proper positioning of the femoral head and surgery to minimize the deformity of the articular surfaces of the bone.

The presentation of a slipped capital femoral epiphysis differs from Legg-Calvé-Perthes disease in that it usually occurs between the ages of 10 and 15 in a 2:1 ratio of male to female occurrence. There is an acute onset of pain primarily at the knee and the child will demonstrate an antalgic gait pattern. It is often misdiagnosed as knee pathology. The affected lower extremity may be in externally rotated with ambulation as a result of limited hip internal rotation. The cause of this disease is unknown, but it is suspected that is it related to an abnormal weakening of the femur, possibly as a result of pituitary dysfunction or endocrine abnormalities. Diagnosis is confirmed by x-ray.

3. Answer: E, A

The most likely diagnosis for this scenario is hip joint osteoarthritis. Hip osteoarthritis is most common in older adult males and is characterized by an insidious onset of groin or medial thigh pain that may radiate to the buttocks or knee. The lower extremity may be held in a guarded position and there is significant limitation in joint motion. A positive Patrick's sign or scouring test are indicative of hip osteoarthritis.

Hallmark signs and symptoms of lumbar degenerative joint disease include localized low back pain, spasm and stiffness, decreased lumbar range of motion, and radicular pain to the posterior thigh. Active lumbar extension may aggravate the pain, while lying supine with the knees flexed may alleviate lumbar discomfort. The Slump test will be negative.

4. Answer: M, N

The most likely diagnosis for this scenario is osteomyelitis. Osteomyelitis is an acute or chronic pyogenic bone infection. The infection can either be caused by a contamination of an open fracture or wound or through seeding of the bloodstream. It may also occur in patients with vascular disease secondary to a skin infection. *Staphylococcus aureus* is the bacterial organism most often responsible for osteomyelitis. Iatrogenic bone infections are those that occur as a result of surgery or other treatment. These infections include pin tract infection, septic joints after joint replacement, or a wound infection. Treatment includes the use of antibiotics and surgical intervention if indicated.

Osteonecrosis is the death of a segment of a bone resulting from ischemia, the interruption of blood supply to the marrow, medullary bone, or cortex. It most commonly occurs in the proximal femur, distal femur, and proximal humerus. Osteonecrosis can result from prolonged steroid therapy, hip trauma or surgery, prolonged alcohol abuse, sickle-cell anemia, or as a complicating factor of Legg-Calvé-Perthes disease or a slipped capital epiphysis.

GYNECOLOGY (EVALUATIVE TESTS)

1. Answer: A, B, E
    The appropriate diagnostic tests for this scenario are mammography, needle biopsy, and ultrasonography. Mammography is useful in giving a clinically suspect area definition, but women with increased breast tissue density secondary to fibrocystic disease may require ultrasonography to clarify an inconclusive test. Fine needle aspiration can identify the presence of malignant cells but cannot differentiate types of cancers. Stereotactic needle biopsy uses a large-bore needle to remove a small tissue sample from the tumor. Cells are histologically evaluated with 96% accuracy in detecting cancer.

2. Answer: C, K
    The appropriate diagnostic tests for this scenario are a complete blood count and laparoscopy. Pelvic inflammatory disease (PID) is a bacterial infection of the upper reproductive tract that includes the uterus, fallopian tubes, or the ovaries. Risk factors for PID include an age between 16 and 24, being single or having a history of multiple sexual partners, nulliparity, and previous history of PID. Fever of > 101°F, an increased erythrocyte sedimentation rate, and an elevated white blood cell count may be seen in women with PID, although the woman may not appear to be ill. Laparoscopy is still considered the gold standard for diagnosis of PID.

3. Answer: K, E
    The appropriate diagnostic tests for this scenario are laparoscopy and ultrasonography. Endometriosis is a condition in which endometrial tissue is found in ectopic sites outside the uterus. These areas may include the ovaries, bladder, colon, vagina, vulva, perineum, intestines, or along the pelvic ligaments. Endometriosis may mimic other pelvic disorders and the symptoms do not always correlate with the severity of the disease. Ultrasonography and MRI are helpful in evaluating endometriosis, but laparoscopy is the gold standard for diagnosis of endometriosis.

4. Answer: M
    The appropriate diagnostic test for this scenario is a microscopic examination of the vaginal discharge. Vaginitis is an inflammation of the vagina, which may be caused by a bacterial infection or chemical irritants.

GASTROINTESTINAL (TREATMENT)

1. Answer: J, I, K, F, C
    The appropriate pharmacological agents used to treat hemorrhoids are corticosteroids to decrease inflammation, topical anesthetics to control pain, protectants for the skin, and stool softeners and laxatives to decrease rectal pressure.

2. Answer: D, C, F
    The appropriate pharmacological agents used to treat irritable bowel syndrome (IBS) are antidiarrheals, laxatives, and stool softeners. The use of either the antidiarrheals or laxatives depends on the individual's immediate symptomology. IBS is a functional gastrointestinal disorder characterized by a combination of chronic, recurrent intestinal symptoms that cannot be explained by abnormalities of the visceral structure or biochemistry.

3. Answer: G, H, E
    The appropriate pharmacological agents used to treat gastroesophageal reflux disease (GERD) include an H2-receptor antagonist to suppress gastric acid release, proton pump inhibitors, and antacids. GERD refers to the backward movement of the gastric contents into the esophagus, which causes heartburn. It is thought to be caused by a weak lower esophageal sphincter.

4. Answer: A, G, H, E
    The appropriate pharmacological agents used to treat peptic ulcer disease include antibiotics, H2-receptor antagonists, proton pump inhibitors, and antacids. Peptic ulcer disease describes a group of ulcerative disorders that occur in areas of the upper gastrointestinal tract exposed to acid secretions. The most common peptic ulcers are duodenal and gastric ulcers, which are most commonly caused by *Helicobacter pylori* infection. The second most common cause of peptic ulcer is NSAID or aspirin use.

DERMATOLOGY
(DIFFERENTIAL DIAGNOSIS)

1. Answer: A, J
    The most likely diagnosis for this scenario is impetigo. Impetigo is a superficial bacterial infection caused by staphylococci, group A beta-hemolytic streptococci, or a combination of both organisms. It is a highly contagious skin disease and is treated with a regimen of antibiotics.
    Herpes simplex virus may be categorized as type I or type II. Type I usually affects the oropharynx, whereas type II also causes genital herpes. Recurrent type I lesions usually begin with a burning or tingling sensation of the lips or around the borders of the mouth or nose. Vesicles and erythema occur in a day or 2 followed by the formation of pustules, ulcers, and crusting before healing occurs. It is a contagious virus that can be transmitted to others when the lesion is active. Healing occurs spontaneously in 10 to 14 days.

2. Answer: D, C
    The most likely diagnosis for this scenario is eczema. Atopic eczema is a common skin disorder associated with hypersensitivity reaction. There is usually a history of asthma or allergies. Treatment includes control of the offending allergens, basic skin hygiene, and medications to control itching, such as a topical corticosteroid.
    Psoriasis is an autoimmune disease that occurs most commonly in the fourth decade of life or later. It is characterized by circumcised, red, thickened plaques with overlying silver-white scales. It is a chronic disease that is exacerbated intermittently for no reason at all and persists throughout life. There is no known cure.

3. Answer: L, K
    The most likely diagnosis for this scenario is tinea pedis, or athlete's foot. It is the most common fungal infection of the skin and is usually found between the toes, on the sole of the foot, or on the sides of the feet. It is treated with proper foot hygiene and either a topical or oral antifungal medication.
    Tinea corporis (tinea of the body) primarily involves the upper extremities and trunk. It is manifested by lesions that are ring-shaped, reddish vesicles that are scaly or crusted. It is also treated with topical or oral antifungal medications.

4. Answer: J, A
    The most likely diagnosis for this scenario is herpes simplex, which is caused by the type I herpes virus. Genital herpes is usually caused by the type II herpes

virus. There is no known cause for oropharyngeal herpes simplex; most treatments are palliative.
See Answer #1 regarding the signs and symptoms of impetigo.

ORTHOPEDIC (EVALUATIVE TESTS)

1. Answer: M, A, B, D, E, H
    The most appropriate diagnostic tests for Ewing's sarcoma include a bone biopsy, MRI, bone scan, chest x-ray, CT scan, and a complete blood count. Ewing's sarcoma is the second most common type of primary bone tumor in children and adolescents. It is seen most during the early teenage years. The most frequent site of occurrence is at the diaphysis of the femur. Signs of this type of tumor include pain, range of motion limitations, and tenderness to palpation over the involved bone and soft tissue. It is treated with a combination of chemotherapy, radiation, and surgery.

2. Answer: J, A
    The most appropriate diagnostic tests for a suspected meniscus tear of the knee joint include conventional x-rays and MRI.

3. Answer: K, H, B, E, A, L, M
    The most appropriate diagnostic tests for osteomyelitis include a blood culture, complete blood count, bone and CT scans, MRI, nuclear imaging, and a bone biopsy.

4. Answer: J
    The most appropriate diagnostic test for a suspected fracture is conventional x-ray.

MUSCULOSKELETAL (TREATMENT)

1. Answer: B, C, A, E, F
    The most appropriate modalities that apply to this condition are the use of phonophoresis or iontophoresis to decrease inflammation, ultrasound (during the subacute phase) to promote healing, and electric muscle stimulation and ice packs to decrease pain and inflammation.

2. Answer: G, A, D, L, F
    The most appropriate modalities that apply to this condition are the use of moist heat packs, ultrasound, TENS, massage, and ice packs to decrease pain and muscular spasm.

3. Answer: J, I
    The most appropriate modalities that apply to this condition are the use of the paraffin bath and warm whirlpool to decrease pain. Modalities utilizing heat tend to make arthritic joints more comfortable.

4. Answer: H, F, G
    The most appropriate modalities that apply to this condition are the use of mechanical traction to decompress the nerve and ice and moist heat packs to decrease muscular pain and spasm.

VISCERAL (SIGNS AND SYMPTOMS)

1. Answer: A, B, C
    The signs and symptoms that correlate with a spontaneous pneumothorax are cyanosis, dyspnea, and a deviated trachea.

2. Answer: H, I, J, L, R
    The signs and symptoms that correlate with acute appendicitis include a low-grade fever, abdominal rigidity, rebound pain, nausea/vomiting, and an increased white blood cell count.

3. Answer: G, H, I, L, U
    The signs and symptoms that correlate with gastroenteritis include diarrhea, low-grade fever, abdominal rigidity, nausea/vomiting, and anorexia.

4. Answer: I, J, K, L
    The signs and symptoms that correlate with a spleen injury include abdominal rigidity, rebound pain, Kehr's sign, and nausea/vomiting.

PSYCHOLOGY (DIFFERENTIAL DIAGNOSIS)

1. Answer: A, C
    This athlete is primarily displaying denial. Denial is the first stage of Kübler-Ross' stages of grieving where the individual refuses to acknowledge that the event has occurred ("This cannot be happening to me!"). Bargaining is the second stage of Kübler-Ross' stages of grieving in which the athlete tries to make a promise or a deal with someone to allow him to play.

2. Answer: B, E
    This young gymnast is experiencing depression. Depression may set in once there is the realization that the injury is significant. In an attempt to accept or cope with the injury, she behaves as though she is no longer interested in gymnastics. Dissociation is an effort to separate oneself from a hurtful part/incident in his or her life.

3. Answer: G, H
    This pitcher is displaying classic signs of anger. He is frustrated with the realization that he cannot return to play and is acting out. He cannot accept that he has been replaced on the mound and demonstrates signs of regression, which is child-like behavior.

4. Answer: F, K
    This volleyball player was lacking commitment and a desire to be an active participant in her rehabilitation because she had yet to fully accept her condition. Once she was able to accept her current status, she was able to move forward and rehabilitate her shoulder. Passive aggression is the demonstration of anger through avoidance, stubbornness, sullenness, or intentional inefficiency.

5. Answer: L, F
    This athlete has compensated for his loss by becoming involved in coaching, which allows him to be a part of the game without being an active player. He is using a compensatory coping mechanism to work toward acceptance of his loss.

DOCUMENTATION/ MANAGEMENT STRATEGIES

1. Answer: H, G
    The billing processes used by allied health care professionals are ICD-10 and CPT codes. These are universal codes that aim to allow consistency in charting and billing for medical diagnoses. The ICD code is an abbreviation for the International Statistical Classification of Diseases and Health Related Problems. It provides codes that classify diseases and injuries along with their signs, symptoms, and causes. The ICD is used worldwide for morbidity and mortality statistics, reimbursement systems, and decision making in medicine. CPT, Current Procedural Terminology, is a coding system that allows for standardization of the language used in third-party reimbursement.

2. Answer: A, B

   SOAP notes are a standard method of recording subjective, objective, and assessment of an injury and the plan of action that the health care provider is going to take in response to the information he or she has received. Focus charting is a medical record that reflects the athlete's subjective complaints, the health care practitioner's actions to that complaint, and the athlete's response to that action. The observation of the shoulder deformity that the athletic trainer sees would be recorded in the objective section of the SOAP note.

3. Answer: E, N

   The WOTS UP analysis is a data collection and assessment technique aimed at examining the weaknesses, opportunities, threats, and strengths of an organization in order to facilitate planning. A market analysis is a written description of a business. Competitive advantages, analysis of the competition, pricing structure, and marketing planning are all components of the analysis.

4. Answer: B, C

   Focus charting and charting by exception are 2 methods of documentation that can be used for athletic-related injuries and illnesses. The format supports outcome-based care. Charting by exception uses the norm of expected responses for a specific injury or illness and only documents deviations from the norm. This type of documentation is less time consuming when recording treatments, but is inappropriate for initial injury evaluation.

5. Answer: P, O

   A computer resources needs assessment analysis must be performed to determine if a computerized system is appropriate. A cost-benefit analysis should follow to decide which types of hardware and software will best suit the department.

6. Answer: I, J

   The HCFA 1500 claim form is an insurance form used by private practice clinics and is widely accepted by most third-party payers. A UB-92 (or HCFA 1450) is a similar claim form that is used by hospitals for reimbursement.

BUDGETING

1. Answer: D, G

   The lump-sum budget allocates a specific amount of money for the program. This type of budget model allows the individual responsible for the budget to utilize the money as he or she deems necessary. In the spending ceiling model, justification is only required if the costs exceed the previous budget cycle.

2. Answer: A, E

   A fixed budget model is one in which expenditures and revenues are projected on a monthly basis. The goal of this type of budget is to be able to estimate monthly cash flow of a clinic. Line-item budgeting allocates a fixed amount of money for each subfunction of a program.

3. Answer: E, F

   A line-item budget allocates a specific amount of funding for each subfunction or budget unit of a program. A zero-based budget requires written justification for all spending.

4. Answer: B, H

   Variable budgeting allows monthly adjustments to the budget according to revenues and expenditures that are received throughout the month. Spending reduction is a type of budgeting model that requires the reallocation of funds and reduction of spending levels during a period of financial stress.

References

American College of Sports Medicine. *ACSM's Guidelines for Exercise Testing and Prescription.* 9th ed. New York, NY: Lippincott Williams and Wilkins; 2013.

Anderson M, Parr G, Hall S. *Foundations of Athletic Training.* 4th ed. New York, NY: Lippincott Williams and Wilkins; 2009.

Baechle TR, Earle RW. *Essentials of Strength Training and Conditioning.* 3rd ed. Champaign, IL: Human Kinetics; 2008.

Board of Certification. *Cert Update.* Omaha, NE: Author; 2016.

Board of Certification. *Online Registration for BOC Central.* http://www.bocatc.org. Accessed August 20, 2016.

Board of Certification. *Role Delineation Study/Practice Analysis.* 6th ed. Morrisville, NC: Castle Worldwide; 2016.

Cantu RC. *Neurological Athletic Head and Spine Injuries.* St. Louis, MO: Mosby-Year Book; 2000.

Cartwright L. *Preparing for the Athletic Trainer's Certification Examination.* Champaign, IL: Human Kinetics; 2002-2004.

Casa DJ, Csillan D; Inter-Association Task Force for Preseason Secondary School Athletics Participants, et al. Preseason heat-acclimatization guidelines for secondary school athletics. *J Athl Train.* 2009;44(3):332-333.

Clarkson HM. *Musculoskeletal Assessment.* 2nd ed. New York, NY: Lippincott Williams and Wilkins; 2000.

Crouch JE. *Functional Human Anatomy.* 4th ed. Philadelphia, PA: Lea and Febiger; 1985.

Crowley LV. *An Introduction to Human Disease: Pathology and Pathophysiology Correlations.* Sudbusy, MA: Jones and Bartlett Publishers; 2001.

Cuppett M, Walsh KM. *General Medical Conditions in the Athlete.* St. Louis, MO: Mosby; 2011.

Denegar CR, Saliba E, Saliba SF. *Therapeutic Modalities for Athletic Injuries.* 2nd ed. Champaign, IL: Human Kinetics; 2006.

Epler M, Wainwright S. *Manual Muscle Testing.* Thorofare, NJ: SLACK Incorporated; 1999.

Gall MD, Gall JP, Jacobsen DR, Bullock TL. *Tools for Learning: A Guide to Teaching Study Skills.* Alexandria, VA: Association for Supervision and Curriculum Development; 1990.

Gallaspy JB, May JD. *Signs and Symptoms of Athletic Injuries.* St. Louis, MO: Mosby-Year Book; 1996.

Hedgpeth EG, Gieck J. Psychological considerations for rehabilitation of the injured athlete. In WE Prentice, ed. *Rehabilitation Techniques for Sports Medicine and Athletic Training.* 4th ed. New York, NY: McGraw-Hill; 2004.

Henry ML, Stapleton ER. *EMT Prehospital Care.* Philadelphia, PA: WB Saunders; 1992.

Heyward VH. *Advanced Fitness Assessment and Exercise Prescription.* 3rd ed. Champaign, IL: Human Kinetics; 1998.

Hillman, SK, Perrin, DH, eds. *Core Concepts in Athletic Training and Therapy.* Champaign, Il: Human Kinetics; 2012.

Hoppenfeld S. *Physical Examination of the Spine and Extremities*. Norwalk, CT: Appleton and Lange; 1976.

Hoppenfeld S, Zeide MS. *Orthopaedic Dictionary*. Philadelphia, PA: JB Lippincott; 1994.

Houglum, JE, Harrelson, GL, Seefeldt, TM. *Principles of Pharmacology for Athletic Trainers*. 3rd ed. Thorofare, NJ: SLACK Incorporated; 2016.

Houglum PA. *Therapeutic Exercise for Athletic Injuries*. 2nd ed. Champaign, IL: Human Kinetics; 2005.

Irion G. *Comprehensive Wound Management*. 2nd ed. Thorofare, NJ: SLACK Incorporated; 2010.

Jimenez CC, Corcoran MD, Crawley JT, et al. National Athletic Trainers' Association position statement: management of the athlete with type 1 diabetes mellitus. *J Athl Train*. 2007;42(4):536-545.

Kersey RD, Elliot DL, Goldberg L, et al. National Athletic Trainers' Association position statement: anabolic-androgenic steroids. *J Athl Train*. 2012;47(5):567-588.

Kleiner DM, Almquist JL, Bailes J, et al. *Prehospital Care of the Spine-Injured Athlete: A Document From the Inter-Association Task Force for Appropriate Care of the Spine-Injured Athlete*. Dallas, TX: National Athletic Trainers' Association; 2001.

Konin JG. *Clinical Athletic Training*. Thorofare, NJ: SLACK Incorporated; 1997.

Konin JG, Wiksten DL, Isear J, Brader H. *Special Tests for Orthopedic Examination*. 4th ed. Thorofare, NJ: SLACK Incorporated; 2016.

Magee DJ. *Orthopaedic Physical Assessment*. 6th ed. Philadelphia, PA: WB Saunders; 2012.

McFarlane P, Hodson S. *Studying Effectively and Efficiently: An Integrated System*. Toronto, Ontario, Canada: Governing Council of University of Toronto; 1983.

McMinn RMH, Hutchings RT. *A Colour Atlas of Human Anatomy*. London, England: Wolfe Medical Publications Ltd; 1998.

Mellion MB. *Sports Medicine Secrets*. Philadelphia, PA: Hanley and Belfus; 1993.

Mellion MB, Walsh WM, Shelton GL. *The Team Physician's Handbook*. Philadelphia, PA: Hanley and Belfus; 1990.

Mensch JM, Miller GM. *The Athletic Trainer's Guide to Psychosocial Intervention and Referral*. Thorofare, NJ: SLACK Incorporated; 2008.

Michlovitz SL. *Thermal Agents in Rehabilitation*. 2nd ed. Philadelphia, PA: FA Davis; 1990.

Miller MG, Weiler JM, Baker R, Collins J, D'Alonzo G. National Athletic Trainers' Association position statement: management of asthma in athletes. *J Athl Train*. 2005;40(3):224-245.

Norkin C, Levangie P. *Joint Structure and Function. A Comprehensive Analysis*. 2nd ed. Philadelphia, PA: FA Davis; 1992.

Norkin CC, White DJ. *Measurement of Joint Motion*. 2nd ed. Philadelphia, PA: FA Davis; 1995.

O'Connor DP, Fincher AL. *Clinical Pathology for Athletic Trainers: Recognizing Systemic Disease*. 3rd ed. Thorofare, NJ: SLACK Incorporated; 2014.

Pagana KD, Pagana TJ. *Mosby's Diagnostic and Laboratory Desk Reference*. 6th ed. St. Louis, MO: Mosby; 2003.

Pakel RE, Bope ET. *Conn's Current Therapy*. Philadelphia, PA: Saunders; 2007.

Porth CM. *Pathophysiology: Concepts of Altered States*. 7th ed. Philadelphia, PA: Lippincott Williams and Wilkins; 2005.

Prentice WE. *Principles of Athletic Training: A Guide to Evidence-Based Clinical Practice*. 16th ed. New York, NY: McGraw-Hill; 2017.

Prentice WE. *Rehabilitation Techniques for Sports Medicine and Athletic Training*. 6th ed. New York, NY: McGraw-Hill; 2015.

Prentice WE. *Therapeutic Modalities in Sports Medicine*. 6th ed. New York, NY: McGraw-Hill; 2008.

Prentice WE, Voight MI. *Techniques in Musculoskeletal Rehabilitation*. New York, NY: McGraw-Hill; 2001.

Ray R, Konin J. *Management Strategies in Athletic Training*. 4th ed. Champaign, IL: Human Kinetics; 2011.

Rehberg RS. *Sports Emergency Care: A Team Approach*. 2nd ed. Thorofare, NJ: SLACK Incorporated; 2013.

Rothstein JM, Roy SH, Wolf SL. *The Rehabilitation Specialist's Handbook*. Philadelphia, PA: FA Davis; 1991.

Scifers JR. *Special Tests for Neurologic Examination*. Thorofare, NJ: SLACK Incorporated; 2008.

Sladyk K, McGeary S, Sladyk L, Tufano R. *OTR Exam Review Manual*. 3rd ed. Thorofare, NJ: SLACK Incorporated; 2001.

Starkey C. *Therapeutic Modalities*. 4th ed. Philadelphia, PA: FA Davis; 2013.

Starkey C; American Academy of Orthopedic Surgeons. *Athletic Training and Sports Medicine: An Integrated Approach*. 5th ed. Chicago, IL: Jones and Bartlett Learning; 2012.

Stedman's Concise Medical Dictionary for the Health Professions. 11th ed. Baltimore, MD: Williams and Wilkins; 2011.

Turocy PS, DePalma BF, Horswill CA, et al. National Athletic Trainers' Association position statement: safe weight loss and maintenance practices in sport and exercise. *J Athl Train*. 2011;46(3):322-336.

Valovich McLeod TC, Decoster LC, Loud KJ, et al. National Athletic Trainers' Association position statement: prevention of pediatric overuse injuries. *J Athl Train*. 2011;46(2):206-220.

Van De Graaff K. *Human Anatomy*. 5th ed. New York, NY: McGraw-Hill; 2000.

Van Lunen BL, Hankemeier DA, Welch CE. *Evidence-Guided Practice: A Framework for Clinical Decision Making in Athletic Training*. Thorofare, NJ: SLACK Incorprorated; 2015.

Van Ost L. *Goniometry*. Thorofare, NJ: SLACK Incorporated; 1999.

Vander A, Sherman J, Luciano D. *Human Physiology*. 9th ed. New York, NY: McGraw-Hill; 2003.

Voss DE, Ionta MK, Myers BJ. *Proprioceptive Neuromuscular Facilitation*. 3rd ed. Philadelphia, PA: Harper and Row; 1985.

Walsh KM, Cooper MA, Holle R, Rakov VA, Roeder WP, Ryan M. National Athletic Trainers' Association position statement: lightning safety for athletics and recreation. *J Athl Train*. 2013;48(2):258-270.

Wardlaw GM, Hampl JS. *Perspectives in Nutrition*. 7th ed. St. Louis, MO: Mosby-Year Book; 2006.